Dental Care
and Oral Health
SOURCEBOOK

Fourth Edition

...nce Series

Fourth Edition

Dental Care
and Oral Health
SOURCEBOOK

Basic Consumer Health Information about Caring for the Mouth and Teeth, Including Facts about Dental Hygiene and Routine Care Guidelines, Fluoride Sealants, Tooth Whitening Systems, Cavities, Root Canals, Extractions, Implants, Veneers, Dentures, and Orthodontic and Orofacial Procedures

Along with Information about Periodontal (Gum) Disease, Canker Sores, Dry Mouth, Temporomandibular Joint and Muscle Disorders (TMJ), Oral Cancer, and Other Conditions That Impact Oral Health, Suggestions for Finding and Financing Care, a Glossary of Related Terms, and Directories of Additional Resources

Edited by
Joyce Brennfleck Shannon

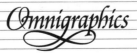

Omnigraphics

155 W. Congress, Suite 200, Detroit, MI 48226

Bibliographic Note

Because this page cannot legibly accommodate all the copyright notices, the Bibliographic Note portion of the Preface constitutes an extension of the copyright notice.

Edited by Joyce Brennfleck Shannon

Health Reference Series

Karen Bellenir, *Managing Editor*
David A. Cooke, MD, FACP, *Medical Consultant*
Elizabeth Collins, *Research and Permissions Coordinator*
Cherry Edwards, *Permissions Assistant*
EdIndex, Services for Publishers, *Indexers*

* * *

Omnigraphics, Inc.

Matthew P. Barbour, *Senior Vice President*
Kevin M. Hayes, *Operations Manager*

* * *

Peter E. Ruffner, *Publisher*

Copyright © 2012 Omnigraphics, Inc.

ISBN 978-0-7808-1273-4

E-ISBN 978-0-7808-1274-1

Library of Congress Cataloging-in-Publication Data

Dental care and oral health sourcebook : basic consumer health information about caring for the mouth and teeth, including facts about dental hygiene and routine care guidelines, fluoride, sealants, tooth whitening systems, cavities, root canals, extractions, implants, veneers, dentures, and orthodontic and orofacial procedures; along with information about periodontal (gum) disease, canker sores, dry mouth, temporomandibular joint and muscle disorders (TMJ), oral cancer, and other conditions that impact oral health ... / edited by Joyce Brennfleck Shannon. -- 4th ed.
   p. cm.
 Summary: "Provides basic consumer health information about dental hygiene, preventive care, and oral health concerns for children and adults, with facts about surgical, orthodontic, and cosmetic dental procedures, and diseases of the mouth and jaw. Includes index, glossary of related terms, and other resources"-- Provided by publisher.
 Includes bibliographical references and index.
 ISBN 978-0-7808-1273-4 (hardcover : alk. paper) 1. Dentistry--Popular works. 2. Mouth--Diseases--Popular works. 3. Mouth--Care and hygiene--Popular works. I. Shannon, Joyce Brennfleck.
 RK61.O66 2012
 617.6--dc23
                                                                        2012024522

This book is printed on acid-free paper meeting the ANSI Z39.48 Standard. The infinity symbol that appears above indicates that the paper in this book meets that standard.

Printed in the United States

Table of Contents

Visit www.healthreferenceseries.com to view *A Contents Guide to the Health Reference Series*, a listing of more than 16,000 topics and the volumes in which they are covered.

Part II: Visiting Your Dentist's Office

Part III: Dental Care for Infants and Children

Part IV: Orthodontic, Endodontic, Periodontic, and Orofacial Procedures

Part VI: Health Conditions That Affect Oral Health

Part VII: Finding and Financing Oral Health in the United States

Part VIII: Additional Help and Information

Preface

About This Book

The Centers for Disease Control and Prevention (CDC) reports that millions of children experience problems from untreated tooth decay and that one-fourth of adults over 65 have lost all of their teeth. Most adults over age 24 have some gum disease which may lead to nutrition problems and may affect health conditions such as diabetes. While researchers seek ways to re-mineralize teeth and disrupt tooth decay processes, prevention is still the best way to maintain optimal oral health. Keys to good oral health include effective hygiene, fluoridated drinking water, fluoride treatments, sealants, and regular dental visits.

Dental Care and Oral Health Sourcebook, Fourth Edition offers updated information about mouth and tooth care guidelines for effective hygiene, nutrition, and decay prevention. Facts about tooth pain, dental fillings, orthodontia, cosmetic procedures, root canals and other endodontic treatments, and dental implants are described. Pediatric preventive treatments, sports injury prevention, and cleft palate treatments are discussed. Disorders such as halitosis (bad breath), temporomandibular joint and muscle (TMJ) disorder, other jaw disorders, mouth sores, and health conditions that impact oral health are also addressed. The book concludes with guidelines for finding and financing dental care, a glossary of dental care terms, and directories with further information about dental care and oral health services.

How to Use This Book

This book is divided into parts and chapters. Parts focus on broad areas of interest. Chapters are devoted to single topics within a part.

Part I: Taking Care of Your Mouth and Teeth describes essential elements of personal oral hygiene. An overview of the mouth and dental structures is provided with information about general oral health. Details are included about home care products to clean teeth and remove dental plaque, including tooth brushes, rinses, irrigation, and whiteners. The impact of nutrition and fluoride is discussed along with information about oral injuries, oral piercings, and how travelers can find safe dental care.

Part II: Visiting Your Dentist's Office explains common procedures, such as x-rays, fillings, sedation, and treatments for tooth pain. Details are offered about types of dental restorations (amalgam and composite fillings, porcelain veneers, and crowns), having a tooth pulled, and the possible choices if dentures are needed.

Part III: Dental Care for Infants and Children offers strategies for initiating and maintaining healthy primary teeth. Fluoride treatments, sealants, and good nutrition with adequate calcium intake are addressed. Other specific concerns for children, such as teething, sports-related orofacial injuries, childhood bruxism, and the impact of sugar-based drinks and snack foods on children's oral health, are discussed.

Part IV: Orthodontic, Endodontic, Periodontic, and Orofacial Procedures offer details about braces, retainers, and treatments of malocclusion for children and adults, along with information about root canals, periodontal (gum) disease treatment, dental implants, and oral surgeries. Facial trauma and corrective jaw surgery are also discussed.

Part V: Oral Diseases and Disorders provides information about bad breath, burning mouth syndrome, cleft palate, dentinogenesis imperfecta, jaw problems, mouth sores, oral cancer, and thrush. Disorders of the tongue, taste, and those that cause dry mouth (xerostomia), such as salivary gland disorders or Sjögren syndrome, are also explained.

Part VI: Health Conditions That Affect Oral Health describes specific conditions that cause—or result in—oral complications, including cancer treatment, celiac disease, diabetes, eating disorders, heart disease, immune system disorders, organ transplantation, osteoporosis, pregnancy, and the use of tobacco or illegal drugs.

Part VII: Finding and Financing Oral Health in the United States provides information on oral health care status and factors that impact access to oral health care. It reviews average dental expenses and private and public sources of coverage that assist in paying for dental care including suggestions for finding low-cost dental care. Specific information is also included about Head Start and other school-based oral health services.

Part VIII: Additional Help and Information provides a glossary of terms related to dental care and oral health. Directories of local dental schools and other dental care and oral health resources are also included.

Bibliographic Note

This volume contains documents and excerpts from publications issued by the following U.S. government agencies: Agency for Healthcare Research and Quality (AHRQ); Centers for Disease Control and Prevention (CDC); Genetics Home Reference; National Cancer Institute (NCI); National Institute of Allergy and Infectious Diseases (NIAID); National Institute of Arthritis and Musculoskeletal and Skin Diseases (NIAMS); National Institute of Child Health and Human Development (NICHD); National Institute of Dental and Craniofacial Research (NIDCR); National Institute of Mental Health (NIMH); National Institute of Neurological Disorders and Stroke (NINDS); National Institute on Deafness and Other Communication Disorders (NIDCD); National Institute on Diabetes and Digestive and Kidney Disorders (NIDDK); National Institute on Drug Abuse (NIDA); National Institute on Aging (NIA); National Institutes of Health (NIH); NIH Office of Science Education; U.S. Environmental Protection Agency (EPA); U.S. Food and Drug Administration (FDA); and the U.S. Department of Health and Human Services (HHS).

In addition, this volume contains copyrighted documents from the following organizations, individuals, and publications: Academy of General Dentistry; A.D.A.M, Inc.; American Academy of Cosmetic Dentistry; American Academy of Oral Medicine; American Academy of Pediatric Dentistry; American Academy of Periodontology; American Association of Endodontists; American College of Rheumatology; American Dental Hygienists' Association; Association of State and Territorial Dental Directors; California Dental Association; Cleft Palate Foundation; Cleveland Clinic; Connecticut Department of Public Health–Office of Oral Health; Dear Doctor, Inc.; Family Gentle Dental Care; Health Physics Society; Indiana Dental Association; *Journal of Clinical Dentistry*; *Journal of Dental Research*; Magic Foundation;

Maryland Department of Health and Mental Hygiene, Office of Oral Health, Family Health Administration; Massachusetts Department of Public Health–Office of Oral Health; Richard Mitchell, BDS; National Academy of Sciences; National Eating Disorders Association; National Marfan Foundation; National Maternal and Child Oral Health Resource Center; Nemours Foundation; North Carolina Department of Health and Human Services–Division of Public Health, Oral Health Section; Organization for Safety, Asepsis and Prevention; Osteogenesis Imperfecta Foundation; Queensland Health; Martin S. Spiller, DMD; and the University of Leeds.

Full citation information is provided on the first page of each chapter or section. Every effort has been made to secure all necessary rights to reprint the copyrighted material. If any omissions have been made, please contact Omnigraphics to make corrections for future editions.

Acknowledgements

In addition to the listed organizations and agencies who have contributed to this *Sourcebook*, special thanks go to managing editor Karen Bellenir, research and permissions coordinator Liz Collins, and prepress services provider WhimsyInk for their help and support.

About the Health Reference Series

The *Health Reference Series* is designed to provide basic medical information for patients, families, caregivers, and the general public. Each volume takes a particular topic and provides comprehensive coverage. This is especially important for people who may be dealing with a newly diagnosed disease or a chronic disorder in themselves or in a family member. People looking for preventive guidance, information about disease warning signs, medical statistics, and risk factors for health problems will also find answers to their questions in the *Health Reference Series*. The *Series*, however, is not intended to serve as a tool for diagnosing illness, in prescribing treatments, or as a substitute for the physician/patient relationship. All people concerned about medical symptoms or the possibility of disease are encouraged to seek professional care from an appropriate health care provider.

A Note about Spelling and Style

Health Reference Series editors use *Stedman's Medical Dictionary* as an authority for questions related to the spelling of medical terms and the *Chicago Manual of Style* for questions related to grammatical structures, punctuation, and other editorial concerns. Consistent adherence is not always possible, however, because the individual volumes within the *Series* include many documents from a wide variety of different producers and copyright holders, and the editor's primary goal is to present material from each source as accurately as is possible following the terms specified by each document's producer. This sometimes means that information in different chapters or sections may follow other guidelines and alternate spelling authorities. For example, occasionally a copyright holder may require that eponymous terms be shown in possessive forms (Crohn's disease *vs.* Crohn disease) or that British spelling norms be retained (leukaemia *vs.* leukemia).

Locating Information within the Health Reference Series

The *Health Reference Series* contains a wealth of information about a wide variety of medical topics. Ensuring easy access to all the fact sheets, research reports, in-depth discussions, and other material contained within the individual books of the *Series* remains one of our highest priorities. As the *Series* continues to grow in size and scope, however, locating the precise information needed by a reader may become more challenging.

A Contents Guide to the Health Reference Series was developed to direct readers to the specific volumes that address their concerns. It presents an extensive list of diseases, treatments, and other topics of general interest compiled from the Tables of Contents and major index headings. To access *A Contents Guide to the Health Reference Series*, visit www.healthreferenceseries.com.

Medical Consultant

Medical consultation services are provided to the *Health Reference Series* editors by David A. Cooke, MD, FACP. Dr. Cooke is a graduate of Brandeis University, and he received his MD degree from the University of Michigan. He completed residency training at the University of Wisconsin Hospital and Clinics. He is board-certified in Internal Medicine. Dr. Cooke currently works as part of the University of Michigan Health System and practices in Ann Arbor, MI. In his free time, he enjoys writing, science fiction, and spending time with his family.

Our Advisory Board

We would like to thank the following board members for providing guidance to the development of this *Series*:

- Dr. Lynda Baker, Associate Professor of Library and Information Science, Wayne State University, Detroit, MI

- Nancy Bulgarelli, William Beaumont Hospital Library, Royal Oak, MI

- Karen Imarisio, Bloomfield Township Public Library, Bloomfield Township, MI

- Karen Morgan, Mardigian Library, University of Michigan-Dearborn, Dearborn, MI

- Rosemary Orlando, St. Clair Shores Public Library, St. Clair Shores, MI

Health Reference Series *Update Policy*

The inaugural book in the *Health Reference Series* was the first edition of *Cancer Sourcebook* published in 1989. Since then, the *Series* has been enthusiastically received by librarians and in the medical community. In order to maintain the standard of providing high-quality health information for the layperson the editorial staff at Omnigraphics felt it was necessary to implement a policy of updating volumes when warranted.

Medical researchers have been making tremendous strides, and it is the purpose of the *Health Reference Series* to stay current with the most recent advances. Each decision to update a volume is made on an individual basis. Some of the considerations include how much new information is available and the feedback we receive from people who use the books. If there is a topic you would like to see added to the update list, or an area of medical concern you feel has not been adequately addressed, please write to:

Editor
Health Reference Series
Omnigraphics, Inc.
P.O. Box 31-1640
Detroit, MI 48231-1640
E-mail: editorial@omnigraphics.com

Part One

Taking Care of Your Mouth and Teeth

Chapter 1

Steps to Dental Health

Healthy teeth and gums make it easy for you to eat well and enjoy good food. There are a number of problems that can affect the health of your mouth, but good care should keep your teeth and gums strong.

Prevent Tooth Decay

Teeth are covered in a hard, outer coating called enamel. Every day, a thin film of bacteria called dental plaque builds up on your teeth. The bacteria in plaque produce acids that can begin to harm enamel. Over time, the acids can cause a hole in the enamel. This hole is called a cavity. Brushing and flossing your teeth can protect you from decay, but once a cavity happens, a dentist has to fix it.

You can protect your teeth from decay by using fluoride toothpaste. If you are at a higher risk for tooth decay (for example, if you have a dry mouth because of medicines you take), you might need more fluoride. Your dentist or dental hygienist may give you a fluoride treatment during an office visit, or the dentist may tell you to use a fluoride gel or mouth rinse at home.

Prevent Gum Diseases

Gum disease begins when plaque builds up along and under the gum line. This plaque causes infections that hurt the gum and bone that hold teeth in place. Sometimes gum disease makes your gums

Excerpted from "Taking Care of Your Teeth and Mouth," National Institute on Aging (NIA), updated October 28, 2011.

tender and more likely to bleed. This problem, called gingivitis, can often be fixed by daily brushing and flossing.

A more severe form of gum disease, called periodontitis, needs to be treated by a dentist. If not treated, this infection can ruin the bones, gums, and other tissues that support your teeth. Over time, your teeth may have to be removed.

To prevent gum disease follow these guidelines:

- Brush your teeth twice a day with fluoride toothpaste.

- Floss once a day.

- Visit your dentist regularly for a checkup and cleaning.

- Eat a well-balanced diet.

- Quit smoking. Smoking increases your risk for gum disease.

Cleaning Your Teeth and Gums

There is a right way to brush and floss your teeth. Every day you need to do the following:

- Gently brush your teeth on all sides with a soft-bristle brush and fluoride toothpaste.

- Use small circular motions and short back-and-forth strokes.

- Take the time to brush carefully and gently along the gum line.

- Lightly brush your tongue to help keep your mouth clean.

People with arthritis or other conditions that limit hand motion may find it hard to hold and use a toothbrush. Some helpful ideas include these:

- Use an electric or battery-operated toothbrush.

- Slide a bicycle grip or foam tube over the handle of the toothbrush.

- Buy a toothbrush with a larger handle.

- Attach the toothbrush handle to your hand with a wide elastic band.

You also need to clean around your teeth with dental floss every day. Careful flossing will take off plaque and leftover food that a toothbrush can't reach. Be sure to rinse after you floss.

See your dentist if brushing or flossing causes your gums to bleed or hurts your mouth. If you have trouble flossing, a floss holder may help. Ask your dentist to show you the right way to floss.

Dentures

Sometimes, false teeth (dentures) are needed to replace badly damaged teeth. Partial dentures may be used to fill in one or more missing teeth. Dentures may feel strange at first. In the beginning, your dentist may want to see you often to make sure the dentures fit. Over time, your gums will change shape and your dentures may need to be adjusted or replaced. Be sure to let your dentist handle these adjustments.

When you are learning to eat with dentures, it may be easier if you:

- start with soft, non-sticky food;
- cut your food into small pieces; and
- chew slowly using both sides of your mouth.

Be careful when wearing dentures because it may be harder for you to feel hot foods and drinks or notice bones from your food in your mouth.

Keep your dentures clean and free from food that can cause stains, bad breath, or swollen gums. Brush them every day with a denture care product. Take your dentures out of your mouth at night and put them in water or a denture-cleansing liquid.

Dry Mouth

Dry mouth happens when you do not have enough saliva, or spit, to keep your mouth wet. Many common medicines can cause dry mouth. That can make it hard to eat, swallow, taste, and even speak. Dry mouth can cause tooth decay and other infections of the mouth.

There are some things you can try that may help with dry mouth. Try sipping water or sugarless drinks. Do not smoke and avoid alcohol and caffeine. Sugarless hard candy or sugarless gum may help. Your dentist or doctor might suggest that you use artificial saliva to keep your mouth wet. Or they may have other ideas on how to cope with dry mouth.

Oral Cancer

Cancer of the mouth can grow in any part of the mouth or throat. It is more likely to happen in people over age 40. A dental checkup is a good time for your dentist to look for signs of oral cancer. Pain is not usually an early symptom of the disease. Treatment works best before the disease spreads. Even if you have lost all your natural teeth, you should still see your dentist for regular oral cancer exams.

You can lower your risk of getting oral cancer:

- Do not use tobacco products—cigarettes, chewing tobacco, snuff, pipes, or cigars.

- If you drink alcohol, do so only in moderation.

- Use lip balm with sunscreen.

Finding Low-Cost Dental Care

Sometimes dental care can be costly. Medicare does not cover routine dental care. Very few states offer dental coverage under Medicaid. You may want to check out private dental insurance. Make sure you are aware of the cost and what services are covered. The following resources may help you find low-cost dental care:

- Some dental schools have clinics where students get experience treating patients at a reduced cost. Qualified dentists supervise the students. Visit www.ada.org online for a list of U.S. dental schools.

- Dental hygiene schools may offer supervised, low-cost care as part of the training experience for dental hygienists. See schools listed online by State at www.adha.org.

- Call your county or state health department to find dental clinics near you that charge based on your income.

- Call toll-free 888-275-4772 to locate a community health center near you that offers dental services, or visit www.hrsa.gov (scroll down to "Find a Health Center").

- United Way chapters may be able to direct you to free or reduced-cost dental services in your community. Call 211 to reach a local United Way chapter.

Chapter 2

Anatomy of the Mouth

Mouth and Teeth

The first thing that comes to mind when you think of your mouth is probably eating—or kissing! But your mouth is a lot more than an input slot for food or a tool for smooching your sweetie.

Where Would We Be without Them?

Your mouth and teeth form your smile, which is often the first thing people notice when they look at you. The mouth is also essential for speech: The tongue (which also allows us to taste) enables us to form words with the help of our lips and teeth. The tongue hits the teeth to make certain sounds—the *th* sound, for example, is produced when the tongue brushes against the upper row of teeth. If a person has a lisp, it means the tongue touches the teeth instead of directly behind them when saying words with the *s* sound.

"Mouth and Teeth," June 2009, and "Your Tongue," June 2010, both reprinted with permission from www.kidshealth.org. Copyright © 2009–2010 The Nemours Foundation. This information was provided by KidsHealth, one of the largest resources online for medically reviewed health information written for parents, kids, and teens. For more articles like these, visit www.KidsHealth.org, or www.Teens Health.org. Images within this chapter, from the North Carolina Department of Health and Human Services, Division of Public Health, Oral Health Section, are cited separately where they appear.

Without our teeth, we'd have to live on a liquid diet or a diet of soft, mashed food. The hardest substances in the body, the teeth, are necessary for mastication—a fancy way of saying chewing—the process by which we tear, cut, and grind food in preparation for swallowing. Chewing allows enzymes and lubricants released in the mouth to further digest, or break down, food. This makes the mouth one of the first steps in the digestive process. Read on to find out how each aspect of the mouth and teeth plays a role in our daily lives.

Basic Anatomy of the Mouth and Teeth

The mouth is lined with mucous membranes (pronounced: myoo-kus mem-branes). Just as skin lines and protects the outside of the body, mucous membranes line and protect the inside. Mucous membranes make mucus, which keeps them moist.

The membrane-covered roof of the mouth is called the palate. The front part consists of a bony portion called the hard palate, with a fleshy rear part called the soft palate. The hard palate divides the mouth from the nose above. The soft palate forms a curtain between the mouth and the throat (or pharynx—pronounced: fa-rinks) to the rear. The soft palate contains the uvula (pronounced: yoo-vyoo-luh), the dangling fleshy object at the back of the mouth. The tonsils are located on either side of the uvula and look like twin pillars holding up the opening to the pharynx.

A bundle of muscles extends from the floor of the mouth to form the tongue. The upper surface of the tongue is covered with tiny projections called papillae. Our taste buds are located here. The four main types of taste buds—sweet, salty, sour, and bitter—are found on the tongue.

Three pairs of salivary glands in the walls and floor of the mouth secrete saliva, which contains a digestive enzyme called amylase that starts the breakdown of carbohydrates even before food enters the stomach.

The lips are covered with skin on the outside and with slippery mucous membranes on the inside of the mouth. The major lip muscle, called the orbicularis oris (pronounced: or-bik-yoo-lar-iss or-iss), allows for the lips' mobility. The reddish tint of the lips comes from underlying blood vessels, which is why the lips can bleed so easily with injury. The inside part of the lips connects to the gums.

All about Teeth

The types of teeth are:

- Incisors are the square-shaped, sharp-edged teeth at the front and middle of the mouth. There are four on the bottom and four on the top.

- To the sides of the incisors are the long, sharp canines, two on the bottom and two on the top. The upper canines are sometimes called eyeteeth.

- Behind the canines are the premolars, or bicuspids. There are two sets, or a total of four premolars, in each jaw—two behind each of the canines on the bottom and two behind each canine on the top.

- The molars, situated behind the premolars, have points and grooves. There are 12 molars in the adult mouth—three sets in each jaw called first, second, and third molars. The third molars are called wisdom teeth. Wisdom teeth get their name because, as the last teeth to erupt, they break through when a person is becoming an adult and is supposedly wiser. Wisdom teeth are not essential today, but some people believe they evolved thousands of years ago when human diets consisted of mostly raw foods that required extra chewing power. Because wisdom teeth can crowd out the other teeth or cause problems like pain and infection, a dentist may need to remove them. This often happens during a person's teenage years.

Each tooth is made of four types of tissue: pulp, dentin, enamel, and cementum. The pulp is the innermost portion of the tooth. Unlike the outer parts of the tooth, the pulp is soft. It is made of connective tissue, nerves, and blood vessels, which nourish the tooth. The pulp has two parts: the pulp chamber which lies in the crown (or top part of the tooth), and the root canal which is in the bottom part of the tooth that lies beneath the gums. Blood vessels and nerves enter the root through a small hole at the very bottom of the tooth and extend through the canal into the pulp chamber.

Dentin surrounds the pulp. A hard yellow substance, dentin makes up most of the tooth. It is the dentin that gives the tooth its slightly yellowish tint.

Both the dentin and pulp cover the whole tooth from the crown into the root. But the outermost layer covering the tooth is different, depending on whether it sits above the gum or below it. Enamel, the hardest tissue in the body, covers the crown. Under the gum line, a bony layer of cementum covers the outside of the root and holds the tooth in place within the jawbone. Cementum is as hard as bone but not as hard as enamel, which enables the tooth to withstand the pressure of chewing and protects it from harmful bacteria and changes in temperature from hot and cold foods.

Normal Development of the Mouth and Teeth

Humans are diphyodont (pronounced: dy-fy-uh-dant), meaning that they develop two sets of teeth. The first set of teeth, the deciduous (pronounced: duh-sid-you-wus) teeth are also called the milk, primary, temporary, or baby teeth. These teeth begin to develop before birth, start to push through the gums between the ages of six months and one year (this process is called eruption), and usually start to fall out when a child is around six years old. They are replaced by a set of 32 permanent teeth, which are also called secondary or adult teeth.

Although teeth aren't visible at birth, both the deciduous and permanent teeth are forming beneath the gums. By the time a child is three years old, he or she has a set of 20 deciduous teeth, ten in the lower and ten in the upper jaw. Each jaw has four incisors, two canines, and four molars.

The deciduous teeth help the permanent teeth erupt in their normal positions; most of the permanent teeth form just beneath the roots of the deciduous teeth above them. When a deciduous tooth is preparing to fall out, its root begins to dissolve. This root has completely dissolved by the time the permanent tooth below it is ready to erupt.

The phase during which permanent teeth develop usually lasts for about 15 years as the jaw steadily grows into its adult form. From age six to nine, the incisors and first molars start to come in. Between ages ten and twelve, the first and second premolars, as well as the canines, erupt. From age 11 to 13 years, the second molars come in.

The wisdom teeth (third molars) erupt between the ages of 17 and 21. Sometimes there isn't room in a person's mouth for all the permanent teeth. If this happens, the wisdom teeth may get stuck (or impacted) beneath the gum and may need to be removed. Overcrowding of the teeth is one of the reasons people get braces during their teenage years.

What Do the Mouth and Teeth Do?

The mouth and teeth play an important role in digesting food. Food is torn, ground, and moistened in the mouth. Each type of tooth serves a different function in the chewing process. Incisors cut foods when you bite into them. The sharper, longer canines tear food. The premolars grind and mash food. Molars, with their points and grooves, are responsible for the most vigorous grinding. All the while, the tongue helps to push the food up against our teeth.

As we chew, the salivary glands secrete saliva, which moistens the food and helps break it down further. As well as containing digestive enzymes, saliva makes it easier to chew and swallow foods (especially dry foods).

Once food has been converted into a soft, moist mass, it's pushed into the pharynx at the back of the mouth and is swallowed. When we swallow, the soft palate closes off the nasal passages from the throat to prevent food from entering the nose.

Things That Can Go Wrong with the Mouth

Proper dental care is essential to good oral health. This includes a good diet, brushing and flossing after eating, and regular dental checkups.

Common mouth diseases and conditions include:

- **Aphthous stomatitis (canker sores):** Canker sores are a common form of mouth ulcer that girls get more often than guys. Although their cause is not completely understood, mouth injuries, stress, dietary deficiencies, hormonal changes (as with the menstrual cycle), or food allergies can trigger them. They usually appear on the inner surface of the cheeks or lips, under the tongue, on the soft palate, or at the base of the gums, and begin with a tingling or burning sensation followed by a painful sore called an ulcer. Pain subsides in seven to ten days, with complete healing usually occurring in one to three weeks.

- **Cleft lip and cleft palate** are birth defects in which the tissues of the mouth and/or lip don't form properly as a fetus is developing in the womb. Children born with cleft lip or cleft palate can have reconstructive surgery in infancy—and sometimes later—to repair the cleft. This surgery can prevent or lessen the severity of speech problems later in life.

- **Enteroviral stomatitis** is a common type of infection. People with this condition have small, painful ulcers inside their mouths that may decrease their desire to eat and drink, putting them at risk of dehydration.

- **Herpetic stomatitis (oral herpes):** Oral herpes causes painful, clustered blisters inside the mouth or on a person's lip. People can get this infection when they have direct contact (such as kissing) with someone with the herpes simplex virus.

- **Periodontal disease:** Periodontal (pronounced: pare-ee-oh-don-tul) disease affects the gums and tissues supporting the teeth. Gingivitis (pronounced: jin-jih-vy-tus), an inflammation of the gums characterized by redness, swelling, and sometimes bleeding, is one common form of periodontal disease. It's usually caused by the accumulation of tartar (a hardened film of food particles and bacteria that builds up on teeth). Gingivitis is almost always the result of not brushing and flossing the teeth properly. When gingivitis isn't treated, it can lead to periodontitis, in which the gums loosen around the teeth and pockets of bacteria and pus form, sometimes damaging the supporting bone and causing tooth loss.

Things That Can Go Wrong with Teeth

Proper dental care is essential to good oral health. This includes a good diet, brushing and flossing after eating, and regular dental checkups.

Common dental diseases and conditions include:

- **Cavities and tooth decay:** When bacteria and food particles are allowed to settle on the teeth, plaque forms. The bacteria digest the carbohydrates in the food and produce acid, which dissolves the tooth's enamel and causes a cavity. If the cavity is not treated, the decay process progresses to involve the dentin. Without treatment, serious infection can develop. The most common ways to treat cavities and more serious tooth decay problems are filling the cavity; performing a root canal procedure, which involves the removal of the pulp of a tooth; crowning a tooth with a cap that looks like a tooth made of metal, porcelain, or plastic; or removing or replacing the tooth. To avoid tooth decay and cavities, get in the habit of good dental care—including proper tooth brushing techniques.

- **Malocclusion** is the failure of the upper and lower teeth to meet properly when you bite down. The types of malocclusion include overbite, underbite, and crowding. Most of these conditions can be corrected with braces. Braces are metal or clear ceramic brackets bonded to the front of each tooth. Wires connecting the brackets are tightened periodically to force the teeth to move into the correct position.

- **Impacted wisdom teeth:** In many people, the wisdom teeth are unable to erupt normally so they either remain below the jawline or don't grow in properly. Dentists call these teeth impacted. Wisdom teeth usually become impacted because the jaw is not large enough to accommodate all the teeth that are growing in and the mouth becomes overcrowded. Impacted teeth can damage other teeth or become painful and infected. Dentists can check if a person has impacted wisdom teeth by taking x-rays of the teeth. If, after looking at the x-rays, a dentist thinks there's a chance that impacted teeth may cause problems, he or she may recommend that the tooth or teeth be removed (extracted).

Your Tongue

Want to find out just how much you use your tongue? Try eating an ice-cream cone or singing your favorite song without it. You need your tongue to chew, swallow, and sing. And don't forget talking and tasting!

Tongue Twister

Has anyone ever told you that the tongue is a muscle? Well, that's only partly true: The tongue is really made up of many groups of muscles. These muscles run in different directions to carry out all the tongue's jobs.

The front part of the tongue is very flexible and can move around a lot, working with the teeth to create different types of words. This part also helps you eat by helping to move food around your mouth while you chew. Your tongue pushes the food to your back teeth so the teeth can grind it up.

The muscles in the back of your tongue help you make certain sounds, like the letters "k" and hard "g" (like in the word "go"). Try saying these letters slowly, and you'll feel how the back of your tongue moves against the top of your mouth to create the sounds.

The back of your tongue is important for eating as well. Once the food is all ground up and mixed with saliva (say: suh-lye-vuh), or spit, the back muscles start to work. They move and push a small bit of food along with saliva into your esophagus (say: ih-sah-fuh-gus), which is a food pipe that leads from your throat to your stomach.

Tongue Held Down Tight

Have you ever wondered what keeps you from swallowing your tongue? Look in the mirror at what's under your tongue and you'll see your frenulum (say: fren-yuh-lum). This is a membrane (a thin layer of tissue) that connects your tongue to the bottom of your mouth. In fact, the whole base of your tongue is firmly anchored to the bottom of your mouth, so you could never swallow your tongue even if you tried.

Tasty Tidbits

Don't put that mirror away yet! Look at your tongue again, but this time look closely at the top of it. Notice how it's rough and bumpy—not like the underside, which is very smooth. That's because the top of your tongue is covered with a layer of bumps called papillae (say: puh-pih-lee).

Papillae help grip food and move it around while you chew. And they contain your taste buds, so you can taste everything from apples to zucchini. People are born with about 10,000 taste buds. But as a person ages, some of his or her taste buds die. (An old person may only have 5,000 taste buds.) That's why some foods may taste stronger to you than they do to an adult. Taste buds can detect sweet, sour, bitter, and salty flavors.

Traveling Tastes

So how do you know how something tastes? Each taste bud is made up of taste cells, which have sensitive, microscopic hairs called microvilli (say: mye-kro-vih-lye). Those tiny hairs send messages to the brain, which interprets the signals and identifies the taste for you.

Identifying tastes is your brain's way of telling you about what's going into your mouth, and in some cases, keeping you safe. Have you ever taken a drink of milk that tasted funny? When the milk hit the taste buds, they sent nerve impulses to your brain: "Milk coming in—and it tastes funny!" Once your brain unscrambled the nerve impulses, it recognized the taste as a dangerous one, and you knew not to drink the milk.

Some things can make your taste bud receptors less sensitive, like cold foods or drinks. An ice pop made from your favorite juice won't taste as sweet as plain juice. If you suck on an ice cube before you eat a food you don't like, you won't notice the bad taste.

Friend of the Tongue

Last time you had a cold and your nose felt stuffed up, did you notice that foods didn't taste as strong as they usually do? Well, that's because your tongue can't take all of the credit for tasting different flavors—it has help from your nose.

Your nose helps you taste foods by smelling them before they go in your mouth and as you chew and swallow them. Strong smells can even confuse your taste buds: Try holding an onion slice under your nose while eating an apple. What do you taste?

Your tongue also gets help from your teeth, lips, and mouth. Your teeth help your tongue grind food as the tongue mixes the food around your mouth. And without your teeth, lips, and the roof of your mouth, your tongue wouldn't be able to form sounds to make words.

Saliva is also a friend of the tongue. A dry tongue can't taste a thing, so saliva helps the tongue by keeping it wet. Saliva moistens food and helps to break it down, which makes it easier for the tongue to push the food back to swallow it.

Fighting Germs

If all that wasn't enough, your tongue even helps keep you from getting sick. The back section of your tongue contains something called the lingual tonsil (say: ling-gwul tahn-sul). Lingual is a medical word that means having to do with the tongue, and tonsils are small masses of tissue that contain cells that help filter out harmful germs that could cause an infection in the body.

But when you have tonsillitis, it's not your lingual tonsil that's infected. Tonsillitis affects the palatine (say: pah-luh-tyne) tonsils, which are two balls of tissue on either side of the tongue. The lingual tonsil, the palatine tonsils, and the adenoids are part of a bigger system that fights infections throughout your body.

The Tongue Is One Tough Worker

With all that talking, mixing food, swallowing, tasting, and germ fighting, does your tongue ever get a rest? No. Even when you are

15

sleeping, your tongue is busy pushing saliva into the throat to be swallowed. It's a good thing, too, or we'd be drooling all over our pillows. Keep your tongue in tip-top shape by brushing it along with your teeth and avoiding super-hot foods. A burned tongue is no fun.

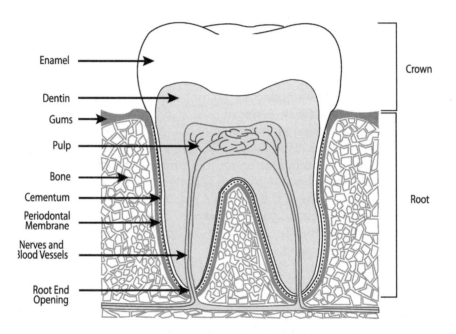

Figure 2.1. *Tooth Anatomy (Source: "Tooth Anatomy," September 2010, reprinted with permission from the North Carolina Department of Health and Human Services, Division of Public Health, Oral Health Section. For additional information, visit http://www.nchhs.gov/dph/oralhealth.)*

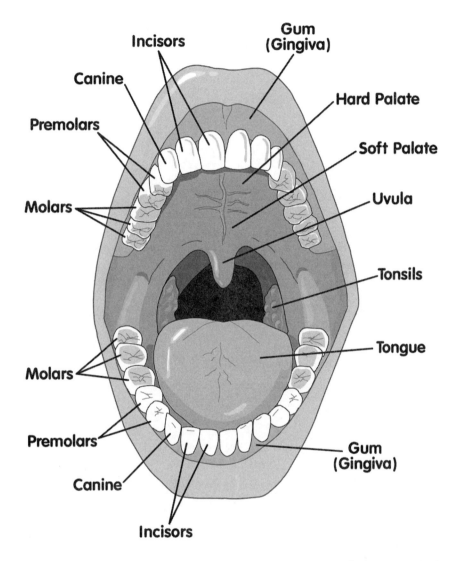

Figure 2.2. Mouth Discovery (Source: "Mouth Discovery," September 2010, reprinted with permission from the North Carolina Department of Health and Human Services, Division of Public Health, Oral Health Section. For additional information, visit http://www.nchhs.gov/dph/oralhealth.)

Chapter 3

Taking Care of Your Teeth

Chapter Contents

Section 3.1

Why Tooth Care Matters

"Taking Care of Your Teeth," November 2009, reprinted with permission from www.kidshealth.org. Copyright © 2009 The Nemours Foundation. This information was provided by KidsHealth, one of the largest resources online for medically reviewed health information written for parents, kids, and teens. For more articles like this one, visit www.KidsHealth.org, or www.TeensHealth.org.

When you get your picture taken, everyone says, "Say cheese! Smile!" So you do—you open your mouth and show your teeth. When you see the picture, you see a happy person looking back at you. The healthier those teeth are, the happier you look. Why is that?

It's because your teeth are important in many ways. If you take care of them, they'll help take care of you. Strong, healthy teeth help you chew the right foods to help you grow. They help you speak clearly. And yes, they help you look your best.

Why Healthy Teeth Are Important

How does taking care of your teeth help with all those things? Taking care of your teeth helps prevent plaque (say: plak), which is a clear film of bacteria (say: bak-teer-ee-uh) that sticks to your teeth.

After you eat, bacteria go crazy over the sugar on your teeth, like ants at a picnic. The bacteria break it down into acids that eat away tooth enamel, causing holes called cavities. Plaque also causes gingivitis (say: jin-juh-vi-tis), which is gum disease that can make your gums red, swollen, and sore. Your gums are those soft pink tissues in your mouth that hold your teeth in place.

If you don't take care of your teeth, cavities and unhealthy gums will make your mouth very, very sore. Eating meals will be difficult. And you won't feel like smiling so much.

Before Toothpaste Was Invented

We're lucky that we know so much now about taking care of our teeth. Long ago, as people got older, their teeth would rot away and be very painful. To get rid of a toothache, they had their teeth pulled out. Finally people learned that cleaning their teeth was important, but they didn't have toothpaste right away. While you're swishing that minty-fresh paste around your mouth, think about what people used long ago to clean teeth:

- ground-up chalk or charcoal
- lemon juice
- ashes (you know, the stuff that's left over after a fire)
- tobacco and honey mixed together

Yuck!

It was only about 100 years ago that someone finally created a minty cream to clean teeth. Not long after that, the toothpaste tube was invented, so people could squeeze the paste right onto the toothbrush. Tooth brushing became popular during World War II. The U.S. Army gave brushes and toothpaste to all soldiers, and they learned to brush twice a day. Back then, toothpaste tubes were made of metal; today they're made of soft plastic and are much easier to squeeze.

Today there are plenty of toothpaste choices: lots of colors and flavors to choose from, and some are made just for kids. People with great-looking teeth advertise toothpaste on television (TV) commercials and in magazines. When you're choosing a toothpaste, make sure it contains fluoride. Fluoride makes your teeth strong and protects them from cavities.

When you brush, you don't need a lot of toothpaste: just squeeze out a bit the size of a pea. It's not a good idea to swallow the toothpaste, either, so be sure to rinse and spit after brushing.

How You Can Keep Your Teeth Healthy

Kids can take charge of their teeth by taking these steps:

- Brush at least twice a day—after breakfast and before bedtime. If you can, brush after lunch or after sweet snacks. Brushing properly breaks down plaque.
- Brush all of your teeth, not just the front ones. Spend some time on the teeth along the sides and in the back. Have your dentist show you the best way to brush to get your teeth clean without damaging your gums.
- Take your time while brushing. Spend at least two or three minutes each time you brush. If you have trouble keeping track of

the time, use a timer or play a recording of a song you like to help pass the time.

- Be sure your toothbrush has soft bristles (the package will tell you if they're soft). Ask your parent to help you get a new toothbrush every three months. Some toothbrushes come with bristles that change color when it's time to change them.

- Ask your dentist if an antibacterial mouth rinse is right for you.

- Learn how to floss your teeth, which is a very important way to keep them healthy. It feels weird the first few times you do it, but pretty soon you'll be a pro. Slip the dental floss between each tooth and along the gum line gently once a day. The floss gets rid of food that's hidden where your toothbrush can't get it, no matter how well you brush.

- You can also brush your tongue to help keep your breath fresh!

It's also important to visit the dentist twice a year. Besides checking for signs of cavities or gum disease, the dentist will help keep your teeth extra clean and can help you learn the best way to brush and floss.

It's not just brushing and flossing that keep your teeth healthy—you also need to be careful about what you eat and drink. Remember, the plaque on your teeth is just waiting for that sugar to arrive. Eat lots of fruits and vegetables and drink water instead of soda. And don't forget to smile!

Section 3.2

Choosing a Toothbrush

"How Do I Choose and Use a Toothbrush?" Reprinted with permission from *General Dentistry*, February 2012. © Academy of General Dentistry. All rights reserved. On the Web at www.agi.org.

How do I choose and use a toothbrush?

Angled heads, raised bristles, oscillating tufts, and handles that change colors with use: you name it, toothbrushes come in all shapes, colors, and sizes, promising to perform better than the rest. But no body of scientific evidence exists yet to show that any one type of toothbrush design is better at removing plaque than another. The only thing that matters is that you brush your teeth. Many people just don't brush long enough. Most of us brush less than a minute, but to effectively reach all areas and scrub off cavity-causing bacteria, it is recommended to brush for two to three minutes.

Which toothbrush is best?

In general, a toothbrush head should be small (one inch by a half inch) for easy access to all areas of the mouth, teeth, and gums. It should have a long, wide handle for a firm grasp. It should have soft nylon bristles with rounded ends so you won't hurt your gums.

When should I change my toothbrush?

Be sure to change your toothbrush, or toothbrush head (if you're using an electric toothbrush) before the bristles become splayed and frayed. Not only are old toothbrushes ineffective, but they may harbor harmful bacteria that can cause infections such as gingivitis and periodontitis. Toothbrushes should be changed every three to four months. Sick people should change their toothbrush at the beginning of an illness and after they feel better.

23

How do I brush?

Place the toothbrush beside your teeth at a 45-degree angle and rub back-and-forth gently. Brush outside and behind the teeth, your tongue, and especially on chewing surfaces and between teeth. Be sure to brush at least twice a day, especially after meals.

How long should I brush my teeth?

You should brush your teeth at least two to three minutes twice a day. Brush your teeth for the length of a song on the radio, the right amount of time to get the best results from brushing. Unfortunately, most Americans only brush for 45 to 70 seconds twice a day.

Which is better, an electric or manual toothbrush?

Electric toothbrushes don't work that much better than manual toothbrushes, but they do motivate some reluctant brushers to clean their teeth more often. The whizzing sounds of an electric toothbrush and the tingle of the rotary tufts swirling across teeth and gums often captivate people who own electric toothbrushes. They are advantageous because they can cover more area faster. Electric toothbrushes are recommended for people who have limited manual dexterity, such as a disabled or elderly person, and those who wear braces. Sometimes, it takes more time and effort to use an electric toothbrush because batteries must be recharged, and it must be cleaned after every use.

How do electric toothbrushes work?

Electric toothbrushes generally work by using tufts of nylon bristles to stimulate gums and clean teeth in an oscillating, or rotary, motion. Some tufts are arranged in a circular pattern, while others have the traditional shape of several bristles lined up on a row. When you are first using an electric toothbrush, expect some bleeding from your gums. The bleeding will stop when you learn to control the brush and your gums become healthier. Children under the age of ten years should be supervised when using an electric toothbrush. Avoid mashing the tufts against your teeth in an effort to clean them. Use light force and slow movements, and allow the electric bristle action to do its job.

Don't Forget

Visit your dentist regularly because tooth brushing and flossing is most effective with periodic checkups and cleanings.

Section 3.3

How to Brush and Floss

This section includes excerpts from "The Use and Handling of Toothbrushes," Centers for Disease Control and Prevention (CDC), 2009; and "How to Brush Your Teeth," and "How to Use Dental Floss," September 2010, reprinted with permission from the North Carolina Department of Health and Human Services, Division of Public Health, Oral Health Section. For additional information, visit http://www.ncchhs.gov/dph/oralhealth.

The Use and Handling of Toothbrushes

Tooth brushing with a fluoride toothpaste is a simple, widely recommended, and widely practiced method of caring for one's teeth. When done routinely and properly, tooth brushing can reduce the amount of plaque which contains the bacteria associated with gum disease and tooth decay, as well as provide the cavity-preventing benefits of fluoride.

Recommended Toothbrush Care

- Do not share toothbrushes. The exchange of body fluids that such sharing would foster places toothbrush sharers at an increased risk for infections, a particularly important consideration for persons with compromised immune systems or infectious diseases.

- After brushing, rinse your toothbrush thoroughly with tap water to ensure the removal of toothpaste and debris, allow it to air-dry, and store it in an upright position. If multiple brushes are stored in the same holder, do not allow them to contact each other.

- It is not necessary to soak toothbrushes in disinfecting solutions or mouthwash. This practice actually may lead to cross-contamination of toothbrushes if the same disinfectant solution is used over a period of time or by multiple users.

- It is also unnecessary to use dishwashers, microwaves, or ultraviolet devices to disinfect toothbrushes. These measures may damage the toothbrush.

- Do not routinely cover toothbrushes or store them in closed containers. Such conditions (a humid environment) are more conducive to bacterial growth than the open air.

- Replace your toothbrush every 3–4 months, or sooner if the bristles appear worn or splayed. This recommendation of the American Dental Association (ADA) is based on the expected wear of the toothbrush and its subsequent loss of mechanical effectiveness, not on its bacterial contamination.

A decision to purchase or use products for toothbrush disinfection requires careful consideration, as the scientific literature does not support this practice at the present time.

Brushing Your Teeth

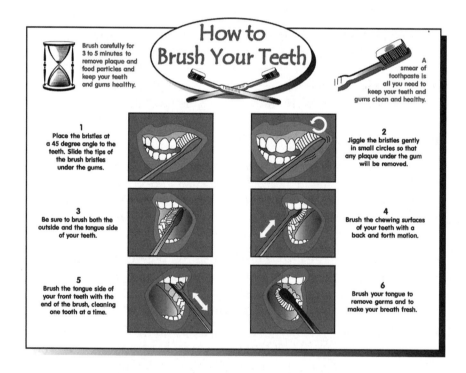

Figure 3.1. How to Brush Your Teeth (September 2010, reprinted with permission from the North Carolina Department of Health and Human Services, Division of Public Health, Oral Health Section. For additional information, visit http://www.ncdhhs.gov/dph/oralhealth.)

Dental Floss

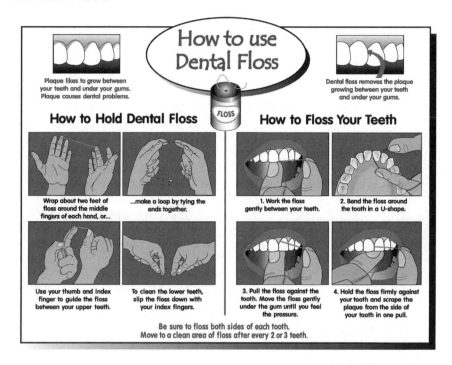

Figure 3.2. *How to Use Dental Floss (September 2010, reprinted with permission from the North Carolina Department of Health and Human Services, Division of Public Health, Oral Health Section. For additional information, visit http://www.ncdhhs.gov/dph/oralhealth.)*

Section 3.4

Mouth Rinses

Mouth rinses are generally classified as either cosmetic or therapeutic.

- **Cosmetic mouth rinses** are commercial, over-the-counter products that help remove oral debris before or after brushing, temporarily suppress bad breath, diminish bacteria in the mouth, and refresh the mouth with a pleasant taste. At the very least, they are effective oral antiseptics that freshen the mouth and alleviate bad breath in the short term.

- **Therapeutic mouth rinses** have the same benefits as cosmetic mouth rinses; however, they also contain an added active ingredient that helps protect against some oral diseases.

Common Mouth Rinses

Common mouth rinses include saltwater, chlorhexidine, essential oils, fluoride, and antibacterial rinses.

- **Saltwater rinse:** Mild, warm saltwater rinses may benefit patients who have ulcers, minor throat irritation, and denture sores by alleviating discomfort and aiding healing. Consult a dental professional if the area continues to be irritated or sore for longer than one week.

- **Chlorhexidine rinse:** Chlorhexidine is very effective in reducing bacteria found in the oral cavity. Long-term use of chlorhexidine rinses may alter perception of taste, cause brown staining on teeth, and increase the formation of calculus (tartar or scale). The use of chlorhexidine should be recommended by a dental professional and used according to their recommendations.

- **Mouth rinse containing essential oils:** The use of essential oils in mouth rinses is proven to be effective in reducing bad breath.

- **Fluoride mouth rinse:** Fluoride mouth rinses are recommended by dental professionals to control and prevent tooth decay. Use of a fluoride mouth rinse, along with fluoride toothpaste, can provide extra protection against tooth decay. However, the use of fluoride mouth rinse is not recommended for children.

- **Antibacterial mouth rinse:** Antibacterial mouth rinses reduce the bacteria in the mouth and alter the bacterial activity in plaque. They are particularly helpful in helping to control gingivitis and minor throat infections.

Practical Advice

While mouth rinses should not be considered substitutes for regular toothbrushing and flossing, they can be useful for a number of different purposes depending on their ingredients. Mouth rinses are unable to penetrate existing plaque, making them ineffective below the gums. A mouth rinse is also unable to reach between the teeth. A dental professional may recommend specific mouth rinses for specific oral conditions. Dental professionals may also recommend rinses for those who can't brush due to physical impairments or medical reasons. Many mouth rinses contain high concentrations of alcohol. Individuals suffering from dry mouth, pregnant women, and children should not use mouth rinses containing alcohol.

Using a Mouth Rinse

- Brush and floss teeth before using a mouth rinse.

- Measure the recommended amount of rinse.

- Rinse or swish the liquid around your mouth for the time recommended on the packaging (or as recommended by your dental professional).

- Spit liquid out of mouth thoroughly.

- To maximize the effects of the mouth rinse, do not rinse, eat, or smoke for thirty minutes after using it.

Section 3.5

Oral Irrigation

Excerpted from "Comparison of Irrigation to Floss as an Adjunct to Tooth Brushing: Effect on Bleeding, Gingivitis, and Supragingival Plaque," by Caren M. Barnes, RDH, MS, Carl M. Russell, DMD, PhD, Richard A. Reinhardt, DDS, PhD, Jeffrey B. Payne, DDS, MDS, and Deborah M. Lyle, RDH, MS. *Journal of Clinical Dentistry, 16(3),* 71–77. © 2005 Journal of Clinical Dentistry. Reprinted with permission. Reviewed by David Cooke, MD, FACP, in April 2012.

Introduction

Research over the last decade has established that the etiology of periodontal disease is a bacterial infection mediated by the host inflammatory response. [1-4] While effective daily removal or disruption of dental plaque is essential, it may not be enough to completely prevent the disease. One oral hygiene device, the oral irrigator, has demonstrated its effectiveness in decreasing the by-products of the host inflammatory response associated with gingivitis and periodontitis when used on a daily basis. [5, 6]

The daily use of oral irrigation has been shown to reduce dental plaque, calculus, gingivitis, bleeding, probing depth, periodontal pathogens, and host inflammatory mediators. [5-20] Of these clinical parameters, all have demonstrated the same consistency in outcomes over the years, with the exception of supragingival plaque reduction. This single incongruence has led some dental professionals to reject irrigation despite evidence that it improves periodontal health.

One reason for this inconsistency may be that traditional dental plaque indices provide a quantitative measure of plaque. Emerging information indicates plaque is a biofilm. Research demonstrates that dental biofilm is a more complex configuration than previously believed, leading many to speculate that traditional indices are inadequate because they fail to evaluate qualitative changes. This may be the case with home irrigation as several researchers have found that irrigation is capable of reducing subgingival pathogens, thus altering biofilm composition. [7, 9, 11, 12, 14, 15, 20, 21] In addition to reducing subgingival pathogens, oral irrigation irreparably damages bacterial cells. Plaque that remains on irrigated teeth contains bacteria that have ruptured cell walls or incomplete cellular contents, rendering the plaque less potent and less pathogenic.[22] Concomitant to damaging bacterial cells, oral irrigation is effective in removing endotoxins that are produced in the immune response to periodontal infections.[23]

The strongest and most consistent evidence for the benefit of home irrigation is its ability to reduce gingivitis and bleeding.[5-8, 10, 12-21] Newman, et al.[8] had subjects add daily irrigation with water to routine oral hygiene (brushing and flossing), and found enhanced gingivitis and bleeding reductions over brushing and flossing alone. Others have found similar findings,[5, 6, 8] including Flemmig[10] who observed a 50% greater reduction in bleeding over routine oral hygiene. Drisko's recent research indicated that when daily irrigation with water was added to a regular oral hygiene home regimen, a significant reduction in probing depth, bleeding on probing, and gingival index was observed. Further, a host modulatory response, as evidenced by changes in the cytokine levels of IL-1β and prostaglandin E$_2$ (PGE$_2$) which are associated with destructive changes in inflamed tissues and bone resorption, also occurs with the use of oral irrigators.[5]

Traditionally, tooth brushing—power or manual—and flossing have been considered the standard for routine plaque removal and gingivitis reduction. One problem with this regimen is that compliance with floss is low.[24] Therefore, the purpose of this study was to assess the efficacy of adding daily oral irrigation to both power and manual tooth brushing, compared to a traditional regimen of manual tooth brushing and flossing, to determine which regimen had the greatest effect on the reduction of bleeding, gingivitis, and supragingival plaque.

Discussion

Although it is universally recognized that interproximal cleaning is essential for controlling periodontal disease, many people have difficulty accomplishing this with traditional dental floss. It has been documented that about 30% of the adult population use floss, and even fewer (22%) use it correctly.[24] Additionally, when given a preference, most patients choose an alternative device over manual floss.[28-30]

This study shows that the addition of oral irrigation to either manual or power tooth brushing provides significant benefits to oral health through greater reductions in bleeding and gingivitis over traditional brushing and flossing, notably with a near two-fold increase in the percent reduction in bleeding in Group 2 compared to Group 1. While oral irrigation studies in the past have allowed subjects who flossed to continue with their regimen, this is the first study to evaluate the use of oral irrigation and brushing compared to a group of subjects that included both brushing and flossing. This finding may be important to individuals who either do not floss, or have significant difficulties flossing. Based on these results, it appears that the manual or power tooth brushing, plus the use of an oral irrigation device once daily with plain water, is as effective as a traditional brushing and flossing routine, and in some cases may provide superior results for reducing bleeding and gingivitis.

The reason oral irrigation is as effective as flossing in this study is not completely understood. Based on previous studies, it is likely related to both the ability of irrigation to reduce subgingival pathogens and to modulate the host response. Cobb and investigators demonstrated via electron microscope that oral irrigation with water reduced periodontal pathogens up to six millimeters (mm), and reduced the fibrin-like network housing the plaque.[9] Likewise, Drisko, et al. demonstrated spirochete reduction up to 6 mm.[11] In 1994, Chaves, et al. found that oral irrigation with either water or 0.04% chlorhexidine reduced subgingival pathogens over tooth brushing plus 0.12% chlorhexidine rinsing and tooth brushing alone.[7] They noted that even though water irrigation reduced subgingival pathogens, it did not significantly change the measurement of supragingival plaque. At the same time, they found that inflammation was reduced independent of plaque removal.

Chaves, et al. further speculated that oral irrigation may produce a change in the host response.[7] In 2000, Cutler, et al. demonstrated the host modulatory effect of oral irrigation by showing that daily irrigation with water reduced the gingival crevicular fluid measures of pro-inflammatory mediators interleukin-13 (IL-13) and PGE_2, while increasing an anti-inflammatory mediatory interleukin-10 (IL-10) and holding stable interferon-gamma (IFNγ) better than routine oral hygiene.[5] Further, Cutler, et al. noted that only the addition of irrigation produced this host modulatory change.[5] Tooth brushing alone did not. Interestingly, the reduction in bleeding could not be linked to plaque removal, but rather was correlated to the reduction of IL-13.[5]

In 2002, Al-Mubarak, et al. found that twice daily water irrigation via a soft subgingival tip (Pik Pocket® subgingival irrigation tip, Waterpik Technologies, Fort Collins, CO) reduced both traditional clinical measures of periodontitis and serum measures of interleukin and PGE_2 in individuals living with diabetes better than tooth brushing alone.[6]

Oral irrigation has a long history of reducing bleeding and gingivitis independent of plaque removal. While this sounds contradictory, emerging information on the virulence of plaque are beginning to provide answers. Full understanding will only come with further research into the complexities of plaque as a biofilm. Socransky and Haffajee[31] noted that hydrodynamics affect both the physical shear stress and the rate at which nutrients are transported to the surface of plaque, and that these impact the structure and growth of plaque. They also state that modification of the host response affects plaque habitat and the colonization of microbiota.[31] These findings have similarities to a 1988 study by Cobb, et al. who found that non-irrigated areas had plaque and debris in fibrin-like mesh, while irrigated sites had little or no fibrin mesh present.[9]

Flossing is a mainstay in the culture of dental professionals. Moving away from traditional devices with concrete methods of removing plaque to products that provide benefits via a host modulatory effect may be difficult. Studies such as this contribute to a healthy professional discourse that paves the road for future research and product development.

The results of this clinical trial support the findings of previous research in that the mechanism by which oral irrigation improves gingival health is not completely understood. A consistent finding in previous research is that the use of an oral irrigator improves bleeding and gingivitis without a direct correlation to a reduction in the amount of plaque, suggesting the disruption of plaque and subsequent removal of endotoxins weakens the pathogenicity of the plaque. Oral healthcare providers are challenged consistently to achieve even 30% patient compliance with flossing,[24] making the selection of alternative interdental cleaning devices all the more important. Significant improvements in oral health occurred regardless of toothbrush type, so it is likely that many patients currently using a power toothbrush may get further improvements in oral health by the addition of oral irrigation. The results of this clinical trial indicate that when combined with tooth brushing, oral irrigation is an effective alternative to traditional dental floss for reducing bleeding and gingival inflammation.

Based upon the findings in this study, further research on the long-term effects of irrigation regimens is warranted.

Conclusions

The results of this study reveal the following:

1. Oral irrigation paired with a manual toothbrush was statistically better at reducing bleeding and gingivitis than manual brushing and flossing. Notably, the group utilizing oral irrigation and manual brushing had a near two-fold increase in the

percent reduction of bleeding, compared to the group utilizing a manual brush and floss.

2. Oral irrigation paired with a power toothbrush was statistically better at reducing bleeding and better at reducing gingivitis than manual brushing and flossing.

3. Oral irrigation and manual brushing removed plaque as well as manual brushing and flossing on lingual surfaces, while oral irrigation plus power brushing was statistically better than manual brushing and flossing on facial surfaces.

References

1. Page RC, Komman KS: The pathogenesis of human periodontitis: An introduction. *Periodontol 2000 14:9–11*, 1997.

2. Komman KS, Page RC, Tonetti MS: The host response to the microbial challenge in periodontitis: Assembling the players. *Periodontol 2000 14:33–35*, 1997.

3. Armitage GC: Periodontal diseases: Diagnosis. *Ann Periodontol 1:37–215*, 1996.

4. Ishikawa I, Nakashima K, Kosedi T, Nagaswa T, Wantabe H, Arakwa S, Nitta H, Nishikara T: Induction of the immune response to periodontopathic bacteria and its role in the pathogenesis of periodontitis. *Periodontol 2000 14:79–111*, 1997.

5. Cutler CW, Stanford TW, Cederberg A, Boardman TJ, Ross C: Clinical benefits of oral irrigation for periodontitis are related to reduction of proinflammatory cytokine levels and plaque. *J Clin Periodontol 27:134–143*, 2000.

6. AI-Mubarak S, Ciancio S, Aljada A, Awa H, Hamouda W, Ghanim H, Zambon J, Boardman TJ, Mohanty P, Ross C, Dandona P: Comparative evaluation of adjunctive oral irrigation in diabetics. *J Clin Periodontol 29: 295–300*, 2002.

7. Chaves ES, Komman KS, Manwell MA, Jones AA, Newhold DA, Wood RC: Mechanism of irrigation effects on gingivitis. *J Periodontol 65: 1016–1021*, 1994.

8. Newman MG, Cattagriga M, Etiene D, Flemmig T, Sanz M, Komman KS, Doherty F, Moore DJ, Ross C: Effectiveness of adjunctive irrigation in early periodontitis: Multi-center evaluation. *J Periodontol 65:224–229*, 1994.

9. Cobb CM, Rodgers RL, Killoy WJ: Ultrastructural examination of human periodontal pockets following the use of an oral irrigation device in vivo. *J Periodontol 59:155–163*, 1988.

10. Flemmig TF, Epp B, Funkenhauser Z, Newman MG, Komman KS, Hawbitz I, Klaiber B: Adjunctive supragingival irrigation with acetylsalicylic acid in periodontal supportive therapy. *J Clin Periodontol 22:427–433*, 1995.

11. Drisko CL, White CL, Killoy WJ, Mayberry WE: Comparison of darkfield microscopy and a flagella stain for monitoring the effect of a Water Pik on bacterial motility. *J Periodontol 58:381–386*, 1987.

12. Ciancio SG, Mather ML, Zambon JJ, Reynolds HS: Effect of a chemotherapeutic agent delivered by an oral irrigation device on plaque, gingivitis, and subgingival microflora. *J Periodontol 60:310–315*, 1989.

13. Flemmig TF, Newman MG, Doherty PM, Grossman E, Meckel AH, Bakdash. MB: Supragingival irrigation with 0.06% chlorhexidine in naturally occurring gingivitis I 6–month clinical observations. *J Periodontol 61:1l2–117*, 1990.

14. Jolkovsky DL, Waki MY, Newman MG, Otono–Corgel J, Madison M, Flemmig TF, Nacknani S, Nowzari H: Clinical and microbiological effects of subgingival and gingival marginal irrigation with chlorhexidine gluconate. *J Periodontol 61:663–669*, 1990.

15. Brownstein CN, Briggs SD, Schweitzer KL, Briner WW, Komman KS: Irrigation with chlorhexidine to resolve naturally occurring gingivitis: A methodologic study. *J Clin Periodontol 17:588–593*, 1990.

16. Felo A, Shibly 0, Ciancio SG, Lauciello FR, Ho A: Effects of subgingival chlorhexidine irrigation on peri–implant maintenance. *Am J Dent 10: 107–110*, 1997.

17. Hugoson A: Effect of the Water Pik device on plaque accumulation and development of gingivitis. *J Clin Periodontol 5:95–104*, 1978.

18. Wolff LF, Bakdash MB, Pihlstrom BL, Bandt CL, Aeppli DML: The effect of professional and home subgingival irrigation with antimicrobial agents on gingivitis and early periodontitis. *J Dent Hyg 63:222–224*, 1989.

19. Lobene RR. The effect of a pulsed water pressure-cleansing device on oral health. *J Periodontol 40:667–670*, 1969.

20. Newman MG, Flemmig TF, Nachnani S, Rodrigues A, Calsin G, Lee Y–S, de Camargo P, Doherty FM, Bakdash MB: Irrigation with 0.06% chlorhexidine in naturally occurring gingivitis. II. 6 months microbiological observations. *J Periodontol 61:427–433*, 1990.

21. Fine JB, Harper DS, Gordon JM, Houliaras CA, Charles CH: Short–term microbiological and clinical effects of subgingival irrigation with an antimicrobial mouthrinse. *J Periodontol 65:30–36*, 1994.

22. Brady JM, Gray WA, Bhaskar SN: Electron microscopic study of the effect of water jet lavage device on dental plaque. *J Dent Res 52:1310–1316*, 1993.

23. Weinberg MA, Westphal C, Froum SJ, Palat M: *Comprehensive Periodontics for the Dental Hygienist, 2nd ed.*, Pearson Prentice Hall, Upper Saddle River, NJ, p. 389, 2006.

24. Lang WP, Ronis DL, Farghaly MM: Preventive behaviors as correlates of periodontal health status. *J Public Health Dent 55:10–17*,1995.

25. Carter HG, Bames GP: The gingival bleeding index. *J Periodontol 45:801– 805*,1974.

26. L6e H, Silness J: Periodontal disease in pregnancy. I. Prevalence and severity. *Acta Odontol Scand 21:533–537*, 1963.

27. Benson BJ, Henyon G, Grossman E, Mankodi S, Sharma NC: Development and verification of the proximal/marginal plaque index. *J Clin Dent 4: 14–20*, 1993.

28. Shibly O, Ciancio SG, Shostad S, Mather M, Boardman TJ: Clinical evaluation of an automated flossing device vs. manual flossing. *J Clin Dent 12: 63–66*, 2001.

29. Pucher J, Jayaprahask P, Aftyka T, Sigmai L, Van Swol R: Clinical evaluation of a new flossing device. *Quintessence Int 26:273–275*, 1995.

30. Christou V, Timmerman MF, Van der Velden U, Van der Weijden FA: Comparison of different approaches of interdental oral hygiene: Interdental brushes versus dental floss. *J Periodontol 69:759–764*, 1998.

31. Socransky SS, Haffajee AD: Dental biofilms: Difficult therapeutic targets. *Periodontol 2000 28:12–55*, 2002.

Section 3.6

Best Whitener to Use at Home

This section includes: "Tooth Whitening Systems," © 2011 American Dental Hygienists' Association (www.adha.org). All rights reserved. Reprinted with permission. Also, "Which Is the Best Teeth Whitener for Use at Home?" reprinted with permission from www.dental-health-advice.com. © 2011 Dr. Richard Mitchell, BDS.

Tooth Whitening Systems

Note: Before using any whitening procedure, American Dental Hygienists' Association (ADHA) recommends that you first be evaluated by an oral health care professional to determine which application and program are best for you.

Why do my teeth have stains and discolorations?

Most stains are caused by age, tobacco, coffee, or tea. Other types of stains can be caused by antibiotics, such as tetracycline; or too much fluoride.

What treatments are used for stained teeth?

Ask your oral health care professional about tooth-whitening options. They include a number of over-the-counter whitening systems, whitening toothpastes, and the latest high-tech option—laser tooth whitening. For maximum whitening, experts agree that peroxide is usually the way to go.

Supervised bleaching procedures that are done in-office and at-home have become among the most popular treatment options. In some cases, the procedure is performed entirely in the office, using a light or heat source to speed up the bleaching process. In other cases, an oral health care professional gets the procedure started during an office visit, and then gives you what you need to complete it at home. Still another popular procedure is one that you complete entirely at home.

At-home procedures, sometimes called nightguard vital bleaching, consist of placing a bleaching solution, usually a peroxide mixture, in a tray (nightguard) that has been custom fitted for your mouth by an oral health care professional. The bleaching solutions may vary in potency and may be worn for an hour, or throughout the night. Your oral health care professional can advise you on the appropriate type of application and the length of time needed to whiten your teeth, based on the severity of tooth discoloration and your specific needs.

How effective are bleaching systems?

Bleaching is effective in lightning most stains caused by age, tobacco, coffee, and tea. Based on clinical studies, 96% of patients with these kinds of stains experience some lightening effect. Other types of stains, such as those produced by tetracycline use or fluorosis (too much fluoride), respond to bleaching less reliably. And one cosmetic dentist points out that bleaching systems are not fully predictable. If you have a tooth-color filling when your teeth are bleached, the filling will stay yellow—dental restorations do not change color when tooth whitener is applied.

Are there any side effects to tooth bleaching?

In some studies, patients have experienced uncomfortable short-term side effects when having teeth bleached. Hydrogen peroxide can increase temperature sensitivity in the teeth, particularly at higher concentrations, and nightguards often cause gum irritation. And over-zealous use of over-the-counter home bleaching products can wear away tooth enamel, especially with solutions that contain acid. Therefore, bleaching is a procedure best done under the care of an oral health care professional. Still, the general health risks of bleaching systems are minimal as far as your body is concerned. Applications are controlled so that you don't swallow hydrogen peroxide.

What's available?

While research continues into all types of bleaching systems, tooth bleaching is sure to continue to grow in popularity. Here's a selection of what's currently available.

- **At-home bleaching kits:** The most popular whitening option. Mouth trays are usually made in one office visit, and your oral health care professional will provide a whitening brand suitable to your needs. Some trays are worn for an hour, others through the night. Kits range in price from $300 to $500.

- **Bonding:** A composite resin that is molded onto the teeth to change their color and to reshape them. The resin material can stain and chip over time. Bonding can usually be done in one office visit for $300-$700 per tooth.

- **Porcelain veneers:** These shell-like facings can be bonded onto stained teeth. They are used to reshape and/or lengthen teeth as well as to whiten. Veneers require at least two office visits and cost $700 to $1,200 per tooth.

- **Whitening toothpastes:** While some whitening toothpastes effectively keep the teeth cleaner and, therefore, looking whiter, some are more abrasive than others. The stronger toothpastes rely on abrasion to remove external stains as opposed to actually changing the color of teeth.

The key is to study a product's ingredients, look at your teeth to see if it changes their color, and consult your oral health care professional for customized advice.

Which Is the Best Teeth Whitener for Use at Home?

(Reprinted with permission from www.dental-health-advice.com. © 2011 Dr. Richard Mitchell, BDS.)

A Review of the Best Home Teeth Whitening Product— Pro-White Teeth

The best teeth whitener for home use is a system that combines the best of two worlds. Normally, at one extreme are teeth whitening products supplied by a dentist. At the other extreme are teeth whitening gels that you can buy over-the-counter at a pharmacy or store and take home. Both methods frequently make claims to be the best home teeth whitening system.

Dentists' teeth whitening products work best but are expensive, while over-the-counter teeth whitening gels are very cheap, but usually do not work very well. Personal experience has shown that Pro-White Teeth is an excellent new product that offers you the best of both worlds. It can whiten teeth just as good as any dentist-supplied teeth whitening products, but it costs a lot less.

It may seem strange for this author, as a dentist, to be recommending a product that does not need a dentist; but, believing in "telling it straight," the Pro-White Teeth system has been found in personal practice to be the best over-the-counter teeth whitener.

Why Dentist Supplied Products Work Well

Looking at why dentist-supplied products work so well, and why over-the-counter teeth whitening gel from a pharmacy or other store just does not work well at all, there are two things that impact effectiveness.

- One of them is the actual teeth whitening gel—how strong is it? Does it lose strength if it is left on the shelf for long? And will it make your teeth sensitive?

- The other one is how the gel is applied to the teeth. Is it protected from saliva? Can it leak out, away from the tooth surfaces?

The dentist-supplied products have both areas covered; they use custom-made splints or trays that fit your teeth very accurately. This concentrates the gel right where you want it for best effect. And because they fit so well, they prevent saliva getting in, diluting the gel, and they prevent any gel from leaking out and getting on your gums. This also means that the gel can be stronger, so it works better. In addition, the gels from a dental office will have a longer shelf-life, and have a lower risk of tooth sensitivity.

On the other hand, the "boil and bite" kits that you can buy over the counter do not fit anywhere near as well as the dentist-supplied splints. This means that over-the-counter whitening gels have to be weaker, because they are going to leak out, and saliva can leak in under the splint, diluting any gel that does remain.

Pro-White Teeth is a clever system that can exploit the advantages of dentist-supplied systems, but without a dentist. And that is the key point. If you take the dentist out of the mix, you are also cutting out the middle man. You deal directly with the manufacturer. And that means lower prices. This combination of "dentist quality whitening" with low prices makes Pro-White Teeth worthy of the title "best teeth whitener".

So how does this all work? Actually, it is surprisingly simple. Here are the steps:

1. First, you go to the Pro-White Teeth website. Have a look at the options available, and decide which kit is right for you. Then you can place your order right there.

2. A few days later, you will receive a package from Pro-White Teeth. This contains the materials you need to take molds (impressions) of your own teeth. The system is easy to use, and comes with full instructions. It is well-explained.

3. After you have taken the molds of your teeth according to the instructions, you mail them back in the envelope provided. Pro-White Teeth have their own specialized dental laboratory, and make up the custom trays themselves. Again, no middle man.

4. A few days after that, you will receive your custom whitening trays in the mail, with a supply of gel. Again, there are full instructions on what to do, which are well-written and very clear.

5. Start whitening.

The only thing this author would not recommend is the "Instant Tray Kit." These trays will just not fit as well as the custom trays. The best options are the Platinum and Titanium kits.

You can also order the gels separately if you want to top-up your whitening later on, perhaps for a special occasion. The 22% strength gel is recommended. If sensitivity proves to be a problem, just wear the custom trays for 30–45 minutes, instead of the normal two hours. Over about 7–10 days, your teeth will gradually become whiter. One of the things about home teeth whitening is that you are in full control. You can start and stop the whitening treatment anytime you want. You can also target individual teeth if there are a couple that are darker than the others. When you think the color is okay, you stop the treatment, and put your spare gel in the refrigerator. (You should always store your gel in the refrigerator.)

Keep the custom whitening trays safe and away from any heat sources. After 12–24 months you may notice a slight loss of whiteness from your teeth. Just get out your gel and trays again—usually 1–2 applications will get your whiteness back to where you want it. Pro-White Teeth has a 30-day money back guarantee. This is unique. There may be some individual dental offices that have a similar guarantee, but it's unusual for a manufacturer to offer a warranty on their teeth whitening gel.

Pro-White Teeth has the vote of many dentists as the best teeth whitener to use at home. It gets great results using professional-quality custom trays and dentist-strength teeth whitening gel, but at a much lower cost.

Section 3.7

Avoiding Tooth Wear

Tooth wear is the irreversible loss of tooth structure, which is often painful, unsightly, and impairs the function of teeth. The damage can also be costly and difficult to repair. There are three types of tooth wear: abrasion, attrition, and erosion. It is sometimes difficult to determine the type of tooth wear present because different types often occur together.

- **Abrasion:** Physical wear of the teeth caused by something other than tooth to tooth contact (for example, overzealous or inappropriate toothbrushing, repeated use of a toothpick, or placing hair pins between the teeth).

- **Attrition:** Loss of tooth structure as a result of tooth to tooth contact, such as grinding of teeth.

- **Dental erosion:** Dissolving of tooth enamel due to the presence of acids in the mouth.

This section discusses how to recognize dental erosion, the causes of dental erosion, and how you can minimize the risk.

What does dental erosion look like?

The first signs of dental erosion include:

- teeth appearing yellow (due to darker colored tissue showing through thinning tooth enamel),

- teeth appearing glazed and smooth (due to the tooth surface being worn away),

- teeth appearing to become shorter,

- fillings sitting higher than the surrounding tooth surface,

- chewing surfaces of the teeth showing smooth, concave craters, and/or

- sensitive teeth.

What causes dental erosion?

The cause of dental erosion is acid attack. Many drinks including soft drinks, energy drinks, sports drinks, alcohol, and fruit juices contain acids. Most of these drinks also have a high sugar content that can cause the teeth to decay.

A diet high in acidic food and drinks can cause tooth wear. The lower the pH of a product, the more acidic it is. Any food or drink with a pH lower than five may cause tooth wear and tooth sensitivity.

Other factors that contribute to erosion include:

- a dry mouth, which increases the risk of damage from acid attack, and/or

- stomach acid coming in contact with teeth due to vomiting from conditions such as bulimia, morning sickness, and gastric reflux.

What should I do to minimize the risk of dental erosion?

- Eat a well-balanced diet, and reduce the amount of acidic and sugary foods and drinks. Try to limit snacking.

Table 3.1. pH of Some Common Foods and Drinks

Milk	pH 6.9
Flavored milk	pH 6.7
Tap water	pH 6.0
Cheddar cheese	pH 5.9
Coffee	pH 5.0
Beer	pH 4.5
Orange juice	pH 3.5
Apple juice	pH 3.4
Grapefruit	pH 3.3
Pickles	pH 3.2
Sports energy drinks	pH 3.0
Common soft drink	pH 2.7
Cola	pH 2.5
Red wine	pH 2.5
Lemon juice	pH 2.2
Vinegar	pH 2.0

- Eat foods that act as a buffer by neutralizing saliva pH more quickly (for example, dairy products contain a protein called casein which protects teeth from acid).

- Avoid holding or swishing acidic drinks around the mouth as this increases the likelihood of tooth decay and tooth wear.

- When drinking, use a straw whenever possible as this minimizes exposure of the drink to your teeth.

- Chew sugar-free gum to stimulate saliva flow and wash acids away.

- Drink plenty of water frequently throughout the day, especially if exercising. If available, drink fluoridated water.

- Avoid caffeinated beverages, as caffeine causes dehydration.

- Do not brush immediately after eating or drinking acidic or sugary foods or drinks as tooth enamel will be softened and could be brushed off.

Chapter 4

Removing Dental Plaque Improves Your Oral Health

Chapter Contents

Section 4.1

What Plaque Is and How to Get Rid of It

"Plaque: What it is and how to get rid of it," National Institute of Dental and Craniofacial Research (NIDCR), NIH Publication No. 99-3245, July 1999. Reviewed by David Cooke, MD, FACP, in April 2012.

Plaque

People used to think that as you got older you naturally lost your teeth. We now know that is not true. By following easy steps for keeping your teeth and gums healthy plus seeing your dentist regularly, you can have your teeth for a lifetime.

Plaque is made up of invisible masses of harmful germs that live in the mouth and stick to the teeth.

- Some types of plaque cause tooth decay.
- Other types of plaque cause gum disease.

Red, puffy, or bleeding gums can be the first signs of gum disease. If gum disease is not treated, the tissues holding the teeth in place are destroyed and the teeth are eventually lost.

Dental plaque is difficult to see unless it is stained, You can stain plaque by chewing red disclosing tablets, found at grocery stores and drug stores, or by using a cotton swab to smear green food coloring on your teeth. The red or green color left on the teeth will show you where there is still plaque—and where you have to brush again to remove it.

- Stain and examine your teeth regularly to make sure you are removing all plaque.
- Ask your dentist or dental hygienist if your plaque removal techniques are okay.

Floss

Use floss to remove germs and food particles between teeth. Rinse after flossing your teeth. Ease the floss into place gently. Do not snap it into place—this could harm your gums.

Brush Teeth

Use any tooth brushing method that is comfortable, but do not scrub hard back and forth. Small circular motions and short back and forth motions work well. Rinse after brushing.

To prevent decay, it is what is on the toothbrush that counts. Use fluoride toothpaste. Fluoride is what protects teeth from decay.

Brush the tongue for a fresh feeling. Rinse again.

Remember: Food residues, especially sweets, provide nutrients for the germs that cause tooth decay, as well as those that cause gum disease. That is why it is important to remove all food residues, as well as plaque, from teeth. Remove plaque at least once a day—twice a day is better. If you brush and floss once daily, do it before going to bed.

Another way of removing plaque between teeth is to use a dental pick—a thin plastic or wooden stick. These picks can be purchased at drug stores and grocery stores.

Section 4.2

Brushing Time and Toothpaste Affect Plaque Removal

Introduction

Routine toothbrushing is perhaps the single most important step an individual can take to reduce plaque accumulation and the consequent risk of plaque-associated diseases, such as periodontitis and caries. Studies of the relationship between time spent brushing and oral hygiene have been inconsistent. However, when the effect of brushing time on plaque removal has been studied on a within-subject basis, a significant effect on plaque removal has been observed.

There have been several studies on the effects of plaque removal concerning the type of brush, brushing technique, and frequency of brushing. However, the authors could find no existing study on the effects time spent brushing had on plaque removal in the general population—that is, when subjects are untutored in brushing technique and are not linked to the oral health profession. Yet this represents the most common situation, and brushing time is important to cleaning the teeth properly and the consequent oral health benefits. Brushing time is the most easily controlled parameter of effective everyday brushing.

The general consensus amongst oral health care professionals is that individuals should spend at least two minutes brushing their teeth with an effective technique at least twice a day, though specific recommendations from national dental associations are frequently lacking. However, most estimates of actual brushing time vary between just over 30 seconds to just over 60 seconds. Some caution regarding these estimates should be exercised as the act of measuring brushing time has been shown to affect brushing behavior. The recent study of Beals et al. determined an average of 46 seconds from a home-use study involving 173 United States adults. It is clear that the average time spent brushing is considerably shorter than two minutes, and a value of about 45 seconds would seem a useful estimate.

Therefore, the aim of this study was to determine whether brushing time is an important determinant of plaque removal during conventional toothbrushing. A sample representative of the general population using their normal brushing technique was tested. Differences in plaque removal could then be related to the possible impact on overall oral health. A specific objective was to compare the effect of brushing for two minutes with brushing for 45 seconds, representing a comparison of the plaque removal benefits of brushing for the consensus minimum time with brushing for the estimated average time. This should assist oral health professionals in encouraging their patients into a more effective oral hygiene routine.

Conclusion

Plaque removal during tooth-brushing, by untutored subjects recruited from the general population local to the study site, was strongly dependent on brushing time. Increasing brushing time increased plaque removal across the period 30 seconds to three minutes. Plaque removal was, however, not influenced by the presence of dentifrice (over 60 seconds brushing), indicating that dentifrice constituents, such as abrasive and surfactant, do not meaningfully assist the action of the brush. A key finding in this study was that brushing for two minutes gave a 26% improvement in plaque removal compared to brushing for 45 seconds. This represents the plaque removal benefit individuals should expect when increasing their brushing time from the average 45 seconds to the consensus minimum of two minutes. Though lower plaque levels as a result of more effective brushing may not always lead to a reduction in gingivitis, this degree of improvement is potentially of clinical significance in reducing the risk of gingival disease. These results reinforce the view that oral health professionals, while coaching their patients in brushing technique, should recommend brushing for at least two minutes.

Section 4.3

Home Test to Identify Dental Plaque

"Dental Plaque Identification at Home," © 2012 A.D.A.M., Inc.
Reprinted with permission.

Dental Plaque Identification at Home

The home dental plaque identification test identifies plaque, a sticky substance that collects around and between teeth. The test helps show how well you are brushing and flossing your teeth. Plaque is the major cause of tooth decay and gum disease (gingivitis). It is hard to see with the naked eye because it is whitish colored, like teeth.

How the Test Is Performed

There are two ways to perform this test. One method uses special tablets that contain a red dye that stains the plaque. One tablet is chewed thoroughly, moving the mixture of saliva and dye over the teeth and gums for about 30 seconds. The mouth is then rinsed with water and the teeth are examined to identify pink-stained areas (plaque that was not removed). A small dental mirror may help to check all areas.

The second method uses a plaque light. A special fluorescent solution is swirled around the mouth. The mouth is rinsed gently with water, and the teeth and gums are examined while shining an ultraviolet plaque light into the mouth. The advantage of this method is that it leaves no pink stains in the mouth.

In the office, dentists are often able to detect plaque through a thorough examination with dental instruments.

How to Prepare for the Test

Brush and floss your teeth thoroughly.

How the Test Will Feel

Your mouth may feel slightly dried out after use of the dye.

Why the Test Is Performed

The test is performed to help identify missed plaque and improve brushing and flossing of the teeth so that areas of plaque are not left. If the plaque is not removed, it can cause tooth decay or cause the gums to bleed easily (gingivitis) and become red or swollen.

Normal Results

No plaque or food debris will be seen on the teeth.

What Abnormal Results Mean

The tablets will stain areas of plaque dark-red.

The plaque light solution will color the plaque a brilliant orange-yellow.

The colored areas show where the brushing and flossing have missed. These areas need to be brushed again to get rid of the stained plaque.

Considerations

The tablets may cause a temporary pink coloring of the lips and cheeks. They may color the mouth and tongue red. Dentists suggest using them at night so that the color will be gone by morning.

Chapter 5

Nutrition Impacts Oral Health

Chapter Contents

Section 5.1

How Food Affects Oral Health

This section includes: "Nutrition and Oral Health," © 2010 Connecticut Department of Public Health, Office of Oral Health, reprinted with permission; and "Foods for Healthy Teeth," Office of Oral Health, Maryland Department of Health and Mental Hygiene, March 2012. Reprinted with permission. For additional information, visit http://fha.dhmh.maryland.gov/oralhealth.

Nutrition and Oral Health

Nutrition affects oral health and oral health affects nutrition. This interdependent relationship sees good nutritional health promoting good oral health (encompassing gum tissue status, the well-being of teeth and jaw, salivary quantity and quality, and sensory dimensions of taste and pain), and vice versa. On the other hand, poor nutritional health is associated with poor oral health, and vice versa.

Malnutrition, Infectious Diseases, and the Immune System

Nutrition is a major factor in infection and inflammation. Several reports emphasize the synergistic relationship between malnutrition, infectious diseases, and the immune system; for example, infections promote malnutrition, the malnutrition elicits dysfunctions of the immune system, and this impaired immunity intensifies the infectious disease. In oral health, cavities and gum disease, as well as many diseases of the mucous membranes, tongue, and salivary glands, are infectious. These oral infections can not only disrupt the integrity of the oral cavity, but can also affect general health.

How Nutrition Affects Oral Health

The foods that you eat come in contact with the germs and bacteria that live in the mouth. If you don't brush, plaque will accumulate on the teeth. Plague thrives on the starches and sugars that are found in a great deal of foods. When plaque combines with the sugars and starches, an acid is produced that attacks enamel on the teeth, and eventually causes decay. According to the American Dental Association, the acid attacks the teeth for 20 minutes or more.

Choosing a Healthy Diet

Choosing a healthy diet may sound easy; however, fruits, milk, cereals, bread, and some vegetables contain sugars and/or starches. Carbonated sodas, sweet fruit drinks, and sugary snack foods should be limited. You don't have to avoid these foods, just keep in mind that you should eat a balanced diet, brush and floss your teeth twice a day.

Healthy Tips

- Drink plenty of water.
- Eat food from all five food groups.
- Limit snacking between meals. (Each time you eat food that contains sugars or starches, the teeth are attacked by acids for 20 minutes.)
- Limit snacks high in sugar and acid (choose nutritious foods, such as cheese, raw vegetables, plain yogurt, or a piece of fruit).
- Brush and floss your teeth twice a day.
- Visit your dentist every six months.

Remember, a well-balanced diet, consisting of a complex mixture of good quality carbohydrates, lipids, proteins, vitamins, and minerals, is required for maintenance of optimal general and oral health.

Foods for Healthy Teeth

Fun Foods for Teeth

Whether you are old or young, good oral health includes good nutrition. What vitamins make a healthy mouth?

- **Vitamin D** is found in dairy foods and strengthens teeth and bones.
- **Vitamin B** is found in breads and cereals along with iron and helps make healthy blood and gums.
- **Vitamin C** is found in fruits and keeps gums healthy.

Food and Tooth Decay

Tooth decay starts with plaque. It is a sticky substance that forms on your teeth after eating. Plaque can also cause gum disease because it irritates the gums and makes them red and swollen. Each time you eat or drink sugary foods, the germs in plaque make acids that destroy the tooth surface. Hard candies, mints, or sticky foods like caramels or jellybeans, stay in the mouth longer and increase the risk for tooth decay. Drinking sugary liquids, including 100% juice, also increase the risk for tooth decay and should be limited. Eating starches or sugars at mealtimes is better than eating them in between meals.

How much juice? The American Academy of Pediatrics recommends:

- Infants over six months and toddlers (ages 1–3) need four to six ounces per day, but not as a pacifying drink.

- Older children and adolescents need two servings a day, six ounces per serving.

Ways to Avoid Tooth Decay

- Limit the amount of sugary liquids and hard candy you eat throughout the day.

- Eat and drink at one sitting instead of sipping and snacking all day long. Avoid frequent snacking.

- Drink water in between meals instead of sugary drinks.

- Brush your teeth with fluoridated toothpaste after every meal.

- End meals with a crunchy and nutritious snack such as apple slices or a carrot to help scrub your teeth.

- Remember the next time you reach for a snack, pick a food that is low in sugar and low fat. Your teeth and your body will thank you.

Teeth Healthy Foods

- Fruits
- Vegetables
- Yogurt
- Milk
- Salad
- Cereal (low sugar)
- Sugar-free gum with xylitol

Foods to Eat in Moderation

- Whole Wheat Pasta
- Potato chips
- Pretzels
- Peanut butter
- Juice (including 100% juice)
- Breads and crackers
- Chocolate milk

Shopping tip: Look for products containing xylitol. Xylitol is an all-natural sweetener used in chewing gum and candies that doesn't cause tooth decay. It's also available at health food stores.

Section 5.2

Minerals and Nutrients Are Important for Oral Health

Nutrition plays an important role in overall wellness, including oral health. Eating well and maintaining a healthy diet can help reduce the risk of developing problems in your mouth, including periodontal disease. In fact, including certain foods as part of a nutritious diet has actually been shown to play a role in the prevention of periodontal disease.

Lactic Acid and Calcium

A recent study determined that individuals who regularly consume 55 or more grams of foods containing lactic acid, commonly found in dairy products such as yogurt, have a lower instance of gum disease. Dairy products are also a good source of calcium which has been shown to lower the risk of severe periodontal disease. The American Dietetic Association advises that adults should consume at least three servings of calcium each day to help keep your jaw bone strong and your teeth in place.

Vitamin C

According to a study, consuming less than 60 milligrams (mg) of vitamin C each day can put you at slightly higher risk for developing certain types of periodontal disease. According to the Institute of Medicine, the recommended dietary allowance for vitamin C is 60 mg per day—or about one orange.

Vitamin D

Sometimes known as the "sunshine vitamin," vitamin D can help lessen inflammation associated with periodontal disease. Research shows that foods fortified with vitamin D such as milk, eggs, sardines, and tuna fish, as well as moderate exposure to sunlight, can provide you with the amount of vitamin D required to stay healthy.

Healthy Diet

Obesity can be the result of an unbalanced diet, which may lack the nutrients known to help prevent gum disease. Also, excessive consumption of sugary drinks such as soft drinks and foods high in sugars, trans-fats, and sodium are often associated with increased tooth decay and can have a negative impact on periodontal health.

Without the proper nutrients from a healthy diet, the body can have a hard time fighting off infections such as periodontal diseases. And routinely including such things as lactic acid, calcium, and vitamins C and D in your diet have been shown to possibly reduce the occurrence of gum disease. So next time you go to the grocery store or sit down for a meal, remember: eat right to smile bright.

Section 5.3

Sugar Intake Affects Oral Health

Excerpted from "The Healthy Journey: Do You Have a Sweet Tooth,"
Healthy Aging in Neighborhoods of Diversity across the Life Span,
Winter 2009, National Institute on Aging (NIA).

Do You Have a Sweet Tooth?

If you do, you're not alone. In 2007 the average person consumed 100 pounds of sugar and other caloric sweeteners. Sugar itself is not bad. In fact, it can be an important ingredient to help with the flavor and texture of many foods we eat, and eating a treat now and again is okay too. Problems arise when we consume too much, often without realizing it. Any excess calories we take in are stored in the body as fat. Tooth decay is another problem that can happen when eating foods high in sugar. Bacteria in the mouth use sugar to produce acid that harms teeth. So, oral hygiene is extremely important after eating, especially after consuming sweets, soft drinks, and other sugar containing beverages. Like all other types of food, the key for eating sweets is moderation.

Sugar Comes in Many Forms

When people hear the word sugar, most automatically think of table sugar. The familiar white sugar, called sucrose, is only one of many types of sugar found in our foods. Others forms of sugar occur naturally in foods such as fruits, vegetables, and dairy products.

Food Labels Can Be Puzzling

You can look at the food label to see how much sugar is in a particular item. But when you read the ingredients on a food label, don't just look for the word sugar. Other ingredients on food labels are also a form of sugar. Look for the following ingredients to know if you are eating added sugar:

- Brown sugar

- Corn sweetener
- Corn syrup
- Dextrose
- Fructose
- Fruit juice concentrates
- Glucose
- High-fructose corn syrup
- Honey
- Invert sugar

- Lactose
- Maltose
- Malt syrup
- Molasses
- Raw sugar
- Sucrose
- Sugar
- Syrup

When possible look for foods that do not have these names listed as one of the first three ingredients. This will help reduce the added sugar in your diet.

Foods with added sugars in American diets include these:

- Regular soft drinks
- Candy
- Cakes
- Cookies
- Pies
- Fruit drinks, such as fruitades and fruit punch
- Milk-based desserts and products, such as ice cream, sweetened yogurt, and sweetened milk
- Grain products such as sweet rolls and cinnamon toast

Ways to Limit Your Intake of Added Sugars

Become knowledgeable about the sugar content in foods. Figure 5.1 displays the amount of sugar in foods commonly eaten.

- Drink water instead of sweetened beverages; add a twist of lemon or lime.
- Try diet sodas, sugar free iced teas, and 100% fruit juices without added sugars.
- Substitute for soda with a mixture of one-half 100% fruit juice and one-half seltzer water, or just seltzer water.

- Try fresh fruit or raisins in cereal instead of sugar.

- When you can, eat fresh fruit, or fruits canned in their own juice. Many canned fruits have added sugars or syrups that contain a lot of sugar.

- When baking, try your recipe with one-third the amount of the sugar in the original recipe.

- Top pancakes or waffles with fruit and powdered sugar instead of syrup.

- Try dairy products such as yogurts and ice creams sweetened with non-caloric sweeteners.

- Make your own salad dressing—many commercial ones contain added sugar.

- Try fresh fruit, vegetables, or popcorn for a healthy snack without the added sugar.

- Look for peanut butter without added sugar

Food	Amount	The amount of sugar in these foods =	
		# Of individual sugar packets	Teaspoons of sugar
Regular soda	12 ounce can	12	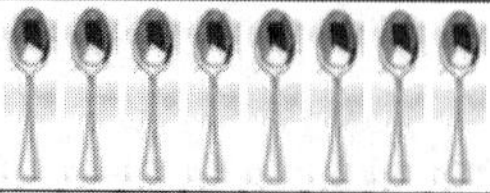
Gatorade	20 ounce bottle	12	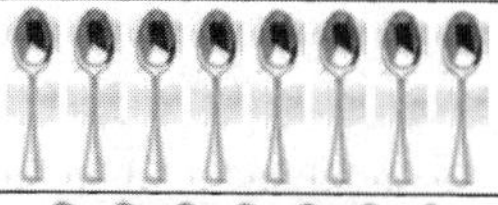
Snickers bar	Regular size	10	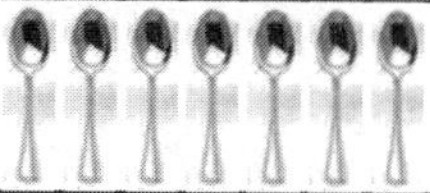
Fruit juice drink	8 ounces (1 Cup)	9	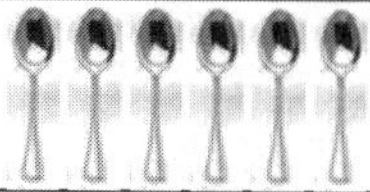
Glazed doughnut	1 medium 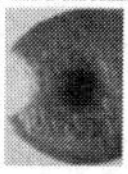	5	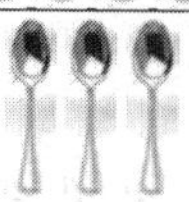

Figure 5.1. *Amount of Sugar in Some Common Snack Foods (Source: USDA National Nutrient Database for Standard Reference)*

Diabetics beware: If you are diabetic, you still need to watch your added sugars. Just because a sugar is natural does not mean it is safe to consume in high amounts.

Flavor your food without using sugar: To lower your use of sugar, you can increase the sweetness of some foods by adding different spices instead of sugar such as the following:

- Add cinnamon to hot cereals.
- Use spices such as nutmeg, cinnamon, allspice, mace, or ginger to mix in your coffee.
- Add nutmeg to cookies and rice.
- A touch of vanilla can sweeten coffee, puddings, and baked goods.
- Season carrots with ginger, or sweet potatoes with cinnamon.

You can experiment with flavors by starting with a small amount, and then increasing it if you enjoy the taste. Another idea is to mix the spices, again starting with small amounts. This can enhance the flavor of your foods without adding calories.

Section 5.4

Xylitol:
Decay-Preventive Sweetener

"Xylitol: The Decay-Preventive Sweetener," © 2005 California Dental
Association (CDA) (www.cda.org). Reprinted with permission. The CDA
states that this information is current as of April, 2012.

What is xylitol?

Xylitol is a natural sugar alcohol that helps prevents cavities. You
may recognize other sugar alcohols used in sugarless products, such
as mannitol and sorbitol. Xylitol is the sugar alcohol that shows the
greatest promise for cavity prevention. It is equal in sweetness and
volume to sugar and the granular form can be used in many of the ways
that sugar is used, including to sweeten cereals and hot beverages and
for baking (except when sugar is needed for yeast to rise).

How does xylitol prevent cavities?

Xylitol inhibits the growth of the bacteria that cause cavities. It
does this because these bacteria (*Streptococcus mutans*) cannot utilize
xylitol to grow. Over time with xylitol use, the quality of the bacteria in
the mouth changes and fewer and fewer decay-causing bacteria survive
on tooth surfaces. Less plaque forms and the level of acids attacking
the tooth surface is lowered.

Studies show that *Streptococcus mutans* is passed from parents
to their newborn children, thus beginning the growth of these decay-
producing bacteria in the child. Regular use of xylitol by mothers has
been demonstrated to significantly reduce this bacterial transmission,
resulting in fewer cavities for the child.

What products contain xylitol and how do I find them?

Xylitol is found most often in chewing gum and mints. You must look
at the list of ingredients to know if a product contains xylitol. Generally,
for the amount of xylitol to be at decay-preventing levels, it must be

listed as the first ingredient. Health food stores can be a good resource for xylitol containing products. Additionally, several companies provide xylitol products for distribution over the internet.

How often must I use xylitol for it to be effective?

Xylitol gum or mints used 3–5 times daily, for a total intake of five grams, is considered optimal. Because frequency and duration of exposure is important, gum should be chewed for approximately five minutes and mints should be allowed to dissolve. As xylitol is digested slowly in the large intestine, it acts much like fiber and large amounts can lead to soft stools or have a laxative effect. However, the amounts suggested for cavity reduction are far lower than those typically producing unwelcome results.

Has xylitol been evaluated for safety?

Xylitol has been approved for safety by a number of agencies, including the U.S. Food and Drug Administration, the World Health Organization's Joint Expert Committee on Food Additives, and the European Union's Scientific Committee for Food.

Xylitol has been shown to have decay-preventive qualities, especially for people at moderate to high risk for decay, when used as part of an overall strategy for decay reduction that also includes a healthy diet and good home care. Consult your dentist to help you determine if xylitol use would be beneficial for you.

Section 5.5

Calcium Is Important for Oral Health

This section includes an excerpt from "Calcium and Bone Health," Centers for Disease Control and Prevention (CDC), April 6, 2011; and excerpts from "Calcium Supplements: What to Look For," National Institute of Arthritis and Musculoskeletal and Skin Diseases (NIAMS), January 2011.

Calcium and Bone Health

Calcium is a mineral needed by the body for healthy bones, teeth, and proper function of the heart, muscles, and nerves. The body cannot produce calcium; therefore, it must be absorbed through food. Good sources of calcium include:

- Dairy products: low fat or nonfat milk, cheese, and yogurt
- Dark green leafy vegetables: bok choy and broccoli
- Calcium fortified foods: orange juice, cereal, bread, soy beverages, and tofu products
- Nuts: almonds

Vitamin D also plays an important role in healthy bone development. Vitamin D helps in the absorption of calcium (this is why milk is fortified with vitamin D).

Table 5.1. Recommended Calcium Intakes

Ages	Amount mg/day
Birth–6 months	210
6 months–1 year	270
1–3	500
4–8	800
9–18	1300
19–50	1000
51–and older	1200

Source: Dietary Reference Intakes for Calcium, National Academy of Sciences, 1997

Calcium Supplements: What to Look For

Calcium is a mineral found in many foods. Getting enough of this nutrient is important because the human body cannot make it. Even after you are fully grown, adequate calcium intake is important because the body loses calcium every day through the skin, nails, hair, and sweat, as well as through urine and feces. This lost calcium must be replaced daily through the diet. Otherwise, the body takes calcium from the bones to perform other functions, which makes the bones weaker and more likely to break over time.

Experts recommend that adults get 1,000–1,300 milligrams (mg) of calcium each day. Although food is the best source of calcium, most Americans do not get enough of it from food sources. Calcium-fortified foods (such as orange juice, bread, cereals, and many others on grocery shelves) and calcium supplements can fill the gap by ensuring that you meet your daily calcium requirement.

Calcium exists in nature only in combination with other substances. These substances are called compounds. Several different calcium compounds are used in supplements, including:

- calcium carbonate,
- calcium phosphate, and
- calcium citrate.

These compounds contain different amounts of elemental calcium, which is the actual amount of calcium in the supplement. Read the label carefully to determine how much elemental calcium is in the supplement and how many doses or pills to take.

Calcium supplements are available without a prescription in a wide range of preparations and strengths, which can make selecting one a confusing experience. Many people ask which calcium supplement they should take. The best supplement is the one that meets your needs.

Other Important Things to Consider

Purity: Choose calcium supplements with familiar brand names. Look for labels that state purified or have the USP (United States Pharmacopeia) symbol. Avoid supplements made from unrefined oyster shell, bone meal, or dolomite that do not have the USP symbol because they may contain high levels of lead or other toxic metals.

Absorbability: The body easily absorbs most brand-name calcium products. If you are not sure about your product, you can find out how well it dissolves by placing it in a small amount of warm water for 30 minutes and stirring it occasionally. If it has not dissolved within this time, it probably will not dissolve in your stomach. Chewable and liquid calcium supplements dissolve well because they are broken down before they enter the stomach.

The body best absorbs calcium, whether from food or supplements, when it is taken several times a day in amounts of not more than 500 mg, but taking it all at once is better than not taking it at all. Calcium carbonate is absorbed best when taken with food. Calcium citrate can be taken anytime.

Tolerance: Some calcium supplements may cause side effects, such as gas or constipation, for some people. If simple measures (such as increasing your intake of fluids and high-fiber foods) do not solve the problem, you should try another form of calcium. Also, it is important to increase the dose of your supplement gradually: take just 500 mg a day for a week, and then slowly add more calcium. Do not take more than the recommended amount of calcium without your doctor's approval.

Calcium interactions: It is important to talk with a doctor or pharmacist about possible interactions between calcium supplements and your over-the-counter and prescription medications. For example, calcium supplements may reduce the absorption of the antibiotic tetracycline. Calcium also interferes with iron absorption. So you should not take a calcium supplement at the same time as an iron supplement—unless the calcium supplement is calcium citrate or the iron supplement is taken with vitamin C. Any medications that need to be taken on an empty stomach should not be taken with calcium supplements.

Combination Products

Calcium supplements are available in a bewildering array of combinations with vitamins and other minerals. Calcium supplements often come in combination with vitamin D, which is necessary for the absorption of calcium. However, calcium and vitamin D do not need to be taken together or in the same preparation to be absorbed by the body. Minerals such as magnesium and phosphorus also are important but usually are obtained through food or multivitamins. Most experts recommend that nutrients come from a balanced diet, with multivitamins used to supplement dietary deficiencies.

Getting enough calcium—whether through your diet or with the help of supplements—will help to protect the health of your bones. However, this is only one of the steps you need to take for bone health. Exercise, a healthy lifestyle, and for some people, medication are also important.

Chapter 6

Fluoride Prevents Tooth Decay

Chapter Contents

Section 6.1

Fluoridation Basics

This section includes: "Fluoridation Basics," and excerpts from "Using Fluoride to Prevent and Control Tooth Decay in the United States," both from the Centers for Disease Control and Prevention (CDC), January, 2011.

Overview

Nearly all naturally occurring water sources contain fluoride—a mineral that has been proven to prevent, and even reverse, tooth decay.

Tooth decay is caused by certain bacteria in the mouth. When a person eats sugar and other refined carbohydrates, these bacteria produce acid that removes minerals from the surface of the tooth. Fluoride helps to remineralize tooth surfaces and prevents cavities from continuing to form.

Fluoridation Beginnings

In the 1930s, dental scientists documented that the occurrence and severity of tooth decay was lower among people whose water supplies contained higher levels of natural fluoride. Extensive studies followed and discovered that fluoride, when present in the mouth, can become concentrated in plaque and saliva, helping to prevent the breakdown of enamel minerals. In 1945, the city of Grand Rapids, Michigan, added fluoride to its municipal water system. Community water fluoridation—adjusting the amount of fluoride in an area's water supply to a level that helps to prevent tooth decay and promote oral health—had begun. Since then, numerous scientific studies and comprehensive reviews have continually recognized fluoridation as an effective way to prevent tooth decay.

Benefits of Fluoridation

Water fluoridation prevents tooth decay mainly by providing teeth with frequent contact with low levels of fluoride throughout each day and throughout life. Even today, with other available sources of fluoride, studies show that water fluoridation reduces tooth decay by about 25% over a person's lifetime.

Community water fluoridation is not only safe and effective, but it is also cost-saving and the least expensive way to deliver the benefits of fluoride to all residents of a community. For larger communities of more than 20,000 people, it costs about fifty cents per person to fluoridate the water. It is also cost-effective because every dollar invested in this preventive measure yields approximately $38 savings in dental treatment costs.

This method of fluoride delivery benefits all people regardless of age, income, education, or socioeconomic status. A person's income and ability to get routine dental care are not barriers since all residents of a community can enjoy fluoride's protective benefits just by drinking tap water and consuming foods and beverages prepared with it.

Fluoride from other sources prevents tooth decay as well, whether from toothpaste, mouth rinses, professionally applied fluoride treatments, or prescription fluoride supplements. These methods of delivering fluoride, however, are more costly than water fluoridation and require a conscious decision to use them.

Fluoridation Today

Currently, more than 195 million people in the United States are served by public water supplies containing enough fluoride to protect teeth. Even so, approximately 100 million Americans do not have access to fluoridated water. The current population with access to fluoridated water is approximately 72%. The widespread availability of fluoride through water fluoridation, toothpaste, and other sources, however, has resulted in the steady decline of dental caries throughout the United States.

Using Fluoride to Prevent and Control Tooth Decay in the United States

Although there have been notable declines in tooth decay among children and adults over the past three decades, tooth decay remains the most common chronic disease of children aged 6–11 years (25%), and of adolescents aged 12–19 years (59%). Tooth decay is four times more common than asthma among adolescents aged 14–17 years (15%).

Guidance of how to achieve protection from tooth decay throughout life:

- Drink tap water with optimal amounts of fluoride.

- Brush at least twice daily with fluoride toothpaste.

- Use prescription fluoride supplements and high concentration fluoride products wisely.

- Know factors that can increase children's risk for tooth decay such as genetic predisposition, eating a lot of sugar-based foods and drinks, not brushing teeth daily, not using fluoride toothpaste, drinking water with a low fluoride content, not visiting a dentist regularly, and wearing braces.

Section 6.2

Questions about Community Water Fluoridation

This section includes excerpts from "Community Water Fluoridation: Questions and Answers," Centers for Disease Control and Prevention (CDC), January 2011.

What is community water fluoridation?

Almost all water contains some naturally occurring fluoride, but usually at levels too low to prevent tooth decay. Many communities choose to adjust the fluoride concentration in the water supply to a level beneficial to reduce tooth decay and promote good oral health. This practice is known as community water fluoridation. Given the dramatic decline in tooth decay during the past 65 years, the Centers for Disease Control and Prevention (CDC) named water fluoridation one of "Ten Great Public Health Interventions of the 20th Century."

Why is the Department of Health and Human Services (HHS) developing new recommendations for community water fluoridation?

Sources of fluoride have increased since the early 1960s. At that time, drinking water and food and beverages prepared with fluoridated water accounted for nearly all of an individual's fluoride intake. Today, water is just one of several sources of fluoride. Other sources include dental products such as toothpaste and mouth rinses, prescription fluoride supplements, and professionally applied fluoride products such as varnish and gels. Recognizing that it is now possible to receive enough fluoride with slightly lower levels of fluoride in water, the HHS set out to develop new recommendations for community water fluoridation.

How is HHS developing new recommendations?

In September 2010, the Department of Health and Human Services scientists reviewed the best available information on: the prevalence and trends in dental caries, water intake in children in relation to outdoor air temperature, changes in the percentage of U.S. children and adults with dental fluorosis, and the U.S. Environmental Protection Agency's (EPA) new assessments of cumulative sources of fluoride exposure and risks of children developing severe dental fluorosis. This new information led HHS to propose changing the recommended level for community water systems to 0.7 milligrams per liter.

How were the recommended levels previously set for fluoride in drinking water?

In 1962, based on scientific studies showing that fluoride reduces tooth decay, the U.S. Public Health Service recommended the amount of fluoride in drinking water range from 0.7 to 1.2 milligrams per liter.

How does fluoride get into tap water?

Fluoride can occur in drinking water naturally as a result of the geological composition of soils and bedrock. Some areas of the country have high levels of naturally occurring fluoride. Fluoride can also be added to public drinking water supplies as a public health measure for reducing cavities.

Since the optimal level of 0.7 milligrams per liter of fluoride is a recommended level (for example, not a nationwide level or Environmental Protection Agency (EPA) enforceable level) in community drinking water systems, how do I know whether my community has or will reduce the level of fluoride in my drinking water? Does it have to?

This optimal level recommendation is voluntary. If your local water system adds fluoride to the water, reducing the level is a simple process that can be completed almost immediately, although it may be several days before the entire water system is at the new level. If you want the most up-to-date information about the current fluoride level in your water, contact your local water system.

Why has exposure to fluoride increased?

Exposures to fluoride have increased since the early 1960s. At that time, drinking water and food and beverages prepared with fluoridated water accounted for nearly all of an individual's fluoride intake. Today, exposure to fluoride comes from more sources including fluoridated dental products such as toothpaste and mouthwash, as well as the voluntary addition of fluoride to drinking water, which some systems do as a public health measure for reducing tooth decay.

In addition to water, what are other specific sources of fluoride?

Fluoridated toothpaste is another main source of fluoride intake. Other fluoride-containing dental products are applied or prescribed by a health care professional such as gels, varnishes, pastes, and restorative materials. These products are used only occasionally on the outside of the tooth and do not contribute much to the total intake of fluoride. Small amounts of fluoride can also come from industrial emissions, pharmaceuticals, and pesticides.

What are the adverse health effects of excessive fluoride exposure?

Children under age eight years and younger exposed to excessive amounts of fluoride have an increased chance of developing pits in the tooth enamel. Excessive consumption of fluoride over a lifetime may increase the likelihood of bone fractures, and may result in effects on bone leading to pain and tenderness, a condition called skeletal fluorosis. Severe skeletal fluorosis is a rare condition in the United States. The EPA exposure analysis suggests that the effects on bone in adults are of greatest concern for those living in areas with high natural background levels of fluoride and favoring beverages, such as tea, that are high in fluoride.

Section 6.3

Bottled Water and Fluoride

Excerpted from "Bottled Water and Fluoride,"
Centers for Disease Control and Prevention (CDC), January, 2011.

Consumers drink bottled water for various reasons, including as a taste preference or as a convenient means of hydration. Bottled water may not have a sufficient amount of fluoride, which is important for preventing tooth decay and promoting oral health.

Some bottled waters contain fluoride, and some do not. Fluoride can occur naturally in source waters used for bottling or it can be added. This section answers common questions about bottled water and fluoride.

Who regulates fluoride in bottled water?

The *Federal Food, Drug, and Cosmetic Act* provides the U.S. Food and Drug Administration (FDA) broad regulatory authority over food, including bottled water, which is introduced or delivered for interstate commerce (produced and sold in more than one state). Bottled water that is in intrastate commerce is under the jurisdiction of the state in which the bottled water is produced and sold. Contact the manufacturer to ask if their product is under FDA jurisdiction or state jurisdiction.

What FDA regulations apply to bottled water?

The FDA has strict regulations on standards of quality, identity, and good manufacturing practices that bottled water must meet. Its regulations for governing the standards of "quality and identity" for bottled water are found in the *Code of Federal Register 21* CFR 165.110. The FDA standards of quality state that domestic bottled water with no added fluoride may contain between 1.4 and 2.4 milligrams per liter (mg/L) fluoride, depending on the annual average daily air temperatures at the location where the bottled water is sold. Domestic bottled water with added fluoride can contain between 0.8 and 1.7 mg/L fluoride, depending on the annual average daily air temperatures where the bottled water is sold. Imported bottled water with no added fluoride may not contain more than 1.4 mg/L fluoride, and imported bottled water with added fluoride may not contain more than 0.8 mg/L fluoride.

Is the amount of fluoride in bottled water always listed on the label?

The FDA does not require bottled water manufacturers to list the fluoride content on the label, but it does require that fluoride additives be listed. In 2006, the FDA approved labeling with the statement, "Drinking fluoridated water may reduce the risk of tooth decay," if the bottled water contains from 0.6 mg/L to 1.0 mg/L.

How can I find out the level of fluoride in bottled water if it's not on the label?

Contact the bottled water's manufacturer to ask about the fluoride content of a particular brand.

Does drinking bottled water without fluoride lead to more cavities?

Your oral health—specifically, how many cavities you have—depends on many factors, one of which is how much fluoride you receive in the form of toothpaste, mouthwash, water, food, and professional fluoride products applied by dental professionals. Other factors include how often and how thoroughly you brush your teeth and floss, what you eat, and whether you receive regular dental care. If you mainly drink bottled water with no or low fluoride, and you are not getting enough fluoride from other sources, you may get more cavities than you would if fluoridated tap water were your main water source.

Will the fluoride content change if the bottled water is stored for a long time?

Fluoride will not react with other minerals present in the water during storage, nor will it react with its plastic or glass container. The FDA considers bottled water to be safe indefinitely if produced in accordance with quality standard regulations, and if stored in an unopened, undamaged, and properly sealed container.

Can I use bottled water for mixing infant formula?

Yes, you can reconstitute (mix) powdered or liquid concentrate formulas with bottled waters, but be aware that the fluoride content in bottled water varies. If your child is exclusively consuming infant formula reconstituted with water that contains fluoride, there may be an increased chance for mild dental fluorosis. To lessen this chance, parents can use low-fluoride bottled water some of the time to mix infant formula. These bottled water products are labeled as de-ionized, purified, demineralized, or distilled, unless they specifically list fluoride as an added ingredient.

Section 6.4

Private Well Water and Fluoride

This section includes excerpts from "Private Well Water and Fluoride," Centers for Disease Control and Prevention (CDC), January, 2011.

How do I know if my water is from a public water system or a private well?

The U.S. Environmental Protection Agency (EPA) defines a public water system as a system that serves 25 or more people per day. If you have water service from a well that has a limited delivery, such as to your house but not to your neighbor's house, then you likely have a private well.

My home gets its water from a private well. What do I need to know about fluoride and groundwater from a well?

Fluoride is present in virtually all waters at some level, and it is important to know the fluoride content of your water, particularly if you have children. A 2008 U.S. Geological Survey study found that 4% of sampled wells had natural fluoride levels above the EPA secondary maximum contaminant level (SMCL) of two milligrams per liter (mg/L). A smaller set of 1.2% of all wells exceeded the maximum contaminant level (MCL) of four mg/L. If you have a home well, the EPA recommends having a sample of your water analyzed by a laboratory at least once every three years. Check with your dentist, physician, or public health department to learn how to have your home well water tested.

What should I do if the water from my well has less fluoride than the recommended level of 0.7 mg/L? Can I add fluoride?

The recommended fluoride level in drinking water for good oral health is 0.7 mg/L. If fluoride levels in your drinking water are lower than 0.7 mg/L, your child's dentist or pediatrician should evaluate whether your child could benefit from daily fluoride supplements. It is not feasible to add fluoride to an individual residence's well.

What should I do if the water from my well has fluoride levels that are higher than the recommended level of 0.7 mg/L?

If your home is served by a water system that has fluoride levels exceeding this recommended guideline, but lower than 4.0 mg/L, currently EPA recommends that children should be provided with alternative sources of drinking water. Continue to test your well water's quality every three years as recommended by EPA.

What should I do if my well water was measured as having too much fluoride (level greater than 4 mg/L)?

It is unusual to have the fluoride content of water exceed 4 mg/L. If a laboratory report indicates that you have such excessive fluoride content, it is recommended that the water be retested. At least four samples should be collected, a minimum of one week apart, and the results compared. If one sample is above 4 mg/L and the other samples are less than 4 mg/L, then the high value may have been an erroneous measurement. If all samples register excessive levels greater than 4 mg/L, then you may want to consider investigating alternate sources of water for drinking and cooking, or installing a device to remove the fluoride from your home water source. Physical contact with high fluoride content water, such as bathing or dishwashing, is safe since fluoride does not pass through the skin.

What are the health risks of consuming water with fluoride levels greater than 4 mg/L?

Children aged eight years and younger have an increased chance of developing severe tooth dental fluorosis. Consumption over a lifetime may increase the likelihood of bone fractures, and may result in skeletal fluorosis, a painful or even crippling disease.

Will using a home water filtration system take the fluoride out of my home's water?

Removal of fluoride from water is difficult. Most home point-of-use treatment systems that are installed at single faucets use activated carbon filtration, which does not remove the fluoride. Reverse osmosis point-of-use devices can effectively remove fluoride, although the amount may vary given individual circumstances. For a home point-of-use device to claim a reduction in fluoride, it must meet National Sanitation Foundation (NSF) Standard 58 criteria for fluoride removal. Standard 58 requires that a device must achieve a 1.5 milligrams per liter (mg/L) concentration in the product water if the original concentration was 8.0 mg/L, or approximately 80% removal. This percentage removal may not be consistent at lower concentrations of fluoride. Check with the manufacturer of the individual product for specific product information.

Fluoride is not released from water when it is boiled or frozen. One exception would be a water distillation system. These systems heat water to the boiling point and then collect water vapor as it evaporates. Water distillation systems are typically used in laboratories. For home use, these systems can be expensive and may present safety and maintenance concerns.

Can I use water with fluoride for preparing infant formula?

Yes, you can use well water for preparing infant formula. It is important, however, to ensure that the well water has been recently tested to verify safety.

For more information on private well testing, contact your local health department or visit the EPA website. Parents and caregivers should speak with their pediatrician to review the results of the private well testing and to determine if the well water should be boiled prior to mixing the formula. If you are advised to boil the water, be sure to boil the water only one time so that you don't concentrate substances by the boiling process itself.

Chapter 7

Oral Injuries

Chapter Contents

Section 7.1

Mouth Guards and Who Should Wear Them

"Mouth Guards: What are they and why are they important?" reprinted with permission from the Massachusetts Department of Public Health, Office of Oral Health (www.mass.gov/dph/oralhealth), © 2012.

Mouth Guards

Facts about Mouth Guards

- More than five million teeth are lost each year due to accidental injury.

- Mouth guard use prevents 200,000 oral-facial injuries per year.

- An athlete is 60 times more likely to suffer a dental injury while not wearing a mouth guard.

- Only 49% of Massachusetts middle school students wear a mouth guard while playing team sports.

What are mouth guards?

Mouth guards are specialized rubber-like devices that typically fit over the upper teeth and help prevent injury to the teeth, lips, cheeks, and tongue. When used during sports, mouth guards can help prevent tooth loss and may reduce the risk and severity of jaw fractures and concussions.

Who should wear a mouth guard?

In Massachusetts, mouth guards are mandated for all persons participating in football, field hockey, ice hockey, soccer, lacrosse, and wrestling. However, mouth guards are strongly recommended for all those participating in any sports where there may be a risk of injury to the jaw, teeth, or head.

Mouth guards are especially important for those who wear braces. Trauma to the face can cause damage to fixed orthodontic appliances and brackets. Mouth guards also provide a barrier between these devices and the soft tissues of the mouth lessening the risk of trauma and injury.

Types of Mouth Guards

There are three basic types of mouth guards that all provide protection with varying levels of cost and comfort. An ideal mouth guard is tear-resistant, comfortable, easy to clean, and does not inhibit breathing.

Stock mouth guards: Stock mouth guards are inexpensive, standard sized guards that can be purchased at most sporting goods stores. They come pre-formed and ready to wear, however some may find them slightly bulky and they may interfere with speech.

Boil and bite mouth guards: Boil and bite mouth guards are designed to be immersed in hot water and then shaped to the form of the teeth using the fingers or biting pressure. This type of mouth guard tends to be more comfortable than a stock mouth guard and provides a better fit when made properly. This type of guard can also be purchased over-the-counter at most sporting goods stores.

Custom made mouth guards: Custom made mouth guards can be obtained from a dentist's office. They are made in a dental office or at a dental laboratory from an impression of the teeth. This type of mouth guard is designed to specifically fit the user's teeth.

How to Care for a Mouth Guard

Before and after each use, mouth guards should be cleaned with cool, soapy water or a mouth rinse. Guards can also be cleaned using toothpaste and a soft-bristled toothbrush. Guards should also be checked for tears or any other kind of damage following each use. Damaged guards have the potential to cause oral irritation and can have a diminished effect. For this reason, damaged or worn out mouth guards should be replaced.

When not in use, clean mouth guards should be stored in plastic wrap or in a vented container. Athletes are encouraged to minimize handling of their mouth guards during games. Whenever the guard contacts the player's hands, players are encouraged to rinse the guard off with water to reduce contamination.

Also, over time the user's jaw size and tooth position may change causing the guard to no longer fit properly. This may require an updated guard to ensure maximum protection at all times. It is also recommended that all guards avoid contact with high temperatures, such as direct sunlight and hot water, to avoid possible distortion.

Remember—mouth guards should never be shared between players.

References

American Dental Association. "ADA: American Dental Association–Mouthguards." ADA: American Dental Association–Home. <http://www.ada.org/2970.aspx#protector>.

"Grin and Wear It–Massachusetts Dental Society." Massachusetts Dental Society. Web. 25 Mar. 2011. <http://www.massdental.org/awarness/grin-and-wear-it.aspx?id=1160#>.

Massachusetts Department of Public Health Office of Oral Health. *The Status of Oral Disease in Massachusetts: The Great Unmet Need.* Boston, MA: Commonwealth of Massachusetts, Department of Public Health Office of Oral Health, 2009.

Section 7.2

First Aid for Dental Emergencies

"First Aid for Dental Emergencies," September 2010, reprinted with permission from the North Carolina Department of Health and Human Services, Division of Public Health, Oral Health Section. For additional information, visit http://www.ncdhhs.gov/dph/oralhealth.

Follow these instructions for a dental emergency.

- In all situations, reassure the injured person.
- If any blood is involved, it is recommended that you wear gloves.
- Do not administer any pain relievers until consulting with a parent if a child is injured.

Bleeding after Losing a Baby Tooth

- Place a clean, folded, gauze pad, cloth, or paper towel over the bleeding area.
- Have the child bite on the gauze with pressure for 15 minutes. This procedure may be repeated.
- Make sure the child refrains from frequent rinsing.

- If bleeding persists, see a dentist.

Broken Braces and Wires

- Broken wires can be covered with wax or gauze until an orthodontist can be seen.
- Do not remove wire embedded in the cheek, tongue, or gums.
- The patient should see their orthodontist immediately.

Broken Tooth

- Gently clean dirt from the injured area with warm water.
- Place a cold compress on the face over the injured area.
- Locate and save any broken tooth fragments if possible.
- See a dentist immediately.

Cut or Bitten Tongue, Lip, or Cheek

- Clean area with a clean, wet cloth.
- Apply pressure with a cloth to stop the bleeding.
- Apply ice to the swollen or bruised areas. If bleeding does not stop after 15 minutes, or with pressure, a dentist or doctor should be seen.

Knocked Out Permanent Tooth

- Find the tooth.
- Handle the tooth by its crown, not the root.
- Gently replace the tooth in its socket and hold the tooth in place.
- A tooth that is quickly reimplanted has a good chance of being saved.
- If the tooth cannot be reinserted into the socket, put the tooth into "Sav-A-Tooth" or a cup of fresh milk. Do not put the tooth into tap water.
- See a dentist immediately.

Possible Broken Jaw

- The jawline may appear distorted.

- Immediately call your local emergency medical service (911).

- Keep the injured person still and calm.

- Make sure the patient can breathe.

- Try to keep the person from moving.

Toothache or Abscess

- Rinse the mouth vigorously with warm salt water to remove any food debris.

- Do not place aspirin on the site of the toothache because it may cause burning to the gum tissue. If the face is swollen, place a cold compress on the outside of the cheek.

- Encourage the patient to see a dentist as soon as possible.

Chapter 8

Caring for Oral Piercings

Mouth Jewelry, Oral Piercings, and Your Health

Piercing the tongue, lip, or cheek—Is this an innocent teenage fad of fashion and self-expression or a prelude to oral health problems? Before piercing this area of your anatomy, it is wise to have a complete understanding of the health-related risks. If you still wish to go through with the procedure, consider what to look for in an oral piercing studio and learn how to care for the pierced area.

What health risks are associated with oral piercings?

There are numerous potential risks. Among them:

Infection: There's a risk of infection associated with oral piercing due to the wound created, the vast amount of bacteria in the mouth, and the introduction of additional bacteria from handling the jewelry.

Transmission of diseases: Oral piercing is a potential risk factor for the transmission of herpes simplex virus and hepatitis B and C.

Endocarditis: Because of the wound created by the piercing, there's a chance that bacteria could enter the bloodstream and lead to the development of endocarditis—an inflammation of the heart or its valves—in certain people with heart health problems.

Nerve damage/prolonged bleeding: Numbness or loss of sensation at the site of the piercing or movement problems (for pierced tongues) can occur if nerves have been damaged. If blood vessels are punctured, prolonged bleeding can occur. Tongue swelling following piercing can be severe enough to block the airway and make breathing difficult. An increase in salivary flow—stimulated by the jewelry—might result in temporary or permanent drooling.

Gum disease: People with oral piercings—especially long-stem tongue jewelry (barbells)—have a greater risk of gum disease than those without oral piercings. The jewelry can come into contact with gum tissue causing injury as well as a recession of the gum tissue—which can lead to loose teeth and tooth loss.

Damage to teeth: Teeth that come into contact with mouth jewelry can chip or crack. One study in a dental journal reported that 47% of people wearing barbell tongue jewelry for four or more years had at least one chipped tooth.

Difficulties in daily oral functions: Tongue piercing can result in difficulty chewing and swallowing food, and speaking clearly. This is because the jewelry stimulates an excessive production of saliva. As noted, temporary or permanent drooling is another consequence. Taste can also be altered.

Allergic reaction to metal: A hypersensitivity reaction—an allergic contact dermatitis—to the metal in the jewelry can occur in susceptible people.

Jewelry aspiration: Jewelry that becomes loose in the mouth can become a choking hazard and, if swallowed, can result in injury to the digestive tract or lungs.

What should I look for in an oral piercing studio?

If you have decided to go through with the oral piercing procedure, here's what to look for:

- Ask friends who have had their tongue, lips, or cheeks pierced—and have suffered no ill consequences—to recommend the name of the studio they visited.

- Visit the studio. Ask to look at the studio's photo portfolio.

- Ask to see the studio's health certificates.

- Does the studio have a clean appearance, especially the area where the piercing is done? Ask if they use hospital-grade autoclaves for sterilization and/or use disposable instruments. Does the staff use disposable gloves?

- Are all the needles, as well as the studs, hoops, and barbells, kept in sterilized packaging?

- Are all staff involved in the piercings vaccinated against hepatitis B? They should be; ask.

- Staff should be friendly and willing to answer all of your questions.

What can I do at home to best care for my new oral piercing?

A pierced tongue can take four to six weeks to heal. Pierced lips take between one and two months to heal. During this healing period, here's what you should do:

- Avoid alcohol, spicy foods, and hard and sticky foods.

- Don't smoke or use tobacco-based products.

- Brush after every meal and rinse with a mouthwash, such as Listerine.

- Rinse your mouth frequently with warm salt water.

- Eat soft foods. Consult your dentist about taking vitamins to promote faster healing.

- Make an appointment with your dentist if you suspect a problem or have a concern. It is critical for dentists to check your teeth, gums, tongue, and soft tissues for early signs of any problems.

Chapter 9

Traveler's Guide to Safe Dental Care

Congratulations! You've decided to finally visit that corner of the world you've always dreamed of seeing. The flights are booked, the hotel reservations made. Most likely, dental care is not on any traveler's "Top 10" list of "Things to Do," but what should you do if you get a toothache, or crack a filling?

Most of us are aware of the high United States' standards for infection control and safety in health care. But in many parts of the world, gloves, sterile instruments, disposable needles, and safe water are not routine elements of dental practice. Furthermore, the standards for educating and licensing dental professionals vary widely.

In case of a dental emergency, knowing what to look for when seeking dental care in a foreign country can help a traveler avoid unnecessary risks.

Take Steps to Ensure a Healthy Trip, Free of Dental Emergencies

No one wants to have a trip ruined by a toothache. To minimize the risk of a dental emergency, visit your dentist for a check-up before your trip. Schedule your appointment to allow enough time to complete any necessary or outstanding dental work before your departure date.

"Traveler's Guide to Safe Dental Care," © 2003 Organization for Safety, Asepsis and Prevention (www.osap.org). Reprinted with permission. Reviewed by David Cooke, MD, FACP, in April 2012.

- Before you leave on your trip, tend to decayed teeth, broken fillings, and other dental problems. Inform your dentist of your travel plans and ask about any other potential dental problems.

- Have your teeth cleaned by the dentist or hygienist. This is particularly important if you have periodontal (gum) disease.

- If you will be away for an extended time, consider having partially exposed lower wisdom teeth removed. The fleshy covering over the tooth creates a food trap that can cause pericoronitis, a potentially serious infection that can spread to parts of the head and neck.

- All root canal treatment should be completed before travel to avoid potential infections and pain due to pressure changes during air travel. If the work cannot be completed, ask your dentist to insert a temporary paste filling to reduce the risk of problems.

Most insurance policies don't provide coverage for care delivered overseas, so it makes sense to take care of any potential problems before leaving home.

Vaccinations

In the United States, most dentists have been vaccinated against hepatitis B virus, a serious blood borne infection affecting the liver. In the developing world, however, hepatitis B infection rates remain high. Immunization requires three injections given over a six-month period, so plan far enough ahead to receive the complete series. Consult the Centers for Disease Control and Prevention, an agency of the U.S. Department of Health and Human Services, for hepatitis B and other immunization recommendations before traveling outside U.S. borders. Call 877-FYI-TRIP (394-8747) or visit www.cdc.gov/travel for more information.

Finding a Dentist

Even with the most thorough examination, no dentist can guarantee a dental emergency will not arise. So what should a traveler do if a dental problem occurs far from home?

- If staying in a hotel, the concierge or senior management staff may be able to suggest a dentist. American Embassy or military personnel—or even other American expatriates living in the area—also may be good sources for a recommendation.

- If you do not speak the local language, a dentist proficient in English is preferred to allow effective communication of the dental problem and treatment as well as questions about infection control practices.

Assessing Infection Control Practices in the Dental Office

Once you have found a dental office, examine its level of compliance with basic infection control and safety standards. "Infection control" seeks to prevent the transmission of disease-causing organisms by:

- reducing their numbers (for example, through cleaning, disinfection, and sterilization of instruments or surfaces);

- preventing exposure by using barriers like gloves, masks, gowns, and protective eyewear, or by covering surfaces to keep them from becoming contaminated; or

- improving a person's ability to resist disease causing agents through the use of vaccines and antibiotics.

The most successful approaches use a combination of all three.

Practicing universal precautions means that the dentist and staff wear a new pair of rubber or vinyl gloves for each patient and wear face masks and protective eyewear for all procedures that generate spatter or splash. It also means that all instruments used on patients are either disposed of or are properly cleaned, then disinfected or sterilized after use.

In the developed world, most dental offices apply the principles of universal precautions, which are based on the assumption that any patient could be infected with a blood borne virus such as the human immunodeficiency virus (HIV), or hepatitis B and C viruses. As such, the highest standards of protection are always applied.

Basic hygiene remains important. Experts in medicine and dental infection control agree: Handwashing is the single most important element in preventing the spread of infection. Dentists and staff should always wash their hands immediately before donning gloves as well as immediately after removing them.

Gloves protect both patients and healthcare workers from disease transmission. The dentist and all assistants involved in treatment should use new gloves for each patient. Gloves should never be washed and reused. It degrades the material and compromises its ability to provide an effective barrier.

Injection needles are no longer reused in most parts of the industrialized world because they pose a high risk of spreading blood borne viruses. Unfortunately, because disposable needles are more expensive, re-usable needles may still be in use in some developing countries.

Heat-sterilizing instruments in an autoclave or dry-heat sterilizer kills all potential disease-causing agents that might remain after patient treatment. All heat-stable instruments that are exposed to a patient's blood should be processed in this manner, including the dental drill. Any instruments that cannot tolerate high temperatures should be thoroughly cleaned and soaked in disinfectant chemicals.

All instruments used for surgery, including tooth extraction, must be heat sterilized and should be stored in a sterile wrap or container until it is used.

Items that are used only outside the mouth, or that never contact blood, can be cleaned and then wiped or soaked in less powerful disinfectant chemicals.

High speed dental drills and other devices used in dental treatment need water to work properly. In many parts of the world, safe drinking water is not always a fact of life. Water that is unsafe to drink is also unfit for dental treatment, especially surgery. In areas that lack potable water, dentists can use bottled water delivered using a bulb syringe. Boiled water is considered acceptable, although bottled sterile water is preferred for surgery.

Choosing Medications

Protection against potentially harmful drugs is nonexistent in some countries. Do not buy medications "over-the counter" unless you're familiar with the product.

Checklist for Obtaining Safe Dental Care

Before you leave:

- Visit your dentist for a check-up to reduce the chances you will have a dental emergency.
- Consider appropriate vaccinations.

When seeking treatment for a dental emergency during your trip:

- Consult hotel staff or the American Embassy or consulate for assistance in finding a dentist.
- If possible, consider recommendations from Americans living in the area or from other trusted sources.

If the answers to any of the following asterisked (*) items are "No," you should have reservations about the office's infection control standards. If the answer to a two-star item (**) is "No," consider making a swift, but gracious, exit.

When making the appointment, ask:

- Do you use new gloves for each patient?*

- Do you use an autoclave (steam sterilizer) or dry heat oven to sterilize your instruments between patients?**

- Do you sterilize your handpieces (drills)?* (If not, do you disinfect them?)**

- Do you use new needles for each patient?**

- Is sterile (or boiled) water used for surgical procedures? ** (In areas where drinking water is unsafe, the water also may cause illness if used for dental treatment.)

Upon arriving at the office, observe the following:

- Is the office clean and neat?

- Do staff wash their hands, with soap, between patients?**

- Do they wear gloves for all procedures?**

- Do they clean and disinfect or use disposable covers on surfaces touched during treatment?

While it is important to be sensitive to cultural differences when making inquiries about the safety of dental care, remember that it is your health and wellbeing that are at stake.

Part Two

Visiting Your Dentist's Office

Chapter 10

Routine Dental Visits

Chapter Contents

Section 10.1

What to Expect

Dental hygienists are licensed oral health care professionals who have completed extensive educational and clinical preparation in preventive oral health care. In all states but one, to become licensed, dental hygienists must graduate from an accredited dental hygiene education program, pass the National Board Dental Hygiene Examination, and pass a state/regional clinical licensure examination.

Accredited education programs are offered at universities and community and technical colleges, with programs varying from two to four years in length, but including prerequisites averaging three years. Graduates may obtain a bachelor's degree, an associate degree, or a certificate, depending on the program. Some dental hygienists go on to earn Master's and Doctorate degrees.

In addition, continuing advances in the dental hygiene field and changing laws in many states have encouraged virtually all registered dental hygienists to participate in continuing education courses, keeping them up to date on the latest trends in dental hygiene practice and legislation regarding the profession.

So what should you expect from your dental hygienist?

Registered dental hygienists can provide a wide range of services as determined by laws in each state. These services include the following:

- After assessing a patient's individual oral health condition and incorporating the most current scientific research, including consideration of the impact of oral health on diseases such as heart disease and diabetes, dental hygienists plan a specific treatment plan designed to make sure each patient has the best oral health possible.

- Targeted and specific dental hygiene treatment for children, adolescents, adults, older adults, and patients who are medically compromised.

- Because targeted and specific systemic diseases like heart disease and diabetes, as well as other conditions, have signs and symptoms that appear in the mouth first, dental hygienists monitor for evidence of disease, and where they find suspicious conditions, inform the patient and recommend a visit to a physician.

- While assessing a patient's overall health, they also look for problems such as caries (cavities) and periodontal (gum) disease.

- Dental hygienists perform thorough head and neck examinations to look for oral cancer and other problems.

- To prevent and treat disease, they remove plaque (a stubborn film that contains bacteria), and calculus, both above and below the gum line.

- To prevent caries, dental hygienists provide nutrition counseling, apply fluorides or pit-and-fissure sealants, and in some states, polish and contour fillings.

- Because dental hygienists specialize in preventive oral health care, they educate their patients, the community, and schools on oral health and its effect on overall health, as well provide dietary education and counseling.

- They expose, develop, and interpret oral x-rays.

- In many states, registered dental hygienists administer local anesthesia and/or nitrous oxide.

- Dental hygienists also evaluate how their recommendations are working and, when necessary, revise treatment as it progresses to help patients achieve their oral health goals.

Who's taking care of your oral health?

When you go for your oral health appointment, make sure you are receiving care from a properly educated and licensed oral health prevention specialist—a registered dental hygienist.

- Ask the person delivering care if he or she has graduated from an education program accredited by the American Dental Association Commission on Dental Accreditation.

- Look to see if the dental hygienist's registered dental hygienist (RDH) license is in plain view.

- Get to know your dental hygienist by name.

- Ask your dental hygienist for treatment and at-home-care plans.

- Ask your dental hygienist to recommend oral health products that are specially formulated for your oral health care needs.

- Prevention is the key: discuss any questions or concerns you have about oral health as part of total health with your dental hygienist.

Long-Term Dental Visiting Patterns and Adult Oral Health

To date, the evidence supporting the benefits of dental visiting comes from cross-sectional studies. We investigated whether long-term routine dental visiting was associated with lower experience of dental caries and missing teeth, and better self-rated oral health, by age 32. A prospective cohort study in New Zealand examined 932 participants' use of dentistry at ages 15, 18, 26, and 32. At each age, routine attenders (RAs) were identified as those who (a) usually visited for a check-up, and (b) had made a dental visit during the previous 12 months. Routine attending prevalence fell from 82% at age 15 to 28% by 32. At any given age, routine attenders had better-than-average oral health, fewer had teeth missing due to caries, and they had lower mean deciduous surfaces (DS) and decayed, missing, filled scores (DMFS). By age 32, routine attenders had better self-reported oral health and less tooth loss and caries. The longer routine attendance was maintained, the stronger the effect. Routine dental attendance is associated with better oral health.

Section 10.2

Easing Dental Phobia

Easing Dental Phobia in Adults

If you fear going to the dentist, you are not alone. Between 9% and 15% of Americans say they avoid going to the dentist because of anxiety or fear.

People with dental anxiety have a sense of uneasiness about the upcoming dental appointment. They may also have exaggerated worries or fears.

Dental phobia is a more serious condition that leaves people panic-stricken and terrified. People with dental phobia have an awareness that the fear is totally irrational but are unable to do much to change this. They exhibit classic avoidance behavior; that is, they will do everything possible to avoid going to the dentist. People with dental phobia usually go to the dentist only when forced to do so by extreme pain.

Other signs of dental phobia include the following:

- Trouble sleeping the night before the dental exam
- Feelings of nervousness that escalate while in the dental office waiting room
- Getting to the dental office but being unable to enter
- Crying or feeling physically ill at the very thought of visiting the dentist
- Intense uneasiness at the thought of, or actually when objects are placed in your mouth during the dental appointment or suddenly feeling like it is difficult to breathe

Fortunately, there are ways to get people with dental anxiety and dental phobia to the dentist.

What causes dental phobia and anxiety?

There are many reasons why some people have dental phobia and anxiety. Some of the common reasons include:

Fear of pain: Fear of pain is a very common reason for avoiding the dentist. This fear usually stems from an early dental experience that was unpleasant or painful or from dental pain and horror stories told by others. Thanks to the many advances in dentistry made over the years, most of today's dental procedures are considerably less painful or even pain free.

Fear of injections or fear the injection won't work: Many people are terrified of needles, especially when inserted into their mouth. Beyond this fear, others fear that the anesthesia hasn't yet taken effect or wasn't a large enough dose to knock out any pain before the dental procedure begins.

Fear of anesthetic side effects: Some people fear the potential side effects of anesthesia such as dizziness, feeling faint, or nausea. Others don't like the numbness or fat lip associated with local anesthetics.

Feelings of helplessness and loss of control: It's common for people to feel these emotions considering the situation—sitting in a dental chair with your mouth wide open, unable to see what's going on.

Embarrassment and loss of personal space: Many people feel uncomfortable about the physical closeness of the dentist or hygienist to their face. Others may feel self-conscious about the appearance of their teeth or possible mouth odors.

Should I talk to my dentist about my dental phobia?

Absolutely! In fact, if your dentist doesn't take your fear seriously, find another dentist. The key to coping with dental anxiety is to discuss your fears with your dentist. Once your dentist knows what your fears are, he or she will be better able to work with you to determine the best ways to make you less anxious and more comfortable.

If lack of control is one of your main stressors, actively participating in a discussion with your dentist about your own treatment can ease your tension. Ask your dentist to explain what's happening at every stage of the procedure. This way you can mentally prepare for what's to come. Another helpful strategy is to establish a signal—such as raising your hand—when you want the dentist to immediately stop. Use this signal whenever you are uncomfortable, need to rinse your mouth, or simply need to catch your breath.

Nitrous oxide gas or intravenous (IV) sedation is also used to help control anxiety. Many dentists have anesthesia licenses for this very reason.

Section 10.3

Questions to Ask about Infection Control

"Want Some Life-Saving Advice? Ask your dental hygienist about protecting against disease transmission in the dental office," © 2010 American Dental Hygienists' Association (www.adha.org). All rights reserved. Reprinted with permission.

Although experts agree it is extremely rare, it may be possible to get an infectious disease during a routine visit to the dental office.

Infected microorganisms live in blood and oral fluids, on contaminated instruments and counter tops, and sometimes even in the air. Patients may be exposed to diseases such as hepatitis B and C, herpes simplex virus, human immunodeficiency virus (HIV), tuberculosis, staphylococci, and other viruses and bacteria that thrive in the oral cavity and respiratory tract. However, there has only been one report of possible HIV transmission in a dental setting and that was in 1991, and last transmission of hepatitis B was in 1987. There have been no documented cases of hepatitis C being transmitted in a dental setting.

But, all of these diseases can be avoided if proper infection control is used in dental offices. Keep an eye out for improper infection control procedures and ask your dental hygienist about the procedures your dental office uses. Many offices post a list of the infection control procedures they follow in a reception area or elsewhere. If you don't see this information, ask about it.

In addition, the Centers for Disease Control and Prevention (CDC) recommends standard precautions that should be used in the care of all patients, regardless of their infection status. The precautions are intended to prevent or reduce the potential for disease transmission among patients and oral health care personnel.

Infection Control Patrol

Your oral health care provider should adhere to all of the following standard infection control procedures:

- Wear protective clothing and gear, including gloves, masks, gowns, or laboratory coats, and protective eyewear for all treatment procedures.

- Change gloves after each patient contact. Whenever possible, complete all work on one patient before re-gloving and performing procedures on another patient.

- Even though gloves are worn, wash hands thoroughly before and after each patient is treated. An alternative to hand washing between each patient is to hand wash before the first patient and then use an alcohol rub between patients. However, alcohol hand rubs have limitations. For instance, they are ineffective if there is visible dirt on hands, and they cannot be used for a sterile procedure. In the case of the latter, a surgical hand scrub is required. The rationale for using gloves despite the fact that hand washing and alcohol rubs are used is that gloves may become perforated, knowingly or unknowingly, during use. The perforations may allow fluids to pass through the gloves to contaminate hands. These fluids could contain infectious microorganisms.

- Use coverings to protect surfaces like light handles or x-ray unit heads that may be contaminated and are difficult or impossible to disinfect.

- Heat sterilize all non-disposable instruments and devices—heat-resistant needles, syringes, and other sharp instruments and devices—and disinfect surfaces and equipment after treatment of each patient.

- Discard disposable syringes and other sharp instruments in puncture-resistant containers. Needles must not be recapped, bent, or broken before disposal because this increases the risk of an unintentional needle stick injury.

- Place all potentially infectious waste in closable, leak-proof containers or bags that are color-coded, labeled, or tagged in accordance with applicable federal, state, and local regulations.

Many infection control precautions oral health care workers take to protect their patients and themselves are not easily apparent to patients, so feel free to ask your oral healthcare professionals to explain the policies and procedures in place in your office.

Chapter 11

Dental Caries
(Cavities) in Adults

Tooth Decay Facts

Tooth decay, known formally as dental caries, has been a serious health problem for all nations since time immemorial. For centuries, tooth decay was thought to be the handiwork of an elusive and, in some cultures, evil tooth worm that gnawed holes into the white, highly mineralized enamel and left all those in its wake in pain. But superstition has yielded to science and its explanation that certain oral bacteria discharge mineral eroding acid onto the enamel, starting the gradual process of decay. Over the last several decades, dental researchers have made tremendous progress in defining and learning to thwart the decay process. This work has involved the three-pronged strategy of discovery, innovation, and prevention—and produced one of the major public health success stories of the 20th century.

Yesterday

Few people were spared the ordeal of losing teeth, often early in life. The combination of tooth decay and periodontal diseases left 17 million people age 45 and older—about three out of ten Americans—with none of their natural teeth. In fact, the most common cause of World War II (WWII) draft rejection was too few teeth because of tooth decay. Until the 1970s, the cause of tooth decay continued to be a subject of debate,

---

Text in this chapter is from "Tooth Decay Fact Sheet," National Institute of Dental and Craniofacial Research (NIDCR), May 2011; and, excerpts from "Dental Caries (Tooth Decay) in Adults (Age 20 to 64)," NIDCR, March 2011.

with some believing dietary deficiencies were the culprit and others focusing on oral bacteria. This uncertainty made effective prevention strategies difficult, if not impossible, to create. Moreover, brushing one's teeth each day was a fairly recent hygienic step forward in dental care, reportedly popularized by returning soldiers from World War II.

The National Institutes of Health (NIH) completed the first water fluoridation study that established the benefits of fluoride in fighting tooth decay. Several years would pass before fluoride, the mainstay of modern prevention strategies, would become a common ingredient in water, toothpaste, and other products. Tooth decay was considered an irreversible disease process—once a cavity started, the only remedy was to drill out the decay and fill the tooth with a restorative material.

Today

Tooth decay is no longer the national epidemic it was a few generations ago. Millions of American children now have little or no decay, and total tooth loss or edentulism is now much less common. Without research progress in the fight against dental caries and periodontal diseases, there would be an additional 18.6 million Americans age 45 and older with none of their natural teeth.

Prevention is now the mantra in American dentistry. In addition to improved products to fight tooth decay, more people benefit from preventive dentistry, including the use of fluorides and dental sealants to prevent decay. Compared to previous years, these techniques have made it possible for millions more people to keep their natural teeth for a lifetime. It is estimated that from 1979 through 1989 alone, the American public saved more than $39 billion in dental expenditures due to the power of prevention. Since the 1950s, the total federal investment in NIH-funded oral health research has saved the American public at least three dollars for every dollar invested.

Tomorrow

New technologies will further prevent tooth decay. Research is underway to develop powerful imaging tools that can detect the earliest demineralization of tooth enamel. These tools will allow the application of special solutions to remineralize the tooth and reverse early decay.

The bacteria that cause tooth decay live in complex communities called biofilms. Great strides have been made in learning how the bacteria communicate with one another within this biofilm. By jamming the communication signals among the bacteria, it may be possible one day to disrupt the biofilm and end the threat of tooth decay.

Dental Caries in Permanent (Adult) Teeth of Adults Age 20–64

Dental caries, both treated and untreated, in all adults age 20 to 64 declined from the early 1970s until the most recent (1999–2004) National Health and Nutrition Examination Survey. The decrease was significant in all population subgroups. In spite of this decline, significant disparities are still found in some population groups. (Note: Approximately 5% of adults age 20 to 64 have no teeth. This survey applies only to those adults who have teeth.)

Prevalence

- 92% of adults 20 to 64 have had dental caries in their permanent teeth.

- White adults and those living in families with higher incomes and more education have had more decay.

Unmet Needs

- 23% of adults 20 to 64 have untreated decay.

- Black and Hispanic adults, younger adults, and those with lower incomes and less education have more untreated decay.

Severity

- Adults 20 to 64 have an average of 3.28 decayed or missing permanent teeth and 13.65 decayed and missing permanent surfaces.

- Hispanic subgroups and those with lower incomes have more severe decay in permanent teeth.

- Black and Hispanic subgroups and those with lower incomes have more untreated permanent teeth.

Chapter 12

Dental Imaging

Chapter Contents

Section 12.1

Dental Radiography and Patient X-Ray Doses

Dental Patient Issues

Is there anything like a computed tomography (CT) scan for teeth?

A couple of years ago a dental CT scan was introduced into this country. There are only a few machines in use, mainly in California, and the one is at the University of North Carolina. There are some ultra-high-resolution dental CT units that are being developed in Japan, but they are not yet licensed for sale in the United States.

Is there residual radiation in a room after a dental radiograph has been taken?

X-rays cease to exist when the machine is switched off, much like the light from a light bulb when it is turned off. No residual radiation remains.

How much has dental x-radiation been studied and how concerned should I be about having dental x-rays done? Is there a limit on how many I can have?

We now have very complete information on patient radiation doses from dental x-rays. They are among the lowest radiation dose exams of any diagnostic radiologic procedure in the healing arts. Current practices deliver patient doses from a full-mouth series of intraoral films (usually 14–18 films) that are less than what a person receives in a month from natural environmental sources (commonly called background exposure). Doses from bitewing or panoramic films are even less. New technology is reducing the doses still further.

There is no limit on how many dental x-rays you can have. The decision to have a dental x-ray is based on the benefit of knowing whether or not there is a cavity, crack, or some other abnormality. So the decision to have them is based on what you and your dentist think.

Dental Patient Doses Information

In dental radiography, the part of the head that receives the greatest dose is the skin in the area where the x-rays enter. A recent study was performed at the Department of Diagnostic Sciences at the University of North Carolina School of Dentistry in Chapel Hill, North Carolina, using a realistic head phantom and state-of-the-art imaging systems (Ludlow et al. 2008). In Table 12.1 are some typical skin and thyroid doses received for the exams indicated. The effective dose is explained. Of course, these doses vary somewhat from different machines, but the figures listed are probably within 10%–20% of the actual amounts received by the patient.

To put these values in perspective, background radiation from naturally occurring radionuclides in our environment and from cosmic rays is approximately 3,100 µSv (National Council on Radiation Protection [NCRP] 2006) every year. Furthermore, differences in background levels between different parts of the country are larger than the effective dose for a bitewing. For example, moving from a lower-background region such as Minneapolis, Minnesota, to a higher-background region, such as Denver, Colorado, for a year would result in an increase in effective dose for that year that is about the same as 30 bitewing exams, or approximately 150 µSv.

Table 12.1. Patient Doses from Dental X-Ray Exams (Ludlow et al. 2008)

Exam	Skin Dose (microsievert [µSv])	Thyroid (µSv)	Effective Dose (µSv)
Full mouth (18 exposures)	90–122	117–550	34.9–170.7
Bitewing	26	0	5
Panoramic	4–6	25–67	14.2–24.3

Epidemiological studies comparing cancer rates in high- and low-background radiation regions have repeatedly failed to show any association with background levels in the United States or in other countries. It also appears that radiation doses at levels of as much as several times natural background do not play a significant role increasing cancer above the natural incidence rate. The fact that routine dental exams listed previously are significantly lower than background radiation exposures leads to the idea that there is no increased risk from such exams.

To predict the probability of radiation causing harm, we calculate a quantity called the effective dose in units of the millisievert (mSv) or microsievert (µSv), where 10 mSv equals one rem in the older radiation dose units. The effective dose takes into account the type of radiation, which is x-rays in this case, and the body parts or organs involved, for example, the skin, salivary glands, bone marrow, mandible, thyroid, and so forth. The absorbed doses to the individual organs are, unfortunately, also expressed in mSv or µSv. The old unit for organ doses was the rad, where 100 millirad (mrad) equals one mSv. Doses to individual organs, however, do not represent the risk or harm to the organ, as various cellular repair mechanisms attenuate the radiation effects. Rather, each organ or body part is assigned a tissue weighting factor (wT) determined by the International Council on Radiation Protection and Measurements (ICRP 2007). For example, the wT values for the thyroid and skin are 0.04 and 0.01, respectively, and do not have any measurement unit associated with them. The sum of the individual organ wT values equals 1.0. Organs that do not receive radiation do not contribute to the effective dose.

The wT values are derived from review of the epidemiological data that exist for humans exposed to large amounts of radiation, primarily the survivors of the atomic weapon detonations in Hiroshima and Nagasaki. The factors indicate the relative likelihood of harm, such as cancer, birth defects, or increased risk of genetic disorders in future generations, per unit dose. Since the dose to reproductive tissue is much less than one µSv for all of the dental exposures here, the only health issue considered is cancer induction.

It is important to point out that in epidemiological studies of humans, no actual increase in cancer incidence has ever been found in groups of humans who have received effective doses below 100 mSv. The effective doses associated with dental exposures are much, much smaller than this. Nevertheless, in order to come up with some estimate of harm for purposes such as setting standards for reasonable levels of exposures in medicine, it is assumed that the probability of harm seen at high doses decreases proportionally with dose and never becomes zero.

In 1995, a joint study on the role of medical radiation in thyroid cancer was conducted in Sweden by the United States and Swedish National Cancer Institute. Sweden was a better country for this type of study than the United States because its entire health care system, including its medical records, is more centralized and standardized. The study showed that patients with thyroid cancer had received the same number of diagnostic x-ray studies, including dental x-rays, as the general population. If it had been found that people with thyroid cancer had had more exposure, it could have indicated some connection between the radiation exposure and thyroid cancer. Of course, it's tough to prove that something is totally unrelated to something else, but this was pretty good evidence that there isn't much of an association between medical x-rays and thyroid cancer (Inskip et al. 1995).

There is also a 1988 study funded by the National Cancer Institute and conducted in Los Angeles by a team at the University of California, Los Angeles, that found a positive correlation between cancer of the parotid gland and previous dental x-ray exposure. It didn't seem to be as definitive a study as the Swedish study. The Los Angeles study information was obtained strictly from interviews with parotid cancer patients, whereas the Swedish study used actual medical records. The Los Angeles study population included only about 400 cancer patients compared with over 4,000 for the Swedish study. Also, U.S. citizens tend to move around the country during their lifetimes, which causes a bigger difference in their lifetime effective doses than is caused by variation in dental radiography practices. So there is probably some controversy in this area (Preston-Martin et al. 1998).

There are reports of epidemiologic studies showing associations between dental x-ray and certain head and neck cancers. Most of these reports, however, were published years ago and are based on the results of dental exposures before World War II, when equipment was much cruder and doses much greater than they are today. In addition, these epidemiological studies show only associations and do not establish a cause-and-effect relation between exposures and cancers. No such reports are associated with recent dental exposures. Risks from dental x-rays are very small when compared with other medical exams involving radiation exposures.

—Written by E. Russell Ritenour and S. Julian Gibb;
revised and updated by John P. Jacobus in July 2010.

References

International Commission on Radiological Protection. *The 2007 recommendations of the International Commission on Radiological Protection.* New York: Pergamon Press; ICRP Publication 103, Ann ICRP 37(2–4); 2007.

Inskip PD, Ekbom A, Galanti MR, Grimelius L, Boice JD Jr. Medical diagnostic x rays and thyroid cancer. *Journal of the National Cancer Institute 87*:1613–1621; 1995.

Ludlow JB, Davies-Ludlow LE, White SC. Patient risk related to common dental radiographic examinations: The impact of 2007 International Commission on Radiological Protection recommendations regarding dose calculation. *Journal of the American Dental Assoc 139*:1237–1243; 2008.

National Council on Radiation Protection and Measurements. Ionizing radiation exposure of the population of the United States. Bethesda, MD: *National Council on Radiation Protection and Measurements; NCRP Report No. 160*; 2006.

Preston-Martin S, Thomas DC, White SC, Cohen D. Prior exposure to medical and dental x-rays related to tumors of the parotid gland. *Journal of the National Cancer Institute 80*:943–949; 1988.

Section 12.2

Newer Technologies Find Tooth Decay Early

This section includes "Advantages and Disadvantages of Digital Imaging," and "Efficacy Studies," © 2011 American Dental Hygienists' Association (www.adha.org). All rights reserved. Reprinted with permission.

Advantages and Disadvantages of Digital Imaging

Advantages

One of the biggest advantages of digital imaging is the ability of the operator to post-process the image. Post-processing of the image allows the operator to manipulate the pixel shades to correct image density and contrast, as well as perform other processing functions that could result in improved diagnosis and fewer repeated examinations. With the advent of electronic record systems, images can be stored in the computer memory and easily retrieved on the same computer screen and can be saved indefinitely or be printed on paper or film if necessary. All digital imaging systems can be networked into practice management software programs facilitating integration of data. With networks, the images can be viewed in more than one room and can be used in conjunction with pictures obtained with an optical camera to enhance the patients' understanding of treatment. Digital imaging allows the electronic transmission of images to third-party providers, referring dentists, consultants, and insurance carriers via a modem. Digital imaging is also environmentally friendly since it does not require chemical processing. It is well known that used film processing chemicals contaminate the water supply system with harmful metals such as the silver found in used fixer solution. Radiation dose reduction is also a benefit derived from the use of digital systems. Some manufacturers have claimed a 90% decrease in radiation exposure, but the real savings depend on comparisons. For example, the dose savings will be different if Insight film (F speed film) with rectangular collimation is used versus Ultra-Speed film (D speed film) with round collimation. Clearly, a much greater dose reduction will result from the change of Ultra-Speed film with round collimation to Insight film with rectangular collimation.

Disadvantages

There are also disadvantages associated with the use of digital systems. The initial cost can be high depending on the system used, the number of detectors purchased, and so forth. Competency using the software can take time to master depending on the level of computer literacy of team members. The detectors, as well as the phosphor plates, cannot be sterilized or autoclaved, and in some cases charge coupled device (CCD)/complementary metal oxide semiconductor (CMOS) detectors pose positioning limitations because of their size and rigidity. This is not the case with phosphor plates; however, if a patient has a small mouth, the plates cannot be bent because they will become permanently damaged. Phosphor plates cost an average of $25 to replace, and CCD/CMOS detectors can cost more than $5,000 per unit. Finally, since digital imaging in dentistry is not standardized, professionals are unable to exchange information without going through an intermediary process. Hopefully, this will change within the next few years as manufacturers of digital equipment become Digital Imaging and Communications in Medicine (DICOM) compliant.

Efficacy Studies

In order for a new technology to be embraced by the scientific oral health community, it must be shown that using it results in at least the same diagnostic outcome as what is currently being used. The scientific oral health community is actively engaged in research to answer questions related to new technologies, like digital radiography. A review of the literature revealed an abundance of studies demonstrating that digital radiography performs as well as conventional film in the diagnosing of caries and periodontal disease. In addition, many scientific studies have looked at more advanced imaging techniques for specific tasks, such as file length measurement, detection of bone loss around dental implant sites, the use of algorithms to optimize contrast and density, and so forth. In most cases, the results overwhelmingly have demonstrated that digital radiography could be substituted for film without any loss in diagnostic information.

Chapter 13

Tooth Pain

Chapter Contents

Section 13.1

Hypersensitive Teeth

Hypersensitivity affects 45 million adults in the United States and 10 million are chronically affected with sensitive teeth. Tooth sensitivity is tooth discomfort after eating cold or hot foods or liquids or even breathing cold air.

This problem often happens when gums recede and/or cementum is not presence. The gum tissue acts like a protective blanket to cover the roots of the teeth. As the gums recede the underlying tooth roots are exposed. They are not covered by hard enamel. Thousands of tiny dentinal tubules (channels) leading to the tooth's nerve center (pulp) are then exposed. These tubules allow more stimuli like heat, cold, or pressure to reach the nerve in the tooth and you feel pain. Think of your gums and the enamel on your teeth as a down comforter covering protecting your body from the cool winter air. Over time, the gums may recede, or the enamel or dentin on your teeth may wear down, creating the condition for tooth sensitivity.

Tooth sensitivity is caused by the following:

- Brushing too hard or with too much pressure which removes gum tissue. Two out of three people brush too hard.

- Aging, sensitivity is highest between the ages of 25–30.

- Using a hard toothbrush instead of a soft one.

- Poor oral hygiene which leads to plaque build-up around the teeth and gums. This plaque hardens into tartar. The bacteria that live in plaque cause gum disease and gum recession.

- The exposed roots contain small pores or tubules which lead directly to the nerve of the tooth. Pain, pressure, and cold stimuli can travel down the tubules and trigger the tooth nerve causing pain and discomfort.

- Stimulation from hot beverages or foods.

- Tooth whitening, often beautiful, but sometimes uncomfortable, at least for a few days.

- Hypersensitivity

- Cracked teeth

- Grinding your teeth

- Long-term use of mouthwashes such as Listerine or Oraldene damage dentine and cause dentin sensitivity and reverse the beneficial effects of toothpaste.

- Enamel erosion by acidic foods

- Root sensitivity can occur after having your teeth cleaned, following root planning , crown placement, or even having fillings. The good news is this sensitivity will disappear in about four to six weeks.

- People with sensitivities to sight, hearing, taste, smell, and touch also usually have sensitive teeth.

- Decreased saliva flow: A simple test is to invert the lower lip, dry the mucous membrane off and see how long it takes for small droplets of saliva to flow from the minor salivary glands. If it takes more than a minute, the saliva flow is down.

- pH test resulting in an "acidic mouth"

- Dental treatments: Simple cleanings, orthodontics, or restoration

- Dehydration due to diuretics such as alcohol beverages, caffeine-containing drinks like coffee and Mountain Dew.

There are many other causes, some of which can require a more comprehensive treatment plan.

1. Broken, chipped, or fractured teeth

2. Nerve damage in the root may require a root canal

3. Grinding and/or clenching the teeth may need a mouthguard

4. Gum disease, needs to begin a comprehensive oral hygiene regimen

5. Receding gums may indicate gum disease and/or oral habits

The key to preventing tooth sensitivity is to keep your gums healthy by reducing the pressure you use while brushing, use a soft toothbrush, and to maintain good oral health habits. This means brushing all your teeth for 2–3 minutes, not the usually 30–45 seconds that most people brush. Flossing is crucial in order to reach the 35% of the tooth surfaces where brushing cannot reach.

What Can You Do If You Already Have Sensitive Teeth?

- Use a toothpaste for sensitivity. This works in a cumulative fashion to cover the open tubules. It contains strontium chloride and/or potassium nitrate which act to remineralize the tooth surface by diffusing into the open pores (tubules) on the enamel. This process helps block transmission of sensation from the tooth surface to the tooth nerve. It needs to be used 4–6 weeks before any changes can be noted.

- Continue to practice brushing gently and carefully around the gum line so you do not remove more gum tissue or continue demineralize the tooth surface.

- Avoid highly acidic foods like citrus or soda pop that can work against the sensitivity toothpaste.

- Brush gently with a soft toothbrush twice a day using a low abrasion desensitizing toothpaste.

- Use fluoride mouth rinse to help remineralize the tooth surface. Fluoride gels and varnish are effective also.

- Don't use a tartar control toothpaste, use a fluoridated toothpaste or desensitizing toothpaste.

- Try spreading a thin layer of desensitizing toothpaste on the exposed roots with your finger or a Q-tip before you go to bed.

- Avoid very cold foods.

- Monitor intake of fruit drinks and sports drinks that are high in sugar and/or acid such as tomatoes, pickles, citrus, pop, or tea.

- Always use a de-sensitizing toothpaste for 2–3 weeks prior to having your teeth cleaned or before having root planning and scaling.

- Avoid teeth grinding and clenching by using a night-guard.

- Have professional tooth cleaning, oral hygiene instructions and fluoride treatments. Some dentists use ultrasonic scaling to help minimize dentin sensitivity

- Home care must be evaluated and adjusted as necessary.

- Chemical desensitization (for example: Gluma, HurriSeal, Pain-Free) provided by your dentist is the most common method of treatment for hypersensitivity.

- Surface sealers or self-etch primers (Seal and Protect, Clearfil SE Bond) can be a costly solution.

- If you drink orange juice in the morning and then brush soon after, you may want to either wait at least an hour before brushing, or at least use water only when brushing, then rinse with mouthwash. This gives give time for your saliva to remineralize the enamel.

If these suggestions do not give you relief please see your dentist. One way your dentist can gauge the severity of your sensitive teeth is by using the air test. The dentist sprays the air gum across each area of your teeth to pinpoint the exact location of sensitivity. The decision of whether a restoration is needed comes after an in-office desensitizer has been applied and you have been sent home for a week with desensitizing tooth paste to see whether a more aggressive approach is needed. An in-office desensitizer can be painted or sprayed on. This is a quick and relatively painless procedure. Your dentist can apply varnishes; high fluoride mouthwashes and toothpaste or gel; dentin sealer; or white fillings (bonding) to cover exposed surfaces and close the pores of the tooth root.

Delay Brushing after Eating Erosive Foods

If you are at risk for erosive tooth wear, you should avoid brushing your teeth for at least 60 minutes after consuming erosive food or drink such as fruits, salads, and sports drinks.

Instead of brushing right after eating erosive foods try:

- rinsing with water,

- rinsing with a fluoride solution,

- chewing sugarless gum, and

- always remember to brush with a soft bristled toothbrush.

Section 13.2

Toothaches

"Toothaches," © A.D.A.M., Inc. Reprinted with permission.

Toothache is pain in or around a tooth.

Considerations

A toothache is generally the result of dental cavities (tooth decay) or sometimes an infection. Tooth decay is often caused by poor dental hygiene, although the tendency to get tooth decay is partly inherited.

Sometimes, pain that's felt in the tooth is actually due to pain in other parts of the body. This is called referred pain or radiating pain. For example, an earache may sometimes cause tooth pain.

Causes

- Abscessed tooth
- Earache
- Injury to the jaw or mouth
- Heart attack (can include jaw pain, neck pain, or toothache)
- Sinusitis
- Tooth decay

Home Care

Over-the-counter pain medications may be used while waiting to see the dentist or primary health care provider.

For toothaches caused by a tooth abscess, the dentist may recommend antibiotic therapy and other treatments, like root canal.

To prevent tooth decay, use good oral hygiene. A low sugar diet is recommended along with regular flossing, brushing with fluoride toothpaste, and regular professional cleaning. Sealants and fluoride applications by the dentist are important for preventing tooth decay.

When to Contact a Medical Professional

Seek medical care if:

- you have a severe toothache;
- you have a toothache that lasts longer than a day or two;
- you have fever, earache, or pain upon opening the mouth wide.

Note: The dentist is an appropriate person to see for most causes of toothaches. However, if the problem is referred pain from another location, you may need to see your primary health care provider.

What to Expect at Your Office Visit

The dentist will examine you. The physical examination may include an examination of the mouth, teeth, gums, tongue, throat, ears, nose, and neck. You may need dental x-rays. The dentist may recommend other tests, depending on the suspected cause.

The dentist will ask questions about your medical history and symptoms, including:

- When did the pain start?
- How severe is the pain?
- Where is the pain located?
  - Does it involve the jaw or ears?
  - Does it radiate to other parts of the body, such as the neck, shoulder, or arm?
- What makes it worse?
  - Is it worse after cold foods or liquids?
  - Is it worse after sweet foods or liquids?
  - Is it worse after chewing?
  - Is it worse after drinking?
  - Is it worse when you touch the area?
  - Is it worse after physical exertion?
- Does the pain wake you up at night?
- What makes it better?
  - Is it better after you use medications? (Which ones?)

- Is it better after you use a heating pad?
- Is it better after you rest?
- What other symptoms do you have?
  - Fever
  - Nausea
  - Sweating
  - Indigestion
  - Chest pain
  - Bleeding
- What medications do you take?
- Have you been injured?
- When was the last dental checkup?
- Have you had previous dental problems?

Treatment may involve fillings, tooth removal, or a root canal, if the problem is severe. If there is a fever or swelling of the jaw, an antibiotic will usually be prescribed.

Section 13.3

Tooth Abscess

"Tooth Abscess," © 2012 A.D.A.M., Inc. Reprinted with permission.

A tooth abscess is a collection of infected material (pus) resulting from a bacterial infection in the center of a tooth.

Causes

A tooth abscess is a complication of tooth decay. It may also result from trauma to the tooth, such as when a tooth is broken or chipped. Openings in the tooth enamel allow bacteria to infect the center of the tooth (the pulp). Infection may spread out from the root of the tooth and to the bones supporting the tooth.

Infection results in a collection of pus (dead tissue, live and dead bacteria, white blood cells) and swelling of the tissues within the tooth. This causes a painful toothache. If the pulp of the tooth dies, the toothache may stop, unless an abscess develops. This is especially true if the infection remains active and continues to spread and destroy tissue.

Symptoms

The main symptom is a severe toothache. The pain is continuous and may be described as gnawing, sharp, shooting, or throbbing.

Other symptoms may include these:

- Bitter taste in the mouth

- Breath odor

- General discomfort, uneasiness, or ill feeling

- Fever

- Pain when chewing

- Sensitivity of the teeth to hot or cold

- Swollen glands of the neck

- Swollen area of the upper or lower jaw—a very serious symptom

Exams and Tests

The patient will feel pain when the dentist taps the tooth. Biting or closing the mouth tightly also increases the pain. The gums may be swollen and red and may drain thick material.

Treatment

The goals of treatment are to cure the infection, save the tooth, and prevent complications. Antibiotics may be given to fight the infection. Warm salt-water rinses may be soothing. Over-the-counter pain relievers may relieve the toothache and fever.

Do not place aspirin directly over the tooth or gums, because this increases irritation of the tissues and can result in mouth ulcers.

A root canal may be recommended in an attempt to save the tooth. If there is a severe infection, the tooth may be removed, or surgery may be needed to drain the abscess. Some people may need to be admitted to the hospital.

Outlook (Prognosis)

Untreated abscesses may get worse and can lead to life-threatening complications. Prompt treatment usually cures the infection. The tooth can usually be saved in many cases.

Possible Complications

- Loss of the tooth
- Mediastinitis
- Sepsis
- Spread of infection to soft tissue (facial cellulitis, Ludwig's angina)
- Spread of infection to the jaw bone (osteomyelitis of the jaw)
- Spread of infection to other areas of the body resulting in brain abscess, endocarditis, pneumonia, or other complications

When to Contact a Medical Professional

Call your dentist if you have a persistent, throbbing toothache.

Prevention

Prompt treatment of dental caries reduces the risk of tooth abscess. Traumatized teeth should be examined promptly by the dentist.

Section 13.4

Phantom Tooth Pain (Atypical Odontalgia)

Atypical odontalgia, also known as atypical facial pain or phantom tooth pain, is characterized by chronic pain in a tooth or teeth, or in a site where teeth have been extracted, without an identifiable cause. Over time, the pain may spread to involve wider areas of the face or jaws. The pain is called atypical because it is a different type of pain than that of a typical toothache. Typical toothache comes and goes and is aggravated by exposure of the tooth to hot or cold food or drink, and/or by chewing or biting on the affected tooth. There is an identifiable cause, such as decay, periodontal disease, or injury to the tooth and the pain is predictably relieved by treatment of the affected tooth.

With atypical odontalgia, the pain is described as a constant throbbing or aching in a tooth, teeth, or extraction site that is persistent and unremitting, and which is not significantly affected by exposure to hot or cold food or drink, or by chewing or biting. The intensity of the pain can vary from very mild to very severe. There is typically no identifiable cause to explain the pain and it often follows or is associated with a history of some type of dental procedure such as having a root canal or tooth extraction. On occasion, the pain can occur without any reason. The pain is felt in a tooth, or teeth, and persists in spite of treatment aimed to relieve the pain such as a filling, a root canal, or even an extraction. This often presents a frustrating and confusing situation for both the patient and the dentist, and can lead to more and more dental treatment, none of which is effective at relieving the pain.

The diagnosis of atypical odontalgia is made after a thorough history, clinical examination, and radiographic assessment fail to identify a cause for the pain. Once the diagnosis is made, medications can be used to reduce the level of pain.

Questions and Answers about Atypical Odontalgia

What causes atypical odontalgia?

The cause of atypical odontalgia is not known, and therefore, some clinicians refer to the pain as idiopathic. In all likelihood, it is probably due to a variety of factors which may include genetic predisposition, age, and sex. It is more common in women than in men, and is found most often in the middle-aged to older age group. Some studies have found an association between atypical odontalgia and depression and anxiety, however, the significance of this association is unclear. The actual pathologic mechanism seems to be dysfunction or short-circuiting of the nerves that carry pain sensations from the teeth and jaws that is triggered by some type of dental or oral manipulation. Areas of the brain that process pain signals, appear to undergo molecular and biochemical changes that result in a persistent sensation of pain.

Why doesn't dental treatment cure the pain?

In most cases, dental treatment doesn't help. In some cases, it may temporarily lessen or change the severity of the pain, but it will inevitably return. This is because the pain is not caused by any pathology in the teeth or gums, but rather it is due to dysfunction of the nerves or a portion of the brain that processes pain sensation. It is important to recognize this in order to prevent unnecessary and ineffective dental treatment.

How is atypical odontalgia treated?

Atypical odontalgia is a chronic pain condition that is treated by using a variety of medications. Many different medications have been used to treat this condition; however, the tricyclic antidepressants are used most frequently. Although these are antidepressant medications, they are primarily used for their pain relieving properties and not for their antidepressant effects. Amitriptyline is one of the more commonly prescribed tricyclic medications used for atypical odontalgia. In addition to the tricyclics, other drugs used to treat chronic pain conditions, such as gabapentin and baclofen, may be prescribed. Generally, treatment is successful in reducing the pain but not eliminating it completely.

Is this a permanent condition?

Since the exact cause of this problem is not known, it is difficult to say whether this is a permanent condition. There are cases in which the pain goes away spontaneously, as well as cases in which the pain gradually subsides and disappears after prolonged treatment with medications. There are many cases, however, that persist and require the continued use of medications.

Why doesn't my dentist know about this problem?

While atypical odontalgia is not rare, it is uncommon enough that many dentists have not seen the problem and are not familiar with it. Therefore, diagnosis and treatment is best done by a dentist with advanced training and familiarity with the problem, such as a specialist in oral medicine or orofacial pain.

Section 13.5

Cracked Teeth

With their more sophisticated procedures, dentists are helping people keep their teeth longer. Because people are living longer and more stressful lives, they are exposing their teeth to many more years of crack-inducing habits, such as clenching, grinding, and chewing on hard objects. These habits make our teeth more susceptible to cracks.

How do I know if my tooth is cracked?

Cracked teeth show a variety of symptoms, including erratic pain when chewing, possibly with release of biting pressure, or pain when your tooth is exposed to temperature extremes. In many cases, the pain may come and go, and your dentist may have difficulty locating which tooth is causing the discomfort.

Why does a cracked tooth hurt?

To understand why a cracked tooth hurts, it helps to know something about the anatomy of the tooth. Inside the tooth, under the white enamel and a hard layer called the dentin, is the inner soft tissue called the pulp. The loose pulp is a connective tissue that contains cells, blood vessels and nerves.

When the outer hard tissues of the tooth are cracked, chewing can cause movement of the pieces, and the pulp can become irritated. When biting pressure is released, the crack can close quickly, resulting in a momentary, sharp pain. Irritation of the dental pulp can be repeated many times by chewing. Eventually, the pulp will become damaged to the point that it can no longer heal itself. The tooth will not only hurt when chewing but may also become sensitive to temperature extremes. In time, a cracked tooth may begin to hurt all by itself. Extensive cracks can lead to infection of the pulp tissue, which can spread to the bone and gum tissue surrounding the tooth.

How will my cracked tooth be treated?

There are many different types of cracked teeth. The treatment and outcome for your tooth depends on the type, location, and extent of the crack.

Craze lines: Craze lines are tiny cracks that affect only the outer enamel. These cracks are extremely common in adult teeth. Craze lines are very shallow, cause no pain, and are of no concern beyond appearances.

Fractured Cusp: When a cusp (the pointed part of the chewing surface) becomes weakened, a fracture sometimes results. The weakened cusp may break off by itself or may have to be removed by the dentist. When this happens, the pain will usually be relieved. A fractured cusp rarely damages the pulp, so root canal treatment is seldom needed. Your tooth will usually be restored with a full crown by your dentist.

Cracked Tooth: Some cracks extends from the chewing surface of the tooth vertically towards the root. A cracked tooth is not completely separated into two distinct segments. Because of the position of the crack, damage to the pulp is common. Root canal treatment is frequently needed to treat the injured pulp. Your dentist will then restore your tooth with a crown to hold the pieces together and protect the cracked tooth. At times, the crack may extend below the gingival tissue line, requiring extraction.

Early diagnosis is important. Even with high magnification and special lighting, it is sometimes difficult to determine the extent of a crack. A cracked tooth that is not treated will progressively worsen, eventually resulting in the loss of the tooth. Early diagnosis and treatment are essential in saving these teeth.

Split Tooth: A split tooth is often the result of the long-term progression of a cracked tooth. The split tooth is identified by a crack with distinct segments that can be separated. A split tooth cannot be saved intact. The position and extent of the crack, however, will determine whether any portion of the tooth can be saved. In rare instances, endodontic treatment and a crown or other restoration by your dentist may be used to save a portion of the tooth.

Vertical Root Fracture: Vertical root fractures are cracks that begin in the root of the tooth and extend toward the chewing surface. They often show minimal signs and symptoms and may therefore go unnoticed for some time. Vertical root fractures are often discovered when the surrounding bone and gum become infected. Treatment may involve extraction of the tooth. However, endodontic surgery is sometimes appropriate if a portion of the tooth can be saved by removal of the fractured root.

After treatment for a cracked tooth, will my tooth completely heal?

Unlike a broken bone, the fracture in a cracked tooth will not heal. In spite of treatment, some cracks may continue to progress and separate, resulting in loss of the tooth. Placement of a crown on a cracked tooth provides maximum protection but does not guarantee success in all cases.

The treatment you receive for your cracked tooth is important because it will relieve pain and reduce the likelihood that the crack will worsen. Once treated, most cracked teeth continue to function and provide years of comfortable chewing. Talk to your endodontist about your particular diagnosis and treatment recommendations. S/he will advise you on how to keep your natural teeth and achieve optimum dental health.

What can I do to prevent my teeth from cracking?

While cracked teeth are not completely preventable, you can take some steps to make your teeth less susceptible to cracks.

- Don't chew on hard objects such as ice, unpopped popcorn kernels, or pens.

- Don't clench or grind your teeth.

- If you clench or grind your teeth while you sleep, talk to your dentist about getting a retainer or other mouthguard to protect your teeth.

- Wear a mouthguard or protective mask when playing contact sports.

Chapter 14

Medications Used in Dentistry

Many different types of medicines are used in dentistry. Medications are used to control pain that occurs with dental procedures, control anxiety, prevent or treat infections, and manage other oral conditions.

This chapter reviews some of the most common medicines used in dentistry. Many of these medicines are used to treat more than one dental condition.

Medicines to Control Pain

Pain and irritation in the mouth can occur with tooth extractions, root canal treatment, toothache, teething, and sores in or around the mouth (such as cold sores, canker sores, and fever blisters). Dentures or other dental appliances, including braces, can also cause pain and irritation.

Local anesthesia, general anesthesia, nitrous oxide, or intravenous sedation are commonly used to manage pain. These medicines can numb the area to be treated (local anesthesia), put you to sleep (general anesthesia), or put you in a drowsy state (nitrous oxide or intravenous sedation). Under nitrous oxide or intravenous sedation, you are able to follow commands, but once awake, will not remember the dental procedure.

Narcotics are also used to relieve pain. Examples of narcotics include: acetaminophen/codeine (Tylenol #3), acetaminophen/hydrocodone (Vicodin), and acetaminophen/oxycodone (Percocet). Narcotics are prescribed for such procedures as tooth extractions or root canal treatment.

Other pain-relievers include anti-inflammatory medications, such as acetaminophen (Tylenol), and anesthetics. Anesthetics reduce pain and irritation caused by toothaches, teething, and sores in or around the mouth (such as cold sores, canker sores, and fever blisters), dentures, braces, and other dental appliances.

Anesthetics are available both by prescription and over-the-counter. They are available as an aerosol spray, dental paste, gel, lozenges, ointments, and solutions. They are known by such brand names as Anbesol, Chloraseptic, Orajel, and Xylocaine.

Note: Medicines used for teething that include benzocaine as an ingredient (for example, Anbesol) can be given to babies four months of age and older. Most of the other nonprescription medicines that contain a dental anesthetic should only be used in children two years of age and older. Also, because the elderly are more sensitive to the effects of many local anesthetics, they should closely follow the label instructions or those of their dentist. Anesthetics used for toothache pain should not be used long term. They are prescribed for temporary pain relief until the toothache can be treated. New denture wearers who use anesthetics to relieve pain should see their dentist. An adjustment to the appliance may be needed to prevent more soreness.

Medicines to Control Anxiety

In addition to managing pain, local anesthesia, general anesthesia, nitrous oxide, or intravenous sedation can also be used to control anxiety. Medicines such as diazepam, valium, halcyon, and Ativan are other anti-anxiety medications.

Medicines to Control Inflammation

Anti-inflammatory medicines, such as corticosteroids, are used to relieve the discomfort and redness of mouth and gum problems. They are only available by prescription and are available as pastes under such brand names as Kenalog in Orabase, Orabase-HCA, Oracort, and Oralone.

Mild pain and/or swelling caused by dental appliances, toothaches, and fevers can be treated with ibuprofen (Advil, Motrin) or Tylenol.

Note: Never give infants and children aspirin. Aspirin thins the blood, which increases the risk of bleeding.

Medicines to Treat Gingivitis

Chlorhexidine is an antiseptic antibacterial mouth rinse that is used to treat gingivitis. Gingivitis is a gum disease. It is caused by bacteria found in dental plaque. Plaque is the thin film that forms on teeth and gums. Plaque forms due to inadequate oral hygiene (not following tooth brushing, flossing recommendations). Signs of gingivitis are red, swollen, and tender gums, and bad breath. If left untreated, gingivitis can eventually destroy the bone that keeps your teeth in place.

Chlorhexidine is only available by prescription. Over-the-counter antiseptic mouth rinses (such as Listerine) reduce plaque and gingivitis and kill the germs that cause bad breath. Look for the words tartar control on tooth pastes and mouthwashes.

Note: Chlorhexidine may cause an increase in tartar on your teeth. Tartar is a hardened form of plaque, which leads to tooth decay. Chlorhexidine may also cause staining of the teeth, teeth fillings, and dentures or other mouth appliances. Brushing with a tartar-control toothpaste and daily flossing help reduce tartar build-up and staining. In addition, visit your dentist at least every six months for a teeth cleaning and gum examination. Tell your dentist if you have ever had any unusual or allergic reaction to chlorhexidine or to skin disinfectants containing chlorhexidine.

Medicines to Prevent Tooth Decay

Fluoride is used to prevent tooth decay. It is absorbed by teeth and helps strengthen teeth to resist acid and block the cavity-forming action of bacteria. When used as a varnish or a mouth rinse, fluoride also helps reduce tooth sensitivity. Nonprescription fluoride products are found in many types of toothpaste. Prescription-strength fluoride is available as a liquid, tablet, gel, paste, and chewable tablets. It is usually taken once daily. Prescription-strength fluoride is prescribed for children and adults who have not had fluoride added to their home water supply. It is also frequently prescribed for patients with uncontrolled tooth decay and in those who are undergoing radiation therapy.

Note: Before taking fluoride, tell your dentist if you are allergic to fluoride, tartrazine (a yellow dye in some processed foods and drugs), or any other drugs. Do not take calcium, magnesium, or iron supplements while taking fluoride without checking with your dentist. Tell your dentist if you are on a low-sodium, or sodium-free, diet. Do not eat or drink dairy products one hour before or one hour after taking fluoride. Fluoride can cause staining of the teeth.

Medicines for Dry Mouth

Pilocarpine (Salagen) is a medicine used to treat dry mouth. The drug stimulates saliva production. An inadequate flow of saliva can lead to gingivitis and other oral health problems.

Medicines for Teeth Grinding

Muscle relaxants are prescribed to reduce stress, which can help stop teeth grinding. They are also used to treat temporomandibular joint disorders (TMJ). TMJ is the result of a group of problems in the jaw area in front of the ear. Symptoms of TMJ include headaches, ear pain, clicking and popping of the jaw, dizziness, and ringing in the ears.

Other Uses of Antibiotics, Antifungals, and Antiviral Medicines

Antibiotics: Penicillin, amoxicillin, and clindamycin are frequently used antibiotics. Another class of antibiotics, the tetracyclines—which includes demeclocycline, doxycycline, minocycline, oxytetracycline, and tetracycline—are also used in dentistry. Antibiotics may be used either in combination with surgery and other therapies, or alone. They are used to kill bacteria associated with periodontal disease, to maintain the attachment of teeth to the jaw bone, and to reduce the pain and irritation of canker sores. Canker sores are a painful, open sore in the mouth. Dental antibiotics come in a variety of forms including gels, thread-like fibers, microspheres (tiny round particles), and mouth rinses.

Antifungals: Antifungals are prescribed to treat oral thrush. The goal of treatment is to stop the spread of a specific type of fungus (Candida) from the tongue and lining of the mouth to the gums, tonsils, roof of mouth, and throat. Antifungal medicines are available in tablets, lozenges, or liquids that are usually swished around in your mouth before being swallowed.

Antivirals: Antivirals such acyclovir (Zovirax), docosanol (Abreva), and valacyclovir (Valtrex) are used to treat cold sores. Cold sores are a small group of blister-like sores that form on the lip and outer edge of the mouth. They are also called fever blisters.

The dose of medicines used in dentistry and instructions on how to take them may differ from patient to patient, depending on what the drug is being used for, patient age and weight, and other considerations.

Your dentist will give you information about all medicines you need to take. Do not hesitate to ask your dentist questions if you do not fully understand the instructions. You should know the name of your medicines, the reason why you are taking them, the number of times to take the medicines a day, the dosage of the medicines, and how to apply gels or pastes or other-than-pill formulations. Also, be sure to tell your dentist of any other health issues, allergies, and medicines you are taking.

Chapter 15

Sedation Techniques Used by Dentists

Anxiety Just Melts Away

When you are afraid, your threshold for pain is much lower, you become hypersensitive to every sensation, prick, and noise. Fear and anxiety trigger the release of certain chemicals like adrenalin which put your fight-or-flight instincts on high alert. You anticipate that something is going to hurt and so you tense your muscles, even if it is subconsciously. In this heightened state of anxiety, you experience more pain during and even after treatment. However, this response can virtually be eliminated with oral sedation dentistry.

The whole purpose of oral sedation is to make you as comfortable and relaxed as possible. It allows you to let your guard down, relax both your mind and body, and focus on feeling peaceful rather than anxious. Your apprehension and hypersensitivity to pain melt away, yet you remain awake and in control.

Sometimes referred to as *comfortable* or *relaxation* dentistry, these terms are used to describe the feelings most people perceive during their dental visits, which are produced by oral sedation.

"Oral Sedation Dentistry," by Dr. Michael D. Silverman, reviewed by Dr. Garry A. Rayant, Editor-in-Chief, Dear Doctor, Inc., February, 2009. Copyright © 2009 Dear Doctor, Inc. (www.deardoctor.com). All rights reserved. Reprinted with permission. This article is Part Two in a series from Dear Doctor, Comfortable Dentistry in the 21st Century. Part One of this series, "Overcoming Fear and Anxiety" (available at http://www.deardoctor.com/articles/overcoming-dental-fear-and-anxiety/) discussed learning to overcome and cope with negative emotions and become comfortable with modern dentistry.

Safety and Effectiveness

Oral sedation dentistry allows you the confidence and peace of mind to experience dental procedures in a whole new way. Hours seem to pass like mere minutes so that necessary dental treatment can be performed comfortably. When you are relaxed, you allow your dentist to be able to work more efficiently by focusing on the work at hand, with the confidence that you are comfortable.

A variety of oral sedative and anxiolytic medications have been developed especially for these purposes. They have been subjected to rigorous research and testing and have a long safety record after decades of use. In addition several have amnesic properties, meaning that you remember little to nothing after treatment.

The safety of sedation medications is measured by pharmacists and health professionals on a scale called the therapeutic index. The larger the number is on the scale, the safer the drug. Oral sedatives and anxiolytics used in dentistry have the highest numbers possible on the therapeutic index, making them the least likely to cause an adverse reaction.

How to Ensure Safety—What to Let Your Dentist Know

It is critical to provide your dentist with a complete health history including:

- Medical conditions for which you are being treated

- Any and all medications prescribed by a doctor

- Over-the-counter medications, remedies and vitamins (including aspirin)

- Alternative or herbal supplements: Many people seek relief from depression and anxiety symptoms with natural remedies like St. John's wort and kava kava. These may have a mild interaction with oral sedatives, so it's critical that you tell your dentist if you are taking them. The medications and dosages for your oral sedation treatment can be adjusted to compensate for any interactions.

- Certain foods: Even something as seemingly insignificant as drinking grapefruit juice can have an effect on sedation. The enzymes in grapefruit interfere with the systems that metabolize (break down) certain oral sedation medications in your body, so you should not consume grapefruit 72 hours prior to or immediately after a sedation procedure.

- Also, be sure to tell your doctor about factors like smoking and alcohol consumption, since these can influence the effectiveness of sedation medications.

Administer the Medication Yourself

Oral sedation is a popular treatment option for many people because it does not require injection, so if you're afraid of needles, you needn't worry. In fact, once you're comfortable with oral sedatives, it may even be easier to have local anesthesia (numbing shots in the mouth) to further facilitate the ease of dental procedures.

Medications are given orally (by mouth). They are either placed and dissolved under the tongue, or they can just be swallowed whole.

Many dentists prefer the sublingual (under the tongue) route which works even more quickly. Taken this way they are absorbed into the bloodstream more rapidly. Both methods are safe and effective and work in a matter of minutes. You can even try the medication the night before to see how it affects you and also ensure a good night's sleep.

Planning for Your Appointment

Once you and your dentist decide to use oral sedation for your next appointment, you will need to make some preparations:

- Your health history can affect your before-and-after care plans, especially for diabetics and smokers, so make sure your dentist knows about any medical conditions that you may have.

- You may be instructed to take oral sedation medication the night before your appointment to make sure you get a good night's sleep.

- You should not eat or drink anything six hours prior to your appointment unless directed by your dentist.

- Be prepared to take time off from work following your appointment. For short appointments, only half a day may be necessary. If a longer appointment is planned, make arrangements to take the remainder of the day off.

- You will need a companion to drive you to and from your appointment; you should not drive or operate heavy machinery until the medication has worn off; this will vary depending upon what drug has been prescribed—follow the directions exactly.

- Be sure to stay hydrated and drink lots of fluids following your appointment.

Which Medication Is Right for You?

While your dentist will decide which medications are appropriate for your treatment, being familiar with the different drugs available can be helpful for you. Knowledge about oral sedation is not only powerful—it is empowering.

There are several commonly prescribed medications, including, but not limited to Valium, Halcion, Sonata, Ativan, Vistaril, and Versed. With the exception of Vistaril and Sonata they all belong to a class of medications called benzodiazepines. Benzodiazepines are prescribed for the treatment of anxiety, insomnia, agitation, seizures, and muscle spasms. Taken in small doses, they are highly effective at relieving the mentioned conditions.

Each medication has a different duration of action (how long it affects you) and different half-life (how long it remains in your body). Dosages can vary greatly depending on whether swallowed whole or placed under the tongue in addition to the treatment protocols for which the sedation is being used. The drugs take effect anywhere from 20 minutes to an hour. Some varieties of the medication have amnesic properties, meaning that you remember little or nothing of your time in the dental chair after the procedure is completed.

Other Forms of Sedation Dentistry

Inhalation conscious sedation is also known as nitrous oxide/oxygen sedation. Nitrous oxide, commonly and inappropriately called laughing gas, has been used by dentists for nearly 100 years. It is an excellent analgesic (pain reliever), but a less effective anxiolytic (anti-anxiety) medication. It is administered through a nasal hood, which is similar to a small cup placed over your nose. Nitrous oxide is extremely safe because it is mixed directly with oxygen to provide you with a feeling of euphoria or light-headedness. All bodily functions remain essentially normal. You may experience a tingling sensation from the use of nitrous oxide. However, its effects wear off almost immediately so there is no hangover effect.

In combination with an oral sedative, nitrous oxide allows your dentist to fine-tune the exact amount of sedation needed to provide you with the best possible experience.

Intravenous (IV) conscious sedation, also known as deep conscious sedation, is used by some dentists, and surgical specialists like oral surgeons and periodontists who must undertake specialized training and certification in IV use. With this type of sedation, medications are administered directly into the blood stream intravenously (intra-within, venous-vein). The main advantage of this method is that it works immediately and the level of sedation can be adjusted quickly and easily. There is a higher degree of risk associated with IV sedation since normal bodily functions especially heart rate, blood pressure, and breathing can be altered necessitating specialized monitoring equipment. The drugs used for IV sedation are more potent when given this way than when taken orally and amnesia may be more profound.

Finding the Right Dentist

Like any informed consumer, you will want to make sure that your dentist is qualified to provide sedation dentistry. It is a good idea to request information on your dentist's training, credentials, and the techniques that may be used prior to an appointment.

You Are Not Alone

Talk to your dentist about your fears and concerns so that together you can decide on the best treatment for you. It's important to remember that dentistry has come a long way. Years of research have been dedicated to studying and finding methods to alleviate pain and anxiety. There are safe and time-tested options available to ensure that you have a positive and painless experience. Step out from under the shadow of fear and into the calm of sedation dentistry. You are not alone, and you don't have to be afraid anymore.

Chapter 16

Alternatives to Dental Drills

Chapter Contents

Section 16.1

Air Abrasion

Air abrasion is a way to remove decay from a tooth without using a dental drill. It works like a sandblaster removing graffiti from walls. The air abrasion hand piece blows a powerful air stream of tiny aluminum oxide particles out of its tip onto the tooth. The tiny particles bounce off the tooth and blast the decay away.

Air abrasion is most commonly used to prepare teeth for composites, or "white fillings." Air abrasion also helps to repair cracks and discolored teeth, to prepare teeth for bonding procedures such as sealants, and for various other procedures. Air abrasion works well to repair chipped, fractured, or worn teeth; to prepare teeth for cosmetic surgery; remove stains and spots; repair old fillings and sealants; and repair broken crowns and bridges.

Your general dentist, who has been trained in restorative dentistry techniques, will perform any procedures that use air-abrasion technology. Ask your dentist if he or she uses air-abrasion equipment and if this technique is right for you.

What Happens?

Your dentist might ask you to wear protective glasses during the procedure, and a rubber dam might be placed inside your mouth and around the tooth area being treated. Air abrasion procedures may leave some dusty particles in your mouth that make your mouth feel gritty. The particles are harmless and can be rinsed out easily. To reduce dust buildup, the dentist might use a vacuum hose or water spray during the procedure.

The Pros and Cons

Because air abrasion procedures are virtually painless, anesthetic injections are generally unnecessary. Also, no vibrations or heat from friction are produced by air abrasion systems, which are quiet and will not harm soft mouth tissue. Because air abrasion dissolves tooth structure very precisely, the process removes less of your tooth than a drill does; in addition, the risk for breaking the enamel is reduced. During teeth cleanings, a dentist sometimes can spot a shallow cavity and fill it the same day using air abrasion techniques, restoring your tooth with natural-looking materials that strengthen and protect it. Additionally, treatment time is usually shorter than with procedures involving a drill.

Air abrasion is not always totally painless. The air and the abrasives used can cause sensitivity in some teeth. It is well-suited for removing small cavities that form on the surface of teeth, but is not recommended for deep cavities (those close to your tooth's pulp). Only composite filling materials can be used following air abrasion because these materials adhere well to the smooth surface created by the process. For silver fillings, a dentist must use a drill to prepare your tooth in order to prevent the filling from falling out.

Will I Feel Anything?

Air abrasion procedures can leave an accumulation of harmless, dusty particle debris in the patient's mouth, resulting in a gritty feeling that is eradicated by rinsing. Your dentist may require you to wear protective glasses during the procedure, and a rubber dam may be applied inside your mouth and around the tooth area being treated to serve as a particle barrier. To reduce dust build-up, the dentist or dental assistant may use a vacuum hose or a water spray technique while administering air abrasion.

If you have a deep cavity, you may experience some sensitivity. Your dentist will make every effort to make you comfortable and may administer local anesthesia, depending on the depth of your cavity.

Is Air Abrasion for Everyone?

Yes. Air abrasion is an especially good option for children or anyone who may be afraid of the needle, noise, and vibration of a regular dental drill. However, there are some treatments—such as crowns, inlays, onlays, and bridges—which still require a dental drill. Air abrasion is not an alternative for every procedure.

Does Insurance Cover Air Abrasion?

Dental insurance plans change often, so some may cover air abrasion and some may not. It is best to check your plan to see if it covers air abrasion procedures.

Section 16.2

Laser Dentistry

"What is Laser Dentistry?" Reprinted with permission from
General Dentistry, February 2012. © Academy of General Dentistry.
All rights reserved. On the Web at www.agd.org.

What is a laser and how does it work?

A laser is an instrument that produces a very narrow, intense beam of light energy. When laser light comes in contact with tissue, it causes a reaction. The light produced by the laser can remove or shape tissue.

Are lasers used in dentistry?

Yes, lasers have been used in dentistry since 1990. Lasers can be used as a safe and effective treatment for a wide range of dental procedures and are often used in conjunction with other dental instruments.

How are lasers used in dentistry?

Dental lasers can be used to:

- reduce the discomfort of canker and cold sores,
- expose partially erupted wisdom teeth,
- remove muscle attachments that limit proper movement,
- manage gum tissue during impressions for crowns or other procedures,
- remove overgrown tissues caused by certain medications,
- perform biopsy procedures,
- remove inflamed gum tissues and aid in the treatment of gum disease,
- remove or reshape gum and bone tissues during crown lengthening procedures,

- help treat infections in root canals,
- speed up tooth whitening procedures.

What are the benefits of using dental lasers?

There are several advantages. Dentists may not need to use a drill or administer anesthesia in some procedures, allowing the patient to enjoy a more relaxed dental experience. Laser procedures can be more precise. Also, lasers can reduce symptoms and healing times associated with traditional therapies; reduce the amount of bacteria in both diseased gum tissue and in tooth cavities; and control bleeding during surgery.

Are dental lasers safe?

If the dental laser is used according to accepted practices by a trained practitioner, then it is at least as safe as other dental instruments. However, just as you wear sunglasses to protect your eyes from prolonged exposure to the sun, when your dentist performs a laser procedure, you will be asked to wear special eyeglasses to protect your eyes from the laser.

How can I be sure my dentist is properly trained to use a laser?

Ask your dentist questions about the extent of his or her laser education and training. Make sure that your dentist has participated in educational courses and received training by the manufacturer. Many dental schools, dental associations, and the Academy of Laser Dentistry (ALD) offer dental laser education. The ALD is the profession's independent source for current dental laser education and credentialing.

How will I know if treatment with a dental laser is an option for me?

Ask your dentist. Although the laser is a very useful dental instrument, it is not appropriate for every dental procedure.

Chapter 17

Dental Fillings

Chapter Contents

Section 17.1

Dental Amalgam Fillings

This section begins with text excerpted from "About Dental Amalgam Fillings," U.S. Food and Drug Administration (FDA), August 11, 2009. Text under the heading "Amalgam Use Is Declining" is excerpted from "Dental Amalgam Use and Benefits," Centers for Disease Control and Prevention (CDC), May 28, 2010.

About Dental Amalgam Fillings

Dental amalgam is a dental filling material used to fill cavities caused by tooth decay. It has been used for more than 150 years in hundreds of millions of patients. Dental amalgam is a mixture of metals, consisting of liquid mercury and a powdered alloy composed of silver, tin, and copper. Approximately 50% of dental amalgam is elemental mercury by weight. Dental amalgam fillings are also known as silver fillings because of their silver-like appearance.

When placing dental amalgam, the dentist first drills the tooth to remove the decay and then shapes the tooth cavity for placement of the amalgam filling. Next, under appropriate safety conditions, the dentist mixes the powdered alloy with the liquid mercury to form an amalgam putty. (These components are provided to the dentist in a capsule.) This softened amalgam putty is placed in the prepared cavity, where it hardens into a solid filling.

What should I know before getting a dental amalgam filling?

Deciding what filling material to use to treat dental decay is a choice that must be made by you and your dentist. As you consider your options, you should keep in mind the following information.

Potential benefits: Dental amalgam fillings are strong and long-lasting, so they are less likely to break than some other types of fillings. Dental amalgam is the least expensive type of filling material.

Potential risks: Dental amalgam contains elemental mercury. It releases low levels of mercury vapor that can be inhaled. High levels of mercury vapor exposure are associated with adverse effects in the brain and the kidneys. However, the U.S. Food and Drug Administration (FDA) has reviewed the best available scientific evidence to determine whether the low levels of mercury vapor associated with dental amalgam fillings are a cause for concern. Based on this evidence, FDA considers dental amalgam fillings safe for adults and children ages six years and above.

Amalgam Use Is Declining

Amalgam use is declining for several reasons. The main reason is that cavity rates among school children and young adults are dropping. Improved filling alternatives are also now available for certain uses.

Dental amalgam is used:

- in persons of all ages;
- in areas where most chewing is done, mainly in the rear teeth;
- when there is severe damage of tooth structure and cost is a big factor;
- as a foundation for metal, metal-ceramic, and ceramic crowns or caps;
- when a patient commitment to personal oral hygiene is poor;
- when moisture control is a problem when placing the filling; or,
- when cost is a large patient concern.

Dental amalgam is not used when:

- looks are important, such as fillings in the front teeth;
- patients have a history of allergy to mercury or other amalgam parts; or,
- a large filling is needed and the cost of other restorative materials is not a major factor in the treatment decision.

Section 17.2

Mercury in Dental Amalgam

This section begins with text excerpted from "Mercury in Dental Amalgam," Environmental Protection Agency (EPA), August 5, 2011. Text under the heading "FDA Answers to Questions about Dental Amalgam" is excerpted from "About Dental Amalgam Fillings," U.S. Food and Drug Administration (FDA), August 11, 2009.

Mercury in Dental Amalgam

Are dental amalgam fillings safe?

When amalgam fillings are placed in or removed from teeth, they can release a small amount of mercury vapor. Amalgam can also release small amounts of mercury vapor during chewing, and people can absorb these vapors by inhaling or ingesting them. High levels of mercury vapor exposure are associated with adverse effects in the brain and the kidneys.

Since the 1990s, several federal agencies have reviewed the scientific literature looking for links between dental amalgam and health problems. According to the Centers for Disease Control and Prevention (CDC), there is little scientific evidence that the health of the vast majority of people with dental amalgam is compromised, nor that removing amalgam fillings has any beneficial effect on health.

FDA Classification of Dental Amalgam as a Medical Device

Dental amalgam is considered to be a medical device, and is regulated by the Food and Drug Administration (FDA). FDA is responsible for ensuring that dental amalgam is reasonably safe and effective, and that, among other things, the product labeling seen by dentists has adequate directions for use and includes any appropriate warnings.

Are there alternatives to using dental amalgam fillings?

Presently, there are five other types of restorative materials for tooth decay:

- resin composite,
- glass ionomer,
- resin ionomer,
- porcelain, and
- gold alloys.

The choice of dental treatment rests with dental professionals and their patients, so talk with your dentist about available dental treatment options.

FDA Answers to Questions about Dental Amalgam

Why is mercury used in dental amalgam?

Approximately half of a dental amalgam filling is liquid mercury and the other half is a powdered alloy of silver, tin, and copper. Mercury is used to bind the alloy particles together into a strong, durable, and solid filling. Mercury's unique properties (it is the only metal that is a liquid at room temperature and that bonds well with the powdered alloy) make it an important component of dental amalgam that contributes to its durability.

If I am concerned about the mercury in dental amalgam, should I have my fillings removed?

If your fillings are in good condition and there is no decay beneath the filling, FDA does not recommend that you have your amalgam fillings removed or replaced. Removing sound amalgam fillings results in unnecessary loss of healthy tooth structure, and exposes you to additional mercury vapor released during the removal process. However, if you believe you have an allergy or sensitivity to mercury or any of the other metals in dental amalgam (such as silver, tin, or copper), you should discuss treatment options with your dentist.

Section 17.3

Composite Fillings

[Ed. Note: Many dentists have given up use of amalgam restorations in favor of the new generation of composite restoration.] The glass particles give the composite restoration their color (and their stiffness in the unset state). The acrylic is the plastic matrix that holds the glass particles together. Most composite restorations today are "light cured" which means that the acrylic remains fluid until a very bright light is shined on it causing it to harden. Light curing allows the dentist time to work with the material, building and shaping it correctly, and when ready, to harden it immediately with the light. The light curing also makes for a more color stable restoration. The new tooth-colored composite restorations do not get yellow or brown with age as the older ones did.

The porcelain particles also give the restoration a great deal of resistance to wear. Amalgam fillings will probably always wear less than composite restorations; however, the recent advances in particle formulation and shape have made the newest posterior composites quite competitive for filling back teeth. Five to seven years is average. Composites are even stronger than amalgams in shear strength which makes them better for overlaying large biting areas.

Composite fillings have been used in front teeth for years, but only recently has the technology in composite formulation improved enough to allow their common use in back teeth. Prior to acrylic/glass composites, other types of composites were used in areas where esthetics was important. This is why even in the early twentieth century people were not forced to have silver amalgam fillings in their front teeth. However, even in the 1980s the technology had not yet advanced enough to allow the routine use of composite to restore chewing areas of the back teeth.

Composite resins are still not as popular with dentists for repairing back teeth as old-fashioned amalgam. In fact, only about 25% of dentists currently use them routinely for restoring posterior teeth. The reasons for this are that they are not as wear resistant as amalgam restorations, they are more technique sensitive than amalgam, and there is a tendency for more prolonged tooth sensitivity to cold after the restoration is done. On the other hand, as the materials continue to improve, they have become tougher and more wear resistant while improvements in placement technique have reduced cold sensitivity. However, the greater difficulty in placing these restorations remains a deterrent for many dentists, and continues to keep the cost of the service higher than for a comparable amalgam restoration.

Why Dentists Are Abandoning Amalgam

1. When first invented, amalgam was great stuff. It still is, in fact, but it isn't any greater now than it was 150 years ago. Technical improvements in it over the years have made minor differences in its physical properties, but other than the addition of trace elements to the mix for the purpose of reducing tarnishing, speeding the setting time, and changing minor physical parameters, it really hasn't changed much since it was invented. On the other hand, the technology involved in composite formulations has made tremendous strides in improving the wear, strength, appearance, setting characteristics, water miscibility, and numerous other less obvious qualities. They continue to improve yearly. The newest generation of composite filling materials has finally overcome most of the difficulties which prevented their widespread use in restoring back teeth.

2. Composite fillings are routinely bonded to the tooth structure. This takes the place of the water resistant layer of corrosion that seals amalgam fillings. It also helps to retain the filling inside the tooth while amalgam fillings depend on the use of undercuts in the cavity preparation to retain them. Amalgam fillings must engage undercuts within the cavity preparation so they will not dislodge. Amalgam also requires a minimum depth of 1.5 millimeters (mm) in order to form its crystalline structure while composite fillings have no minimum depth. (If they are not deep enough, the amalgam will be too thin and tends to crack.) The use of bonded composites has made possible the use of very small fillings that do not have the mechanical retention necessary to retain an amalgam. It has also made possible the use of shallow and thin cavity preparations which do not require the use of anesthetic to cut due to their very small size.

- Note that it is possible to bond amalgam fillings to the tooth. However, the process takes so long that the cost of such a bonded amalgam filling is actually greater than the cost of the comparable bonded composite. While most U.S. dentists still use amalgam, very few of them bond it to the tooth.

3. There is no comparison between the appearance of a composite filling and an amalgam. The results are so esthetically superior, that most people opt for the slightly more expensive composite over the less expensive amalgam. Since many people have quite a few fillings in their back teeth, the difference between a mouth with composite fillings versus the same mouth with amalgams is striking. After a year or so of offering both to my patients and explaining these differences to them, I discovered that my amalgam was approaching its maximum shelf life, so I discarded it and never bought any more.

4. Composite restorations can be repaired while most amalgam restorations cannot. A tooth has five surfaces that can become decayed. The size (and cost) of a filling is judged by the number of surfaces it encompass. When a filling covers, two surfaces, that leaves three other surfaces untouched. If the patient returns a year or two later with decay in one of those other surfaces, it is usually necessary to replace the entire amalgam that was done previously in order to place one that encompass the new decay. But, since composite bonds reasonably to itself, the dentist can usually simply add the new surface to the old filling and avoid the trauma to the nerve that replacing the entire filling would entail. It is also less expensive to the patient. (In order to save time, many dentists do repair old amalgam fillings, but the interface between the old and new materials is not chemically sealed as it is when repairing composite fillings.)

5. Before the advent of composite filling materials, many damaged teeth could not be repaired unless a root canal, post and core, and crown were done. This was because the working characteristics of amalgam required stringent techniques which were absolutely necessary, but not always achievable under real circumstances. Once modern composites became available, it became possible to repair some of these teeth using "freehand" techniques impossible with amalgam. Repair of these teeth is often not technically perfect, but it offers an affordable alternative to the stark choices of extraction or a very expensive series of steps like root canals, posts, and crowns.

Should I have all my amalgam fillings replaced with composites?

If esthetics is of major concern to the patient, then you should request the replacement of all your amalgams with composites, or porcelain crowns. But beware! Every time you remove one filling and put another in its place, you run the risk of killing the nerve of the tooth and then needing a root canal or extraction. Remember that the presence of mercury in amalgams is not considered a sufficient reason to replace them, and no dentist should ever recommend replacing yours on the basis of mercury poisoning. We do not solicit the replacement of any old filling provided that it is still serviceable and the patient does not object to its appearance.

Section 17.4

Temporary Fillings

"Temporary Filling Materials (ZOE and IRM)," reprinted with permission from http://doctorspiller.com. Copyright © 2010 Martin S. Spiller, D.M.D., updated 2012. All rights reserved.

When a patient presents at my office with pain attributable to a cavity, I sometimes place a temporary filling in the tooth and reappoint the patient for a final permanent filling at another visit. Sometimes, this is done in order to save time, especially if we have slipped the emergency patient between two regularly scheduled patients. Sometimes it is done in order to save money.

Temporaries are the least expensive (and most temporary) way to fill a tooth. Temporary fillings can be done quickly, because they are usually inserted without any of the time consuming rituals associated with a permanent filling. The patient is anesthetized, the decay removed, and the temporary filling is mixed and inserted, generally simply by pushing it into the cavity preparation with a gloved finger. The patient bites into it while it is still soft in order to adjust the height, and the patient leaves the office without even waiting for a final set on the material. In a phrase, a temporary is fast and cheap.

But, there is another reason that may indicate that a temporary is the best way to treat the patient, even if time or money is not an issue. Temporary fillings are different from permanent amalgam or composite fillings because they are sedative fillings. This means that they tend to soothe an inflamed nerve in a tooth, and may make the difference between the tooth needing a root canal (or an extraction), or simply filling the tooth later on, after the nerve has calmed down. Sometimes a temporary filling is the best course to relieve pain.

Temporary fillings are made of two major components: Oil of clove (eugenol), which has been used for centuries to relieve toothaches, and zinc oxide which is the ingredient that makes Desitin diaper rash ointment white. Zinc oxide is an excellent disinfectant. The oil and oxide mix together to make a stiff paste that eventually hardens into a waterproof substance which soothes the nerve of the tooth and kills germs while protecting the cavity like a hard band-aide.

When used as a temporary filling material or cement, this material is called "zinc oxide and eugenol," or ZOE for short. Zinc oxide and eugenol (ZOE) is not very durable, and it wears away after just a few weeks, but it works to relieve pain, calm the nerve, and protect the tooth until an appointment can be made to get it filled permanently. During the Vietnam war, the U.S. Army invented a more durable form of ZOE called intermediate restorative material (IRM) which is fortified with plastic powder. (It originally came in red, white, or blue colors.) IRM is used almost universally in dental offices throughout the world for temporary fillings. The increase in durability allows the temporary to last three to six months (sometimes even longer).

Never plan to keep a temporary filling more than six months. They are not meant to last that long, and while the eugenol lulls the patient into a false sense of security, the restoration wears rapidly and begins to leak. If you wait too long, the nerve could die, the temporary filling will wear away, the tooth will decay further, and then you will need a root canal or extraction.

Section 17.5

Peptide Fluid Stimulates Tooth Regeneration

Filling without Drilling

Researchers at the University of Leeds have discovered a pain-free way of tackling dental decay. The pioneering treatment promises to transform the approach to filling teeth forever.

Tooth decay begins when acid produced by bacteria in plaque dissolves the mineral in the teeth, causing microscopic holes or pores to form. As the decay process progresses, these micro-pores increase in size and number. Eventually, the damaged tooth may have to be drilled and filled to prevent toothache, or even removed.

The very thought of drilling puts many people off going to see their dentist, whether or not they actually need treatment. This tendency to miss check-ups and ignore niggling aches and pains means that existing problems get worse and early signs of decay in other teeth are overlooked.

It's a vicious cycle, but one that can be broken, according to researchers at the University of Leeds who have developed a revolutionary new way to treat the first signs of tooth decay. Their solution is to arm dentists with a peptide-based fluid that is literally painted onto the tooth's surface. The peptide technology is based on knowledge of how the tooth forms in the first place and stimulates regeneration of the tooth defect.

"This may sound too good to be true, but we are essentially helping acid-damaged teeth to regenerate themselves. It is a totally natural non-surgical repair process and is entirely pain-free too," said Professor Jennifer Kirkham, from the University of Leeds Dental Institute, who has led development of the new technique.

The "magic" fluid was designed by researchers in the University of Leeds' School of Chemistry, led by Dr. Amalia Aggeli. It contains a peptide known as P11-4 that—under certain conditions—will assemble together into fibers. In practice, this means that when applied to the tooth, the fluid seeps into the micro-pores caused by acid attack and then spontaneously forms a gel. This gel then provides a scaffold or framework that attracts calcium and regenerates the tooth's mineral from within, providing a natural and pain-free repair.

The technique was recently taken out of the laboratory and tested on a small group of adults whose dentist had spotted the initial signs of tooth decay. The results from this small trial have shown that P11-4 can indeed reverse the damage and regenerate the tooth tissue.

"The results of our tests so far are extremely promising," said Professor Paul Brunton, who is overseeing the patient testing at the University of Leeds Dental Institute. "If these results can be repeated on a larger patient group, then I have no doubt whatsoever that in two to three years' time this technique will be available for dentists to use in their daily practice."

"The main reason that people don't go to the dentist regularly is fear. If we can offer a treatment that is completely non-invasive, that doesn't involve a mechanical drill, then we can change that perceived link between dental treatment and pain. This really is more than filling without drilling, this is a novel approach that enables the patients to keep their natural teeth!"

The study is being funded by Credentis AG who have licensed the technology and are preparing to introduce P11-4 to dentists worldwide.

Chapter 18

Rebuilding and Reshaping Teeth

Chapter Contents

Section 18.1

Porcelain Veneers

Porcelain veneers are thin pieces of porcelain used to recreate the natural look of teeth, while also providing strength and resilience comparable to natural tooth enamel. It is often the material of choice for those looking to make slight position alterations, or to change tooth shape, size, and/or color.

Veneer Consultation

Visiting an American Academy of Cosmetic Dentistry (AACD) member dentist and asking about veneers is the first step in determining if veneers are the right option for you, or if there are alternate solutions available. Communication with your dentist about what you want corrected is critical for a successful result. Spend time clearly identifying what cosmetic improvements you want to accomplish.

You'll often hear people say that celebrities have veneers and this may seem like the best way to replicate picture-perfect teeth, but each mouth is different and veneers need to be carefully researched.

Your dentist will most likely begin with a smile analysis to determine what steps are necessary to achieve the smile you desire. In addition, your dentist may create a diagnostic mock-up that will allow you to "try on" veneers and other procedures to see if the final result is actually what you're looking for.

Your dentist may also show you a photo of how your new smile will look. This is called cosmetic imaging. Deciding that porcelain veneers will create the look you want is only one step in the process. There is much more to learn before proceeding further.

The How and Why of Porcelain Veneers

Porcelain laminate veneers consist of a compilation of several thin ceramic layers, which replace original tooth enamel, and an adhesive layer. To apply a veneer, a very small amount of the original tooth enamel must be removed, usually less than a millimeter. This is essential as it creates room for the porcelain veneer to fit within the mouth and most accurately restore natural tooth function while creating an even better appearance than the original tooth.

The bond between original tooth and porcelain veneer is critical as it not only provides the esthetic perfection desired, but also a strong bond which is essential for correct veneer function. Light-sensitive resin is placed between the original tooth and the veneer and then hardened using a special curing light.

Porcelain veneers are a very successful option in many situations where the original tooth has developed poor color, shape, and contours. It is also a good choice for fractured teeth, gaps between teeth, and in some situations where the tooth position is compromised and there are minor bite-related problems. For some people, superficial stains do not respond well to tooth whitening or bleaching. In these situations, a porcelain veneer may be the best option.

Minimal Prep or No-Prep Veneers

Some patients are looking for an alternative to traditional dental veneers or bonding, but be aware that this treatment option is not appropriate for everyone.

Just as with porcelain veneers, no-prep or minimal preparation veneers—so-called because they typically don't require the dentist to remove as much tooth material—are bonded to the front surface of your teeth. Often, the placement of no-prep veneers can be done more quickly and with less discomfort than traditional veneers.

Your AACD member dentist will let you know if you are a good candidate for minimal preparation or no-prep veneers and if this option makes a sensible treatment plan.

The Benefits of Veneers

Since veneers are individually sculpted for each patient, it is nearly impossible to tell the difference between a veneer and a natural tooth. Unlike natural teeth, custom-made veneers resist coffee and tea stains, and cigarette smoke because they are made of high-tech materials.

With veneers—as opposed to crowns—your natural teeth remain largely intact with only a minimal amount being altered to fit the veneer. For teeth that resist whitening, veneers can make even the darkest teeth appear bright white. Dentists may also recommend veneers to quickly fix minor twists, overlaps, and small gaps.

Potential Veneer Downsides

Because a portion of the original tooth enamel is reduced, a veneer is not considered a reversible treatment. Although adjustments and even new veneers can be made, you can never reliably return to the original condition of the tooth.

Creating porcelain veneers requires some laboratory time, so expect at least a week before they're ready to be applied.

After the porcelain veneers are attached you will probably have some sensitivity to hot and cold temperatures due to the removal of that thin layer of enamel. This typically disappears within a few days. In a healthy mouth properly treated with porcelain veneers—and where destructive forces are minimized or eliminated, a patient should be able to use porcelain veneers like his or her own teeth. Although they're very strong, veneers are also brittle. You should avoid the same excessive stresses you would avoid with non-veneered teeth: don't bite your fingernails, chew ice, or open beer bottles with your veneers.

Maintenance of a Porcelain Veneer

Maintaining porcelain veneers is actually quite simple: Treat them as you would your original teeth, with routine brushing and flossing. Using non-abrasive fluoride toothpaste will typically be suggested by your dental professional.

One week after your veneers are placed, you will be required to return to the office for a follow-up visit and evaluation so the dentist can see how your mouth is reacting to the veneers. Even if you feel the veneers are a success, this appointment is vital to your future oral health.

If you have a habit of grinding or clenching your teeth, your dentist may fit you with a nighttime bite guard so you do not damage your veneers.

You should also return to your dentist for regular professional maintenance because porcelain veneers should be polished with a specially formulated, non-abrasive paste, and because your dentist needs to inspect your dentistry for any sign of potential failure.

Section 18.2

When Should a Tooth Be Crowned, Not Filled?

When is it more appropriate to place a crown on a tooth instead of a filling?

A filling is a repair to an otherwise healthy, intact tooth. The term filling implies that the repair should be contained within the boundaries of that tooth. In other words, the filling should be surrounded by natural tooth structure insofar as it is possible. In practice, of course, dentists frequently replace large sections of teeth with large, bulky fillings. As the filling gets larger and larger, the amount of natural tooth structure necessary to retain the filling decreases. The ultimate consequence of this is that the filling becomes a rickety patchwork of artificial materials that is inherently weak and may break out at any time.

Furthermore, as the natural tooth structure becomes thinner, replaced by more filling material, it becomes more and more likely to break off, necessitating an even larger repair. The larger a filling is, the more technically difficult it is for the dentist to do, and the larger the tooth to filling interface. This means that very large fillings are likely to be unstable and to leak over time, leading to recurrent decay and replacement with even larger fillings. This process of patching or replacing already large fillings is what we call "patchwork dentistry".

In most situations, patchwork dentistry ultimately leads to the loss of the tooth, or at minimum to very expensive methods of repair. If your dentist recommends placing a crown on the tooth, he is attempting to stop this cycle of recurrent decay, breakage, and repair before it becomes necessary to do a root canal and post and core in order to have anything left above gum line to repair.

A crown is a cast metal covering, generally overlain with porcelain, which is placed over the tooth in order to hold it together and to withstand the forces of chewing. Sometimes the entire crown is made out of porcelain in order to attain the greatest esthetic (appearance) value possible. The crown may even be made entirely out of gold if that is the wish of the patient. While no dentist can guarantee that a crown will repair the tooth forever, it is still the very best restoration possible for a severely damaged tooth, and may be the only way that some severely damaged teeth can be repaired at all.

The following is a list of reasons that a crown might be more appropriate than a filling:

- A tooth should be crowned if the filling would make up more than half the bulk of the clinical crown of a tooth (that part above the gum line).

- A tooth should be crowned if the filling would make up more than half of the surface area of the clinical crown.

- A tooth should be crowned if the clinical crown is cracked or seriously mechanically weakened.

- A tooth should be crowned if the filling is very deep under the gum line since a filling under these circumstances is difficult to do and is more likely to leak. This leads to recurrent decay a year or two later.

- All back teeth with root canals should be crowned as the tooth structure tends to become brittle after the living nerve is no longer present.

- All front teeth that have root canals and also have large fillings should be crowned.

- Teeth that are unsightly (ugly) and embarrass the patient should be crowned. This is especially true in front teeth that have root canals.

- Teeth with circumferential decay (decay at the gum line that encircles more than one surface of the tooth) should be crowned in view of the near impossibility of properly repairing this type of decay with simple fillings.

- Teeth that are worn down due to attrition from bruxing (grinding and clenching) are often best crowned.

Consider Doing It

When the dentist says you need a crown, you really ought to think twice before rejecting the advice.

Even though a good dentist can repair almost any tooth with a filling, he or she may recommend a crown instead. Lots of people choose the filling anyway since it is always cheaper. This is often a bad choice. Very large fillings are technically very difficult to do. You may leave the office with what looks and feels like a tooth only to find that a year or two down the line, there is recurrent decay under the filling. It may be near impossible for the dentist to make the filling contact the tooth next to it leaving a gap which jams food between the teeth. Pieces of the tooth or the new filling may break off over time. The filling may even have required just enough removal of tooth structure to cause the nerve to die which will lead to a root canal followed by a crown, or even an extraction. These problems are not the fault of the dentist.

There is a limit to what even the best and most conscientious dentist can accomplish with a very large, difficult filling. Opting for a filling on a tooth that the dentist feels needs a crown may be opting for an extraction a year or two later.

Section 18.3

Dental Crowns

A dental crown is a tooth-shaped "cap" that is placed over a tooth. Crowns restore a tooth's shape and size, strength, and/or improve its appearance. Crowns encase the entire visible portion of a tooth—from top of tooth to the gum line.

Why is a dental crown needed?

A dental crown may be needed to:

- protect a weak tooth (from decay) from breaking or to hold together parts of a cracked tooth;

- restore an already broken tooth or a tooth that has been severely worn down;

- cover and support a tooth with a large filling when there isn't a lot of tooth left;

- hold a dental bridge in place;

- cover misshaped or severely discolored teeth;

- cover a dental implant;

- cover a tooth that has been endodontically treated (had a root canal).

What materials are used to make crowns? Is one type of material better suited for specific dental problems?

Permanent crowns can be made from all metal, porcelain-fused-to-metal, all resin, or all ceramic materials.

- **Metals** used in crowns include gold alloy, other alloys (for example, palladium) or a base-metal alloy (for example, nickel or chromium). Compared with other crown types, less tooth structure needs to be removed with metal crowns, and tooth wear to opposing teeth is kept to a minimum. Metal crowns withstand biting and chewing forces well and probably last the longest in terms of wear down. Also, they rarely chip or break. The metallic color is the main drawback. Metal crowns are a good choice for out-of-sight molars.

- **Porcelain-fused-to-metal** dental crowns can be color matched to your adjacent teeth (unlike the metallic crowns). However, more wear to the opposing teeth occurs with this crown type compared with metal or resin crowns. The crown's porcelain portion can also chip or break off. Next to all-ceramic crowns, porcelain-fused-to-metal crowns look most like normal teeth. However, sometimes the metal underlying the crown's porcelain can show through as a dark line, especially at the gum line and even more so if your gums recede. These crowns can be a good choice for front or back teeth.

- **All-resin** dental crowns are less expensive than other crown types. However, they wear down over time and are more prone to fractures than porcelain-fused-to-metal crowns.

- **All-ceramic or all-porcelain** dental crowns provide the best natural color match than any other crown type and may be more suitable for people with metal allergies. However, they are not as strong as porcelain-fused-to-metal crowns and they may wear down opposing teeth a little more than metal or resin crowns. All-ceramic crowns are a good choice for front teeth.

- **Temporary versus permanent:** Temporary crowns can be made in your dentist's office whereas permanent crowns are made in a dental laboratory. Temporary crowns are made of acrylic or stainless steel and can be used as a temporary restoration until a permanent crown is constructed by the dental laboratory.

How is a tooth prepared to receive a crown?

Today, many dentists are able to make in-office, same-day crowns. An impression (mold) is taken of the tooth needing the crown and wirelessly sent to machine located in the office. Ten to 15 minutes later the crown is ready to be cemented in place. Another advantage of this approach is that the digital impression can be sent to a lab for them to manufacture.

Labs are also offering pressable ceramic crowns. Theses crowns have a hard inner core, which replaces the metal substructure, and uses porcelain material to cap the tooth. Porcelain is a material that best matches the color of the surrounding teeth. This approach for crowning teeth is becoming more common. The pressable ceramic crown is much more durable than the porcelain jacket crown.

If my dentist is unable to make an in-office, same-day crown, what steps are taken to prepare a tooth for a crown?

The more traditional method to prepare a tooth for a crown usually required two dentist visits.

First Visit: Examining and Preparing the Tooth

At the first visit:

1. The tooth is examined and prepared. X-rays may be taken to check the roots of the tooth receiving the crown and the surrounding bone. If the tooth has extensive decay or if there is a risk of infection or injury to the tooth's pulp (the center core of the tooth, which contains blood vessels and nerves), a root canal may be performed first.

2. Next, your dentist will anesthetize (numb) your tooth and the gum tissue around the tooth. The tooth receiving the crown is

filed down along the chewing surface and sides to make room for the crown. The amount removed depends on the type of crown used. For instance, all-metal crowns are thinner, requiring less tooth structure removal than all-porcelain or porcelain-fused-to-metal ones). If, on the other hand, a large area of the tooth is missing (due to decay or damage), filling material is used to build up the tooth to support the crown.

3. After reshaping the tooth, an impression of the tooth to receive the crown is made. Impressions of the teeth above and below the tooth to receive the dental crown will also be made. This is done to make sure that the crown will not affect your bite.

4. The impressions are sent to a dental laboratory where the crown is actually made. The crown is usually returned to your dentist's office in 2–3 weeks. If your crown is made of porcelain, your dentist will also select the shade that most closely matches the color of the neighboring teeth.

5. Your dentist will make a temporary crown to cover and protect the prepared tooth while the crown is being made. Temporary crowns are usually made of acrylic and are held in place using temporary cement.

Second Visit: Receiving the Permanent Dental Crown

At your second visit, your dentist will remove your temporary crown and check the fit and color of the permanent crown. If everything is acceptable, a local anesthetic may be given to numb the tooth and the new crown is permanently cemented in place.

How should I care for my temporary dental crown?

Because temporary dental crowns are just that—a temporary fix until a permanent crown is ready, most dentists would recommend the following:

*   Avoid sticky, chewy foods (for example, chewing gum, caramel) which have the potential of grabbing and pulling off the crown.

*   Minimize use of the side of your mouth with the temporary crown. Shift the bulk of your chewing to the other side of your mouth.

*   Avoid chewing hard foods (such as raw vegetables) which could dislodge or break the crown.

- Slide flossing material out—rather than lifting out—when cleaning your teeth. Lifting the floss out, as you normally would, might pull off the temporary crown.

What problems could develop with a dental crown?

Discomfort or sensitivity: Your newly crowned tooth may be sensitive immediately after the procedure as the anesthesia begins to wear off. If the tooth that has been crowned and still has a nerve in it, you may experience some heat and cold sensitivity. Your dentist may recommend that you brush your teeth with toothpaste designed for sensitive teeth. Pain or sensitivity that occurs when you bite down usually means that the crown is too high on the tooth. If this is the case, call your dentist. He or she can easily fix this problem.

Chipped crown: Crowns made of all porcelain can sometimes chip. If the chip is small, a composite resin can be used to repair the chip with the crown remaining in your mouth. If the chipping is extensive, the crown may need to be replaced.

Loose crown: Sometimes the cement washes out from under the crown. Not only does this allow the crown to become loose, it allows bacteria to leak in and cause decay to the tooth that remains. If your crown feels loose, contact your dentist's office.

Crown falls off: Sometimes crowns fall off. Usually this is due to an improper fit or a lack of cement. If this happens, contact your dentist's office immediately. He or she will give you specific instructions on how to care for your tooth and crown until you can be seen for an evaluation. Your dentist may be able to re-cement your crown in place; if not, a new crown will need to be made.

Allergic reaction: Because the metals used to make crowns are usually a mixture of metals, an allergic reaction to the metals or porcelain used in crowns can occur, but this is extremely rare.

Dark line on crowned tooth next to the gum line: A dark line next to the gum line of your crowned tooth is normal, particularly if you have a porcelain-fused-to-metal crown. This dark line is simply the metal of the crown showing through.

What are onlays and 3/4 crowns?

These are variations on the technique of dental crowns. The difference between these crowns and the crowns discussed previously is their coverage of the underlying tooth—the traditional crown covers the entire tooth; onlays and 3/4 crowns cover the underlying tooth to a lesser extent.

How long do dental crowns last?

On average, dental crowns last between five and fifteen years. The life span of a crown depends on the amount of wear and tear the crown is exposed to, how well you follow good oral hygiene practices, and your personal mouth-related habits (you should avoid such habits as grinding or clenching your teeth, chewing ice, biting your fingernails, and using your teeth to open packaging).

Does a crowned tooth require any special care?

While a crowned tooth does not require any special care, remember that simply because a tooth is crowned does not mean the underlying tooth is protected from decay or gum disease. Therefore, continue to follow good oral hygiene practices, including brushing your teeth at least twice a day and flossing once a day—especially around the crown area where the gum meets the tooth. I would also avoid knowingly biting on hard surfaces with porcelain crowns (like chewing ice and popcorn hulls, to prevent porcelain fracture)

How much do crowns cost?

Costs vary depending on what part of the country you live in and on the type of crown selected (for example, porcelain crowns are typically more expensive than gold crowns, which are typically more expensive than porcelain-fused-to-metal crowns). Generally, crowns can range in cost from $800 to $1,500. The cost of crowns is not generally fully covered by insurance. To be certain, check with your specific dental insurance company.

Chapter 19

Having a Tooth Pulled

Chapter Contents

Section 19.1

Facts about Extraction

"What's Involved in Getting a Tooth Pulled?" reprinted with permission from www.dental-health-advice.com. © 2011 Dr. Richard Mitchell, BDS.

What's involved in getting a tooth pulled?

Getting a tooth pulled is a big decision. The two main reasons why you might need to get a tooth pulled are either toothache, or to make some room for braces. If you are thinking about having a tooth out because of toothache, remember that the tooth does not grow back afterwards, and you will have a gap. It is always possible to get a replacement tooth, such as a bridge or an implant, but these options are never as good as the real thing. Also, they will involve additional expense. So, do not make the decision about getting a tooth pulled quickly or lightly.

If your dentist has told you that you need to get a tooth removed, you are probably wondering what is going to happen, what will it be like, and how sore will it be afterwards.

A tooth can cause you pain for the following reasons:

- Wisdom tooth—where there's no room for it to grow properly
- Infected tooth—and you don't want root canal or the dentist has said it isn't possible
- Cracked or broken tooth—where the tooth is broken beyond repair
- Gum disease—you have a loose tooth

In these situations, the only option is to get the tooth out.

Orthodontics (Braces): If the dentist needs to make some space to straighten your teeth with braces, and a tooth needs to be removed to make that space, the dentist will look to see if there is a tooth with a big filling or some other problem. If you only need to have a tooth out to make room for braces, it obviously makes sense to take out a weak or chipped tooth, rather than one that's completely healthy.

What is the procedure?

The first thing is to get the tooth really numb. First a small amount of anesthetic gel is put on the gum next to the tooth. This should stay in place for 3–5 minutes, and will numb the gum before the shot. After the gel has been in place long enough, the dentist should slowly numb the tooth.

Two important points about dental anesthesia are that: First, the injection should be given very slowly, and then you should get at least one additional injection after the first one has started to work. Second, you need to wait a full ten minutes after that for the anesthetic to really take effect.

Once the tooth is numb, it is time to start. Unless the tooth is really loose, it cannot just be grabbed and yanked out. The dentist will be much more careful than that. So, the best way to remove the tooth is to slowly and gently wiggle it from side to side. It is very similar to how you pulled out your own baby teeth. As the dentist slowly moves the tooth from side to side, you will feel quite a lot of pressure building up. In fact, the pressure on the tooth is what most people notice most. If the tooth is in your lower jaw, and you jaw joint starts to get tired, the dentist can give you a small rubber block to bite on. This lets your strongest jaw muscles work against the pressure, and hold your jaw joint in place so that it does not get tired.

After a few minutes, the tooth will start to become loose. But still, the dentist has to go slowly. He wants to avoid breaking any bits if possible. As the tooth becomes looser, you will feel the pressure easing off.

Finally, the dentist can gently lift the tooth out of its socket. Job done. At this stage, your jaw muscles will be feeling quite tired, and you will be glad to relax. The dentist will put a small piece of gauze over the socket in the gum, and get you to bite down gently to hold the gauze in place.

After about five minutes or so, the gum should have settled enough for you to leave the office. It is best to take it easy for the rest of the day— no sports or exercise. General advice for the first 48 hours after getting a tooth pulled usually includes not smoking and not rinsing your mouth vigorously—only very gently bathing the area with hot salty water, but not swishing it around forcefully.

The best painkillers at this stage are probably ibuprofen (sold under the name Advil) or acetaminophen (Tylenol). You should avoid taking any aspirin at all, as this can stop the gum socket from clotting properly. If you have any questions after getting a tooth pulled, telephone the dentist's office. It is always better to check and be sure if something does not seem right.

Section 19.2

Impacted Teeth

An impacted tooth is a tooth that fails to fully pass through the gums.

Causes

Teeth start to pass through the gums (emerge) during infancy, and again when the primary (baby) teeth are replaced by the permanent teeth. If a tooth fails to emerge, or emerges only partially, it is considered to be impacted. The most common teeth to become impacted are the wisdom teeth (the third set of molars). They are the last teeth to emerge, usually between the ages of 17 and 21.

An impacted tooth remains stuck in gum tissue or bone for various reasons. It may be that the area is just overcrowded and there's no room for the teeth to emerge. For example, the jaw may be too small to fit the wisdom teeth. Teeth may also become twisted, tilted, or displaced as they try to emerge, resulting in impacted teeth.

Impacted wisdom teeth are very common. They are often painless and cause no apparent trouble. However, some professionals believe an impacted tooth pushes on the next tooth, which pushes the next tooth, eventually causing a misalignment of the bite. A partially emerged tooth can trap food, plaque, and other debris in the soft tissue around it, leading to inflammation and tenderness of the gums and unpleasant mouth odor. This is called pericoronitis.

Symptoms

- Bad breath
- Difficulty opening the mouth (occasionally)
- Pain or tenderness of the gums (gingiva) or jaw bone
- Prolonged headache or jaw ache
- Redness and swelling of the gums around the impacted tooth

- Swollen lymph nodes of the neck (occasionally)
- Unpleasant taste when biting down on or near the area
- Visible gap where a tooth did not emerge

Exams and Tests

Your dentist will look for swollen tissue over the area where a tooth has not emerged, or has only partially emerged. The impacted tooth may be pressing on nearby teeth. The gums around the area may show signs of infection such as redness, drainage, and tenderness. As gums swell over impacted wisdom teeth and then drain and tighten, it may feel like the tooth came in and then went back down again. Dental x-rays confirm the presence of one or more teeth that have not emerged.

Treatment

No treatment may be needed if the impacted tooth is not causing any problems.

Over-the-counter pain relievers may help if the impacted tooth causes discomfort. Warm salt water (one-half teaspoon of salt in one cup of water) or over-the-counter mouthwashes may be soothing to the gums.

Removal of the tooth (extraction) is the usual treatment for an impacted tooth. This is usually done in the dentist's office, but difficult cases may require an oral surgeon. Antibiotics may be prescribed before the extraction if the tooth is infected.

Outlook (Prognosis)

Impacted teeth may cause no problems for some people and may never require treatment. Treatment is usually successful when it does cause symptoms.

It is often preferable to have wisdom teeth removed before age 30 due to the flexibility of bone, which will allow an easier removal and better healing. As a person ages, the bone becomes more rigid and complications can develop.

Possible Complications

Complications of an impacted tooth include:

- abscess of the tooth or gums,
- chronic discomfort in the mouth,

- infection,

- malocclusion of the teeth,

- plaque trapped between teeth and gums.

When to Contact a Medical Professional

Call your dentist if there is an impacted tooth (or partially emerged tooth) and pain in the gums or other symptoms have developed.

Chapter 20

Dentures

Chapter Contents

Section 20.1

Types of Dentures

There are five different types of full dentures:

- Standard dentures

- Immediate dentures

- Overdentures

- Implant retained dentures

- Transitional dentures like Cu-Sil partial dentures

The Standard Denture

The back of a standard denture ends just behind the hard bone in the roof of the mouth. Dentures do this because they require as much surface area as possible to maximize retention and stability. In the case of people who gag, the back of the denture can be cut forward making the denture base look more and more like an arch. However, the more it is cut back, the less stable and retentive it will be.

Standard dentures are made for people who are already missing all their teeth. The top denture relies on "suction" to retain it, and the hardness of the underlying tissues for its stability. It generally takes four or sometimes more appointments to make a set of standard dentures.

The first appointment consists of an oral examination, sometimes x-rays, and a set of impressions of the upper and lower edentulous (toothless) ridges (gums). These impressions are poured with plaster to form accurate models of the shape of the edentulous ridges. Other parameters are determined such as the shade, size, and shape of the teeth that will be placed on the new dentures.

Upon occasion, the dentist will recommend surgical alteration of the ridges to remove flabby tissue which will interfere with the stability of the denture, and sometimes to alter the shape of the underlying bone allowing for a better fit. In most cases, such surgery is not essential, but can create the conditions for a much more satisfactory final denture. Alterations like this are generally money well spent.

In some offices, the first set of impressions are used to make custom fitting impression trays for a second, more accurate impression. In this case, there will be one extra appointment in addition to the standard four.

The second appointment consists of deciding how "long" to make the teeth, determining the plane of the tooth setup (when you smile, the teeth should be parallel to a line between the pupils of your eyes), and the correct relationship of the upper and lower teeth so that when you bite together, the upper and lower teeth line up correctly. This is done using a loose fitting denture base and a rim of wax to approximate the position of the teeth. This appointment is often called the CJR (central jaw relation), or the MMR (maximum mandibular retrusion) to denote the relationship of the upper and lower jaws.

Both upper and lower wax rims are adjusted to fit correctly in the patient's mouth so he can speak correctly without the wax rims "clicking" together, and so that the upper and lower rims fit together evenly. Ideally, the wax rim should be visible slightly below the patient's lip when the lip is at rest. When the patient smiles, the position of the lip is marked in the wax to help the lab decide which set of teeth are appropriate for this patient. Once these relationships are correct, the rims are sent to the lab where they are used to fabricate the wax-try-in.

The third appointment is called the "wax try-in." The lab returns the loosely fitting tray from the second appointment with the actual final plastic teeth lined up along the outer edge of the wax rim. The wax try-in looks just like a real denture, except that the base fits loosely on the gums, and the teeth are embedded in wax instead of plastic.

This gives the dentist an opportunity to see how the denture looks and works before we are committed to the setup. At this point, if something is wrong, it can be changed. If the teeth look too long, or the patient clicks when talking, or the midline is wrong, we can send the denture back to the lab where a technician can melt the wax and reset the teeth to specification.

The denture is tried as many times as necessary until the teeth look and function well. What you see is what you get. When everything is perfect, the denture is sent back to the lab to be processed and finished. The old loose-fitting base and all the wax are discarded, and replaced by a tightly fitting plastic denture base.

The fourth appointment is the insertion date when the patient walks out of the office with new dentures. The plastic tends to shrink while being processed, so some adjustment is usually necessary before they will get the suction that you might associate with a new denture.

Immediate Dentures

Immediate dentures (sometimes called temporary dentures) are actually made before the natural teeth are extracted. The patient walks into the office with natural teeth, and walks out with false teeth. The teeth are extracted, and a prefabricated denture is inserted directly over the bleeding sockets. The patient is still numb from the extractions, and nothing hurts until he or she gets home. Generally, most patients do not complain of much pain after their teeth are extracted and the immediate denture is inserted. The denture acts like a band aid and reduces pain.

The construction of an immediate denture requires only one or two preliminary appointments before the insertion date, depending on how many natural teeth the patient has left. They usually work out reasonably well. When the patient leaves, he looks much better than when he walked into the office. The bone that supported the original teeth is still intact, and the gum tissue is firm. For the first week or so, the denture remains stable and reasonably retained.

In a majority of cases, immediate dentures become permanent dentures, but there are a number of problems associated with immediate dentures than may cause the patient to want new dentures made after their gums have healed, in about a year. These problems account for the alternate name; temporary dentures:

1. If the patient has more than one or two remaining front top teeth, it is usually impossible to do a wax try in. The denture teeth are placed in about the same position as the natural teeth before extraction. Even though the denture teeth will be straight, and clean, their position may not be ideal because there is no way to preview them as with a standard denture. For this reason, not everyone will be happy with the final appearance of their immediate denture, and may wish to invest in a new one at the end of about a year when most of the healing has taken place.

2. After the natural teeth are extracted and the immediate denture is inserted, there is a relatively fast loss of the bone that

used to hold the natural teeth in place. By the end of three weeks, enough bone has been lost that there is a lot of space between parts of the denture and the healing gums. This leads to rapidly increasing looseness and sore spots which must be removed frequently. In some offices, the dentist will include a free temporary "soft" reline at about one month after the extraction/insertion date. This is a simple way to tighten the denture against the gums, and since the material is a bit rubbery, and frequently medicated, it makes the denture much more comfortable until enough healing has taken place to do a permanent "hard" reline (at additional charge).

3.   At the end of four to six months, the immediate denture must be relined with the same acrylic that the denture base was made from originally. The longer you wait, (no more than six months), the longer you can expect the denture to remain tight before another reline is needed. The hard reline is a separate procedure and the cost is not generally included in the original price of the immediate denture. Thus the immediate denture ends up costing a bit more than the standard denture when the cost of the reline is taken into account. The hard reline marks the official transition of the immediate denture into a standard denture.

Cu-Sil Transitional Dentures

There are a number of drawbacks associated with full dentures, and not everyone can successfully wear them. In many instances, false teeth are not especially useful because of retention or stability problems. For this reason, even a single healthy tooth left in place can stabilize an otherwise unstable full denture.

Only recently has it become possible to build a denture leaving a hole here and there to allow a few remaining teeth to poke through without ruining the suction which generally holds the denture in the mouth. The Cu-Sil partial denture has holes for natural teeth. These holes are surrounded by a gasket of stable silicone rubber which hugs the natural teeth and allows the rest of the denture to rest against the gums giving the benefit of suction in addition to the mechanical stability offered by the immobility of the natural teeth. These are especially useful in situations in which the remaining teeth are on the same side or area of the arch. Even a single remaining tooth in the arch can increase the stability of the entire denture several hundred percent over a completely edentulous (no teeth) arch.

Cu-Sil partial dentures are not the best solution for people with numerous, evenly distributed, stable natural teeth. They are advertised mostly as transitional dentures meaning that they are especially recommended when the remaining teeth are likely to be lost (eventually) for any reason, or in cases where stable teeth are poorly distributed about the dental arch. A Cu-Sil partial denture can stabilize loose teeth and, with care, can extend their lives. It is also easy to replace lost natural teeth on the Cu-Sil denture, and the denture can be relined like any other standard denture. In other words, the Cu-Sil denture can eventually be transformed into a regular full denture if the patient loses all the natural teeth. This author has found them to be especially useful for upper dentures, but more of a problem for lowers. Lower Cu-Sil partial dentures are prone to breakage if the patient is a heavy bruxer (grinder), especially if the remaining natural teeth are located in the front of the arch. This is because the holes that allow the penetration of the natural teeth weaken the architecture of a lower denture.

An additional problem with Cu-Sil partial dentures is a longer wait to get them relined. Most dentists work with a local lab which can return a relined standard denture within 6–8 hours. Unfortunately, since Cu-Sil is generally offered in specialty labs, the wait to get one back can be as much as a week.

If there are many stable natural teeth remaining, and they are distributed on both sides of the arch with some in front and some in back to lend support, a partial denture may be as good or even better solution. Partial dentures have the added advantage of not having to cover the entire roof of the mouth.

Note: If you wish to find a dentist who will make you a Cu-Sil partial denture, you may be able to get a referral from one of the 125 dental laboratories throughout the U.S. and Canada who make them. In order to find a dental lab that has experience with this product, you may try to contact the manufacturer of the resins:

Present Investment Corporation

700 W. Hillsboro Blvd., Suite 2-206
Deerfield Beach, FL 33441
Phone: 954-426-4666
Fax: 954-427-8535
Website: http://www.cu-sil.com
E-mail: info@cu-sil.com

Overdentures

Overdentures are defined as any removable tooth replacement device that is inserted over existing teeth or their remnants, replacing these teeth with false teeth. Prior to modern dentistry, overdentures were very nearly the universal tooth replacement device since surgical removal of teeth was painful, dangerous, and frequently impossible without modern anesthetics. In those days, dentures were made to fit over the rotting stumps of decayed or broken teeth.

Today, non-restorable teeth are generally removed prior to the placement of a removable prosthesis; however, there are still instances where these teeth can be maintained to the patient's advantage. The most frequently seen overdenture today involves teeth that have had root canal therapy. If the roots of these teeth are still serviceable, the crown may be cut off at gum line and a removable appliance may be placed over the stumps. Sometimes, the stumps are themselves covered with filling material or cast metal copings in order to protect them from decay. The advantage to this is that the roots of these teeth can maintain the bone that supports them. This bone would otherwise resorb away leaving less tissue to support the denture. In addition, the root itself can serve as a rest, or a vertical support for the denture allowing for more stability than would otherwise be available.

The addition of a soft denture material such as Cu-Sil on the denture surface that immediately overlies the rigid root stumps allows the overdenture to nestle more snugly into the soft tissue on the roof of the mouth. This allows for more suction to develop and can frequently improve the retention of an overdenture.

Implant Retained Dentures

Implants are quite expensive (generally about $2000 apiece, not counting the tooth replacement that goes on top of them), but quite effective in retaining an otherwise non-retentive denture. A titanium "screw" is actually placed into a hole drilled into the bone to approximate the position of teeth. After several months, the titanium has integrated (attached) into the bone, and the implant is then uncovered and a post which pokes through the gums into the mouth is attached to the implant. This post may support a porcelain tooth, or it may support an attachment for a denture. If the patient has no teeth at all in any given arch (upper or lower), a full mouth of individual implants, attached to porcelain teeth and bridges, could cost about what an expensive automobile costs.

On the other hand, a minimum of two implants can maintain a lower denture which would not otherwise be tolerated by that patient. More than two implants are needed for upper implant retained dentures. Although the dentures that fit over implants are considerably more expensive than standard dentures, they offer the added advantage of allowing upper dentures to be built in the shape of an arch instead of having to cover the entire palate. This is of special significance to people who otherwise cannot wear full dentures because they make them gag.

Implant retained dentures have special significance for people who cannot wear lower dentures. As an edentulous (toothless) person ages, and the bone continues to resorb away, lower ridges frequently disappear entirely. Thus there is no vertical bone underlying the gums to stabilize a lower denture. These people frequently cannot wear a lower denture at all. The addition of two implants in the front of the lower jaw can make it possible to retain a lower denture which would otherwise be impossible for the patient to tolerate.

Mini Implant Retained Dentures

Since their introduction in the late 1990s, mini implants are beginning to become the standard of care for retaining lower dentures. Unlike the standard implants discussed previously, there is no three to six month waiting period before mini implants can be loaded (support the denture). Mini implants can generally be placed in the lower jaw without cutting an incision in the gums. The only anesthesia used is an injection directly over the site of each implant. The old lower denture can then be retrofitted directly over the newly placed implants, and the patient can use the denture immediately. Furthermore, because the implants are about the size of a standard wooden toothpick (they are made out of a titanium alloy), patients who have been told that there is not enough bone to accommodate standard implants can generally be fitted with minis. The entire procedure (placing the implants and retrofitting the old denture so that it is supported by the newly placed minis) takes about one hour. It is generally painless, and produces very minimal postoperative discomfort. Finally, due to the ease of insertion, this procedure is much less expensive than standard implants for retaining lower dentures.

Duplicate Dentures

When a new full denture is first made, it is possible to make a duplicate, or an exact copy of the denture cheaply and quickly. This is a "quick and dirty" method of obtaining a second denture for emergencies.

Duplicate dentures are made by flowing liquid "agar" around the finished denture and allowing it to harden. (Agar is a gelatin-like material made from seaweed which is liquid when hot, but cools to form a flexible rubbery substance similar to very dense gelatin. When agar is used in dentistry, it is generally called "reversible hydrocolloid." It is one of the oldest, but still one of the most accurate impression materials known.) The original denture is removed from the agar mold (the agar is cast around the denture in two halves) leaving a hole in the agar where the denture used to be. The hole is then filled with liquid plastic; white plastic in the tooth indents and pink to form the base and flanges. The two halves of the agar form are placed back together and the liquid plastic is allowed to harden. Duplicate dentures are not especially high quality since the flowable plastic used to make them tends to be porous and less resistant to wear, and the delineation between the tooth colored plastic in the tooth indents and the pink base plastic may not always be exactly at the margins of the teeth, but these dentures make it possible to keep a spare set of dentures tucked away just in case the regular denture must be sent out for repair, or is lost and a new denture must be made. They are frequently delivered to the patient without adjusting them for sore spots or any other technical modifications to make them more affordable. Duplicate dentures are only an adjunctive service and are not intended to take the place of the real thing. Adjustments cost money, and if the dentist were to spend as much time and effort on them as he did on the primary service, the duplicate could end up costing as much as the primary full denture.

Section 20.2

Partial Dentures

If you are missing only a few teeth scattered over either arch (upper or lower teeth), or even if you have a minimum of two teeth on both sides of the arch, then you can most inexpensively replace the missing teeth with a removable partial denture (RPD). There are several types of RPDs. All of them use standard plastic denture teeth as replacements for the missing natural teeth. The differences between them are the materials that are used to support the denture teeth and retain the RPD in the mouth.

Treatment RPD (Flippers)

Affectionately known in dentistry as a flipper, this is the least expensive of all the removable partial dentures. Two of the natural teeth are clasped with wrought wire clasps which are cured into the structure of the denture base.

The pink plastic of the denture base is brittle acrylic, the same material used to make standard full dentures. The largest single advantage to this type of RPD (aside from the cost) is that new teeth and new denture base can easily be added to an existing treatment RPD. These are frequently fabricated even if the remaining teeth have existing decay or periodontal disease and their prognosis is doubtful. If later in the course of treatment some of the existing natural teeth are extracted for any reason, new false teeth can be added quickly to the partial, maintaining the patient's appearance. In spite of the fact that they are considered a temporary solution, many people keep this type of appliance for many, many years, because as long as they are properly maintained, they look outwardly as good as the more expensive permanent appliances described later.

One of the neatest tricks that a flipper can do is to act as an immediate partial denture. This means that the appliance can be made before the teeth are removed, and inserted immediately after the extraction of the offending teeth. If the patient is presently wearing one of these inexpensive appliances, and needs to have an existing natural tooth extracted, an impression can be taken with the flipper in place. The impression with the flipper embedded in it is sent to the lab and a new denture tooth put in place of the one to be extracted. This can be done in the course of a single day, so a patient can come in with a bad tooth and walk out with a good false tooth in its position.

Flippers do have a number of disadvantages, however:

- The acrylic denture base is somewhat brittle, and due to their irregular shape, these partials tend to break frequently, especially those made for the lower arch. (Full dentures are more regular in shape and tend to be fairly strong as a result.)

- In order to counteract their tendency to break, the acrylic is usually built fairly thick which can take some getting used to.

- The denture base rests only on the gums, and even though they are much more stable than full dentures, they are much less stable than the more permanent RPDs which are "tooth born."

- As the gums resorb, the false teeth tend to sink below their original level making it necessary to reline them frequently, and sometimes even to reset the teeth which adds to their expense.

- Flippers are most frequently retained with wire clasps. These are frequently unsightly due to the limitations that pertain to their placement (they can't interfere with the way you bite).

Cast Metal Removable Partial Dentures (RPD)

Removable partial dentures with cast metal frameworks are probably one of the oldest forms of dentistry. Originally, the frameworks were made out of wrought (hammered) silver. One of the most famous American dentists was Paul Revere who was a silversmith when he wasn't fighting redcoats.

This type of partial denture offers numerous advantages over the treatment RPD described earlier. Since they sit on the teeth, as well as being attached to them, they are extremely stable and retentive. The teeth have been altered slightly beforehand in order that the partial denture can rest upon them without interfering with the way the patient bites the teeth together.

The metal framework does not contact the gums. Thus, as the gums resorb, this type of partial does not sink with them and rarely requires relines. Because the teeth are altered by the dentist beforehand, there are fewer limitations in the placement of clasps, and they are less likely to be seen than the wrought wire clasps of the treatment partial. Modern frameworks are cast from an extremely strong alloy called chrome cobalt which can be cast very thin and are much less likely to break than the all plastic variety. They are also much less noticeable to the tongue.

The largest single advantage that cast metal framework partial dentures have over the newer flexible framework partials (covered later) is that sore spots are almost never an issue since neither the framework, nor the plastic extensions contact the soft oral tissues with any force. Patients who exhibit the symptoms of TMJ, or who are known bruxers are much better off with cast metal partials than with flexible framework partials.

Flexible Framework RPDs

The most recent advance in dental materials has been the application of nylon-like materials to the fabrication of dental appliances. Nylon generally replaces the metal, and the pink acrylic denture material used to build the framework for standard removable partial dentures. Nylon is similar to the material used to build those fluorescent orange traffic cones you sometimes see on highways. It is nearly unbreakable, is colored pink like the gums, can be built quite thin, and can form not only the denture base, but the clasps as well. Since the clasps are built to curl around the necks of the teeth, they are practically indistinguishable from the gums that normally surround the teeth. Brands of this type are: Luciton FRS, Sunflex, TCS, Duraflex, Valplast, and Flexstar.

A second type of flexible partial denture base uses a vinyl composite instead of nylon. The most commonly sold brand is Flexite. A second brand is Ultraflex. These materials are also flexible and can be built with tooth or gum colored clasps. Ultraflex even comes in a clear variety. Unlike nylon partial dentures, they are much easier for the dentist to adjust making them a much more user friendly denture base.

Even though this type of denture does not rest on the natural teeth like the metal framework variety, the clasps rest on the gums surrounding the natural teeth. This tissue, unlike the gums over extraction sites, is stable and changes very little over time which keeps these RPDs stable and unchanging similar to the cast metal variety. This type of partial denture is extremely stable and retentive, and the elasticity of the flexible plastic clasps keeps them that way indefinitely.

A good alternative to the all-nylon partial denture is one made with a combination cast metal framework with nylon clasps. This has the advantage of being tooth supported (like the cast metal framework partial denture discussed previously) and also having gum colored plastic clasps like the nylon partial.

This combination of metal framework and plastic clasp eliminates most of the difficulty of recurrent sore spots, since the framework resists movement and pressure from the clasps, while having the benefit of nearly invisible clasps.

Nesbit RPD

The flexible framework RPD can replace any number of teeth in a dental arch, similar to the flipper and cast metal RPD. There is, however, one type of removable tooth replacement device that can (legally) be built only out of the flexible framework variety of material. This is the single tooth RPD that we refer to as a Nesbit.

Dentists used to build Nesbits for their patients all the time. They were composed of a single denture tooth (usually a back tooth) between two cast metal clasps which attached onto the teeth on either side of the missing one. They looked a little like spiders when out of the mouth. Patients tended to like them, but they came to an abrupt end in the 1970s. Prior to that time, in the rare event that a patient swallowed his appliance, he either waited for it to pass, or sought medical help on his own assuming that the accident was his own fault. In rare instances, the metal clasps were sharp enough to cause damage to the digestive system. After that time, tort lawyers discovered that it was a potential law suit, and it didn't take the dental profession long to abandon this service.

The design of the new flexible plastic framework takes the danger out of an accidental swallowing of the appliance. In the event that someone did swallow one, it is unlikely that any damage could be done to the lining of the digestive system.

Cu-Sil Partial Denture

Full dentures tend to be unstable and difficult to retain in the mouth. However, even the presence of a single remaining tooth in an arch can make the denture much more stable and retentive. A new kind of appliance is now available to allow a patient to retain one or more teeth and still wear a full denture. A Cu-Sil partial denture is essentially a full denture with holes allowing the remaining natural teeth to protrude through. Normally, the key to retaining a full denture is the suction that is obtained by fitting the plastic closely to the gum tissue, but a hole allowing a tooth to protrude through would ordinarily break the suction. The Cu-Sil partial denture is unique because the holes that surround the natural teeth are lined with a Silicone rubber gasket which snugly holds the teeth while allowing a natural suction to form under the denture.

Section 20.3

Information about Denture Care

"Dentures: A New Smile in Days, and Important Information about Denture Care," reprinted with permission from www.dental -health-advice.com. © 2011 Dr. Richard Mitchell, BDS.

You can get new dentures made up really quickly, if you need a new smile for an important occasion. There are a few things you should know about dentures before you choose the express route. Knowing about correct denture care will make sure that your investment lasts as long as possible and an ultrasonic denture cleaner is essential to keeping your dentures hygienically clean. But first, take a look at what you can expect with dentures in general.

Good dentures can sometimes be surprisingly difficult for a dentist to make. A lot depends on the attitude and expectations of the denture wearer. If you are expecting a new set of denture teeth to be just like your natural teeth, you are probably going to be disappointed. If you had lost the lower part of one of your legs, you wouldn't expect to be able to play basketball as well as you could before, even with the best artificial leg. The same thing applies to dentures. You only have about one-third of the bite force that you had with natural teeth. There are two sayings that stick in my mind from dental school:

- "Dentures are not an alternative for natural teeth. They are an alternative to not having any teeth at all."

- "You wouldn't expect to be able to see with a glass eye. You can't expect to be able to chew steak with dentures."

While these phrases sound cute, there is an underlying truth behind them. Dentures can never be as good as the real thing. But, as an alternative to no teeth at all, they can be pretty good.

If you are looking for the best dentures possible, you will need to think about some dental implants to support your denture. Implant-supported dentures are rock-solid. But there are several other advantages, too.

One Day Dentures

One thing a lot of patients ask about is how quickly a new set of dentures can be made. They have seen some advertisements for one-day dentures or "new dentures–a new smile." It may be difficult to imagine how it would be possible for a dentist to make a set of dentures from scratch in a single day. However, the phrase "one day dentures" can have two meanings. The first one means what it says; you get your dentures within 24 hours of walking into the dentists' office.

The second meaning is where you still have some natural teeth left, but want them taken out and full dentures put in. The dentures are made in the usual way, but you only get your remaining teeth out when the dentures are ready to be fitted. So you never have to walk around with no teeth at all. This type of "denture in a day" is usually called an "immediate denture" by dentists, because it is put in immediately after the teeth are removed. An advantage is that the dentures protect the gums where you had the teeth out, preventing bits of food getting in. The gums tend to heal up more quickly.

However, one disadvantage with immediate dentures is that the gums will shrink pretty quickly in the first month or so, as they heal up. This means the denture won't fit as well, and will need to be relined. Initially, it is possible to do this yourself with denture reline kits. After 3–6 months, though, you will really need to have the denture relined professionally by a dentist, to get a long-lasting good fit.

One denture that is quite a bit different from full dentures is the dental flipper. This is for replacing just one or two teeth, and is quite small. It is usually regarded as being a temporary or interim solution for a missing tooth, especially while an implant is healing up, but sometimes it can be satisfactory for some years.

An important consideration for any type of denture will be denture prices. The cost of dentures can vary greatly. At one extreme, there are dental groups such as Affordable Dentures in the U.S.A. who can make inexpensive dentures that are great value for the money. One other option may be to do a little of the work yourself at home. Such information is available online by researching the topic "make your own dentures." At the other extreme, some dentists charge $10,000 for a full set of false teeth.

Why Is There Such a Huge Range of Prices?

It is a bit like buying a car. If you think about a Ford, a Cadillac, and a Mercedes, all of them have four wheels, four seats, and an engine. And all of them will get you from place A to B. The difference is how they get you from there.

- How comfortably?
- How efficiently?
- How reliably?
- How long do they last?

Thinking about full dentures in that way, the big range in price becomes more understandable. The inexpensive dentures will fit reasonably well at first, work well enough, and look okay, but they will be more liable to crack or break, and they will wear down more quickly. However, they will do their job well enough to start with. More expensive dentures should have a better fit, should look natural, work well when you are chewing, be resistant to cracking or breaking, and of course last longer.

Does Lasting Longer Really Matter?

Bearing in mind that your gums are continually changing shape and gradually shrinking, you might wonder how long dentures need to last before they are replaced? That is a good point. For most folks, you should consider getting new dentures every five to seven years. Of course, it depends on how your gums change, and if the dentures are still fitting and working properly. Many dentures still fit well, look good, and show minimal signs of wear at ten or twelve years. So there is no hard-and-fast rule.

Dental Adhesive

Whatever type of denture you have, it may not stay in place quite as well as you would like. Even with the best quality dentures, sometimes the shape of your gums will not give the denture enough grip. It moves around when you try to chew certain foods.

This is where a very thin application of a good quality denture adhesive will make a big difference. These gels and pastes are not just for badly-fitting and old dentures. They actually work even better with newer, well-fitting teeth. The best denture adhesive is a matter of personal preference. You may need to try a few different ones to make up your own mind.

One problem that concerned patients was a possible link between denture adhesives and zinc poisoning. This turned out to affect some people who were using about two or three tubes of adhesive per week, instead of the recommended amount where a single tube should last about eight weeks. Essentially, their dentures fitted so badly that they had to use great wads of the gel to fill in the huge gaps under the denture. The correct solution would have been to get a new set of teeth.

What about Denture Care?

Keeping your dentures clean is very important. You must prevent a build-up of bacteria on the denture surface. Here is a guide to cleaning dentures.

- One mistake a lot of denture wearers make is using a normal toothbrush and normal toothpaste. Normal toothpaste is much too abrasive for dentures. Toothpastes are designed to clean and polish tooth enamel, which is extremely hard. The acrylic used in dentures, even the most expensive, is nowhere near as hard as tooth enamel. Using a normal toothpaste on your dentures will gradually dull the denture surface, leaving microscopic scratches all over the acrylic. This actually makes it easier for bacteria to collect on the denture.

- A great addition for cleaning dentures is an ultrasonic denture cleaner. These clean the whole denture, inside and out, using ultrasonic waves in a small bath. Ultrasonic denture cleaners are great at shifting any tiny deposits in the nooks and crannies of a denture. However, the denture has to be reasonably clean before it goes in the bath. You still need to give it a good brushing to remove any food debris and plaque. Then the ultrasonic cleaner will do the rest.

Dentures can sometimes cause problems, the main one being discomfort or irritation of one sort or another. Dentures may not be a perfect answer to replacing lost teeth, but they can serve very well. One big advantage is that you can pretty much choose how you want your teeth to look. You can have them perfectly straight and level, and as white as you like. Or, you may choose to have them like your own teeth were, with a small gap here and there. It is up to you. New dentures equal a new smile.

Dental Protection

Dental treatment can be expensive. Many traditional dental insurance plans do not cover all procedures, but an alternative is a discount dental plan. Such a plan will usually cover all dental treatments at a lower price.

Section 20.4

Home Use
Denture Reline Kit

"How to Use Denture Reline Kits When Relining Dentures at Home,"
reprinted with permission from www.dental-health-advice.com. © 2011
Dr. Richard Mitchell, BDS.

Denture reline kits are useful when you're thinking about relining dentures yourself at home.

Why would you want to reline your dentures?

There is really only one reason to do a reline—your denture does not fit properly any more—but there are several reasons why you might want to do it yourself at home. There's absolutely no doubt that getting your denture relined at a dentist's office will give you the best fit and the longest lasting result. But, doing it at home has a couple of advantages:

- It is the most economical way to get a reline, much cheaper than going to a dentist.

- You do not have to leave your home.

- You do not have to take any time off work.

However, there are some disadvantages:

- The home kits are really only useful for full dentures, not partial dentures.

- If you do not get it exactly right, you have to go to a dentist anyway to get the denture adjusted.

- The result you get with a home reline kit will not last long.

When is it a good idea to use a denture reline kit at home?

- You need to get your denture relined, but your current budget does not allow you to get it done at a dentist's office.

- You cannot get to a dentist's office due to distance or problems getting out of your home.

- You only want a short-term fix because you are getting a new denture or fixed bridge soon.

For best results, use a kit that requires you to get any loose or soft lining material and denture adhesive out of your denture. Soaking the denture in hot water for a minute can help to soften any of the old materials. Once you have got the denture completely clean of any old stuff, just follow the directions on the packet carefully. In two recommended kits, Acryline2 is a hard acrylic material, whereas PermaSoft is an acrylic material that remains slightly flexible when fully set and it is more porous, and loses its flexibility over a period of time. That is when you need to remove it and apply a new reline.

Tip: The directions will tell you to bite down gently while the liner is setting, but most people bite down way too hard. It is very important to bite gently at first, just to get the dentures into the right position. Then hold it still and after a minute, you can slowly increase the pressure. For lower dentures, it's a good idea to swallow a couple of times during the setting time, because the swallowing action helps to push any excess material away from under your tongue.

Denture reline kits are an inexpensive way of relining dentures, providing you take your time and pay attention to detail.

Section 20.5

Make Your Own Dentures

The advertisements for "make your own dentures" might sound a bit like "how to take out your own tooth" or "do-it-yourself eye tests." Taken literally, it would be just about impossible for someone without any dental training to make their own dentures, all on their own.

It is quite a complicated process to get right, and the tools and equipment you need would cost more than just getting a set of teeth made by a dental professional. But, in the United States it is possible to do some of the work yourself at home. The tricky bits are done by a dental laboratory, and they send you the finished dentures by mail. So, it is possible to make your own dentures—with a bit of help.

How does this work?

One company specializing in this type of work is Denture.com. They have been doing this since 2001, and now have plenty of experience. First, you have to go to their website (www.denture.com) and select the type of job you want—a partial denture, a full denture, or a full set (upper and lower). Then Denture.com will send you a kit by mail. This contains all the things you need to make your own molds. It comes with written instructions and a video to help you along.

You get to tell them how you want the front teeth to look, and also pick the color of the teeth. These days, more folks are picking the lighter colors that give the appearance of having had tooth whitening. Once you are done, you send everything back. Next, you get a "trial run" of your new teeth. These are wax dentures that you can put in your mouth and see how they look. You can check to see if:

- the front teeth are too long or too short,

- you can bite comfortably,

- and how that color you selected looks.

Once you are done, you pack them up and send them back. Finally, you get your finished dentures a week or so later. Denture.com guarantees their work.

What are the advantages of doing things this way?

By doing some of the work yourself, you can reduce the cost of new dentures approximately fifty percent. A full set of upper and lower teeth costs around $900. Also, you can do this no matter where you live. If you have access to the U.S. mail service, you can use denture.com.

It may be possible to get new dentures more cheaply if you are able to attend an office belonging to certain dental groups, such as Affordable Dentures. But you can only do this if there is an office near you. These groups offer services that are of value to a number of people.

So, how does that phrase "make your own dentures" sound now? Maybe not quite so odd as before. It may not be for everyone, but a dentures-by-mail service is definitely worth looking at if you are searching for inexpensive dentures, and live outside the big towns and cities.

Part Three

Dental Care for
Infants and Children

Chapter 21

Oral Health for Infants

Chapter Contents

Section 21.1

A Healthy Mouth for Your Baby

Excerpted from "A Healthy Mouth for Your Baby,"
U.S. Department of Health and Human Services (HHS),
NIH Publication No. 11–2884, September 16, 2011.

Healthy teeth are important—even baby teeth. Children need healthy teeth to help them chew and to speak clearly. And baby teeth hold space for adult teeth. Healthy teeth should be all one color. If you see spots or stains on the teeth, take your baby to a dentist.

Clean Your Baby's Teeth

Clean your baby's teeth as soon as they come in with a clean, soft cloth or a baby's toothbrush. Clean the teeth at least once a day. It's best to clean them right before bedtime.

At about age two (or sooner if a dentist or doctor suggests it), you should start putting fluoride toothpaste on your child's toothbrush. Use only a pea-sized drop of toothpaste.

Young children cannot get their teeth clean by themselves. Until they are seven or eight years old, you will need to help them brush. Try brushing their teeth first and then letting them finish.

Feed Your Baby Healthy Food

- Choose foods without a lot of sugar in them.
- Give your child fruits and vegetables for snacks.
- Save cookies and other treats for special occasions.

What's one of the most important things you can do to keep your baby from getting cavities?

Avoid putting him to bed with a bottle—at night or at nap time. (If you do put your baby to bed with a bottle, fill it only with water.) Here are some other things you can do:

- Between feedings, don't give your baby a bottle or sippy cup filled with sweet drinks to carry around.

- Near his first birthday, teach your child to drink from an open cup.

- If your baby uses a pacifier, don't dip it in anything sweet like sugar or honey.

- Your child should have a dental visit by his first birthday.

Section 21.2

Teething

"Teething Tots," November 2011, reprinted with permission from www.kids health.org. Copyright © 2011 The Nemours Foundation. This information was provided by KidsHealth, one of the largest resources online for medically reviewed health information written for parents, kids, and teens. For more articles like this one, visit www.KidsHealth.org, or www.TeensHealth .org. The text and figure under the heading "When Do Baby Teeth Appear?" from the North Carolina Department of Health and Human Services, is cited separately within the text.

Teething Tots

Teething, the emergence of the first teeth through a baby's gums, can be a frustrating time for little ones and their parents. But knowing what to expect during teething and how to make the process a little less painful can help you manage.

The Teething Process

While teething can begin as early as three months, most likely you'll see the first tooth start pushing through your baby's gum line when your little one is between four and seven months old.

The first teeth to appear usually are the two bottom front teeth, also known as the central incisors. They're usually followed 4–8 weeks later by the four front upper teeth (central and lateral incisors). About a month later, the lower lateral incisors (the two teeth flanking the bottom front teeth) will appear.

Next to break through are the first molars (the back teeth used for grinding food), then finally the eyeteeth (the pointy teeth in the upper jaw). Most kids have all 20 of their primary teeth by their third birthday. (If your child experiences significant delay, speak to your doctor.)

In some rare cases, kids are born with one or two teeth or have a tooth emerge within the first few weeks of life. Unless the teeth interfere with feeding or are loose enough to pose a choking risk, this is usually not a cause for concern.

As kids begin teething, they might drool more and want to chew on things. For some babies, teething is painless. Others may have brief periods of irritability, while some may seem cranky for weeks, with crying jags and disrupted sleeping and eating patterns. Teething can be uncomfortable, but if your baby seems very irritable, talk to your doctor.

Although tender and swollen gums could cause your baby's temperature to be a little higher than normal, teething doesn't usually cause high fever or diarrhea. If your baby does develop a fever during the teething phase, it's probably due to something else and you should contact your doctor.

Easing Teething

Here are some tips to keep in mind when your baby is teething:

- Wipe your baby's face often with a cloth to remove the drool and prevent rashes from developing.

- Give your baby something to chew on. Make sure it's big enough so that it can't be swallowed and that it can't break into small pieces. A wet washcloth placed in the freezer for 30 minutes makes a handy teething aid—just be sure to wash it after each use. Rubber teething rings are also good, but avoid ones with liquid inside because they may break or leak. If you use a teething ring, be sure to take it out of the freezer before it becomes rock hard—you don't want to bruise those already swollen gums!

- Rub your baby's gums with a clean finger.

- Never tie a teething ring around a baby's neck—it could get caught on something and strangle the baby.

- If your baby seems irritable, acetaminophen may help—but always consult your doctor first. Never place an aspirin against the tooth, and don't rub alcohol on your baby's gums.

Baby Teeth Hygiene

The care and cleaning of your baby's teeth is important for long-term dental health. Even though the first set of teeth will fall out, tooth decay can hasten this process and leave gaps before the permanent teeth are ready to come in. The remaining primary teeth may then crowd together to attempt to fill in the gaps, which may cause the permanent teeth to come in crooked and out of place.

Daily dental care should begin even before your baby's first tooth emerges. Wipe your baby's gums daily with a clean, damp washcloth or gauze, or brush them gently with a soft, infant-sized toothbrush and water (no toothpaste!). As soon as the first tooth appears, brush it with water.

Toothpaste is okay to use once a child is old enough to spit it out—usually around age three. Choose one with fluoride and use only a pea-sized amount or less in younger kids. Don't let your child swallow the toothpaste or eat it out of the tube because an overdose of fluoride can be harmful to kids.

By the time all your baby's teeth are in, try to brush them at least twice a day and especially after meals. It's also important to get kids used to flossing early on. A good time to start flossing is when two teeth start to touch. Talk to your dentist for advice on flossing those tiny teeth. You can also get toddlers interested in the routine by letting them watch and imitate you as you brush and floss.

Another important tip for preventing tooth decay: Don't let your baby fall asleep with a bottle. The milk or juice can pool in a baby's mouth and cause tooth decay and plaque.

The American Dental Association (ADA) recommends that kids see a dentist by age one, when six to eight teeth are in place, to spot any potential problems and advise parents about preventive care.

When Do Baby Teeth Appear?

"When Do Baby Teeth Appear?" September 2010, reprinted with permission from the North Carolina Department of Health and Human Services, Division of Public Health, Oral Health Section. For additional information, visit http://www.ncdhhs.gov/dph/oralhealth.

Healthy baby teeth are important for chewing food, for speaking clearly, for normal jaw growth, and a healthy appearance. But most important, baby teeth keep the spacing for the adult teeth, or permanent teeth. Baby teeth are replaced by permanent teeth as your child gets older. Baby teeth lost early because of tooth decay are the leading cause for crowded and crooked permanent teeth.

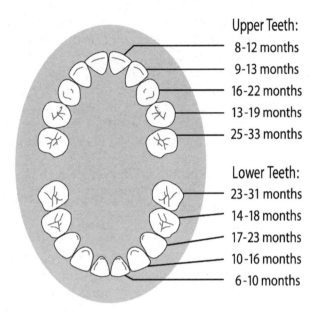

Upper Teeth:
8-12 months
9-13 months
16-22 months
13-19 months
25-33 months

Lower Teeth:
23-31 months
14-18 months
17-23 months
10-16 months
6-10 months

Figure 21.1. There are 20 baby teeth, or primary teeth: ten in the upper jaw and ten in the lower jaw. (Source: "When Do Baby Teeth Appear?" September 2010, reprinted with permission from the North Carolina Department of Health and Human Services, Division of Public Health, Oral Health Section. For additional information, visit http://www.ncdhhs.gov/dph/oralhealth.)

Chapter 22

Routine Care for Children's Teeth

Chapter Contents

Section 22.1

How to Keep Children's Teeth Healthy

This section includes excerpts from "Take Care of Your Child's Teeth," U.S. Department of Health and Human Services (HHS), updated January 12, 2012.

The Basics

Take care of your child's teeth to protect your child from tooth decay (cavities). Tooth decay can cause your child pain, make it hard for your child to chew, and make your child embarrassed to talk or smile. Your child's first teeth (baby teeth) are important. Baby teeth hold the spaces for adult teeth.

Is My Child at Risk for Tooth Decay?

Tooth decay is one of the most common childhood diseases. Almost half of kids ages 2–11 have had decay in their baby teeth. Bacteria in the mouth use the sugar in food to cause tooth decay. Eating and drinking lots of sugary foods and drinks puts your child at risk for tooth decay. Good tooth care can prevent tooth decay.

Take Action

Start with the first tooth: Once your baby's teeth come in, clean them with a clean cloth or a soft children's toothbrush. Clean them after feeding, especially right before bedtime.

Teach your child to brush two times a day: Around age four or five, kids can start to brush their own teeth. Watch to make sure your kids brush all their teeth and use only a pea-sized amount of fluoride toothpaste. Remind your kids not to swallow the toothpaste.

Make brushing fun: Getting kids to brush their teeth can be hard. Following are some ideas that may help.

- Let your child choose a toothbrush in a favorite color or with a character from a television (TV) show or movie. Just make sure it is the right size for your child's mouth.

- Make a checklist and have your child add a sticker after each brushing.

Protect your child's teeth with fluoride: Fluoride is a mineral that helps protect teeth from decay. Here are some ways to make sure your child gets enough fluoride.

- Fluoride is added to the drinking water in many towns and cities. Check with your town or child's doctor if you aren't sure whether there is fluoride in your water.

- If your water doesn't have fluoride in it, a doctor or dentist can give your child fluoride drops. The doctor or dentist may also paint a fluoride varnish on your child's teeth.

- Start brushing your child's teeth with fluoride toothpaste by age two. Use just a pea-sized amount of toothpaste. If young children swallow too much fluoride, their adult teeth may have white spots.

Take your child to the dentist: Take your child to the dentist for a checkup by age one, and at least once every year after that. Ask your child's doctor for the name of a dentist who is good with kids. Talk to your child's dentist about how to clean your child's teeth and other ways to keep your child's mouth healthy.

Section 22.2

From Primary Teeth to Permanent Teeth

Includes "Developing from Primary Teeth to Permanent Teeth," September 2010, and "When Do Molars Come In?" September 2010, reprinted from the North Carolina Department of Health and Human Services, Division of Public Health, Oral Health Section. For additional information, visit http://www.ncdhhs.gov/dph/oralhealth.

Developing from Primary Teeth to Permanent Teeth

There are twenty primary teeth, commonly known as baby teeth. There are ten teeth in the upper jaw, and ten teeth in the lower jaw. As a child gets older, the twenty primary teeth are replaced by twenty permanent teeth. This change to permanent teeth is usually complete by around age 13 years.

Twelve new permanent molars also come in as the child gets older. The first molars appear around the age of six years just behind the primary teeth. Six molars develop in the upper jaw, and six in the lower jaw.

The last molars appear around the age of 20 years, to complete the full set of permanent teeth. There are 32 teeth in a full set of permanent teeth: 16 in the upper jaw and 16 in the lower jaw.

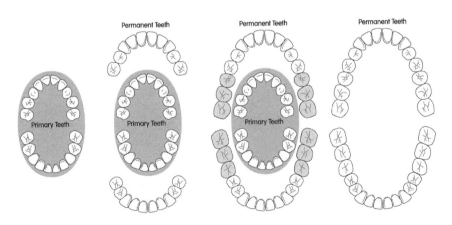

Figure 22.1. Primary and Permanent Tooth Development

When Do Molars Come in?

Molars often need dental sealants to protect them from decay. The best time to put sealants on teeth is just after the molars appear, but before decay starts.

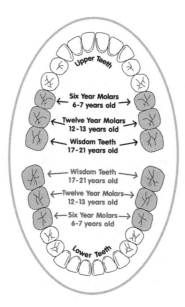

Figure 22.2. *Upper and Lower Molars*

Section 22.3

Calcium Is Critical for Tooth Development

This chapter includes excerpts from "Milk Matters: Calcium Is Critical for Teeth; Milk and Calcium; and Calcium from Other Foods," National Institute of Child Health and Human Development (NICHD), reviewed 2012.

Calcium Is Critical for Teeth

Even before they come in, baby teeth and adult teeth need calcium to develop fully. And after the teeth are in, calcium may also help protect them against decay. Calcium makes jawbones strong and healthy too.

How much calcium do kids need?

Tweens and teens can get most of their daily calcium from:

- three cups of low-fat or fat-free milk (900 mg of calcium); and
- additional servings of calcium-rich foods to get the 1,300 mg of calcium necessary to build strong bones for life.

Milk and Calcium

Low-fat or fat-free milk is a great source of calcium:

- Milk contains a lot of calcium in a form that the body can easily absorb.

Table 22.1. Calcium Needs by Age

0–6 months	210 mg
6–12 months	270 mg
1–3 years	500 mg
4–8 years	800 mg
9–18 years	1300 mg

Source: Dietary Reference Intakes for Calcium, National Academy of Sciences (NAS) 1997

- Milk has other important nutrients that are good for bones and teeth. One especially important nutrient is vitamin D, which helps the body absorb more calcium.

- Milk is widely available and is already a part of many people's diets.

One cup, or eight ounces (oz.) of milk contains 300 milligrams (mg) of calcium.

Is one type of milk better than the other?

Today, tweens and teens have more milk choices than ever before. Most types of milk have approximately 300 mg of calcium per 8-fluid ounces (one cup)—about 25% of the calcium that children and teenagers

Table 22.2. Calcium-Rich Foods

Food	Serving Size	Calories	Amount of Calcium
Plain yogurt, fat-free	1 cup	127	452 mg
Orange juice with added calcium	8 oz. (1 cup)	120	350 mg
Fruit yogurt, low-fat	1 cup	232	345 mg
Ricotta cheese, part skim	½ cup	170	334 mg
American cheese, low-fat or fat-free	2 oz (about 3 slices	188	312 mg
Soybeans, cooked	1 cup	175	298 mg
Cheddar cheese, low-fat or fat-free	½ cup	114	204 mg
Tofu, firm, with added calcium sulfate	½ cup	97	204 mg
Soy beverage with added calcium	8 oz. (1 cup)	100–130	200–300 mg
Cheese pizza	1 slice	240	200 mg
Broccoli, raw	1 medium stalk	106	180 mg
Broccoli, cooked	1 cup	52	94 mg
Bok Choy, boiled	1 cup	20	158 mg
Spinach, cooked from frozen	½ cup	27	139 mg
Frozen yogurt, soft serve vanilla	½ cup	114	103 mg
Macaroni and cheese	1 cup	230	100 mg
Almonds	1 oz (22 nuts)	169	75 mg
Tortilla, flour (7–8 inches)	1 tortilla	150	58 mg
Tortilla, corn (6 inches)	1 tortilla	53	42 mg

need every day. The best choices are low-fat or fat-free milk and milk products. Because these items contain little or no fat, it's easy to get enough calcium without adding extra fat to the diet.

Calcium from Other Foods

Milk is not the only way for tweens and teens to get the calcium they need every day. Lots of calcium-rich foods are available to help them get the 1,300 mg of calcium they need every day. Experts report that the best way to get calcium is by eating calcium-rich foods. But for people who have lactose intolerance or who do not eat dairy products, foods with calcium added are also an option.

Check the ingredient list for added calcium in the following foods:

- Tofu (with added calcium sulfate)
- Calcium-fortified orange juice
- Soy beverages with added calcium
- Calcium-fortified cereals or breads

Calcium supplements are also an alternative way to get calcium for children and adults who don't or can't have milk or milk products.

Chapter 23

Fluoride Consumption during Tooth Development

Chapter Contents

221

Section 23.1

Dental Fluorosis Overview

Text in this section is excerpted from "Dental Fluorosis,"
Centers for Disease Control and Prevention (CDC), January 6, 2011.

The proper amount of fluoride helps prevent and control tooth decay in children and adults. Fluoride works both while the teeth are developing and every day after the teeth have emerged through the gums. Fluoride consumed during tooth development can also result in a range of visible changes to the enamel surface of the tooth. These changes have been broadly termed dental fluorosis, or dental fluorosis.

What is dental fluorosis?

Dental fluorosis is a change in the appearance of the tooth's enamel. These changes can vary from barely noticeable white spots in mild forms to staining and pitting in the more severe forms. Dental fluorosis only occurs when younger children consume too much fluoride, from any source, over long periods when teeth are developing under the gums.

Who develops dental fluorosis?

Only children aged eight years and younger can develop dental fluorosis because this is when permanent teeth are developing under the gums.

- Once the teeth erupt through the gums and are in the mouth, children can no longer develop fluorosis.

- The teeth of children older than eight years, adolescents, and adults cannot develop dental fluorosis.

What does dental fluorosis look like?

- Very mild and mild forms of dental fluorosis—teeth have scattered white flecks, occasional white spots, frosty edges, or fine, lacy chalk-like lines. These changes are barely noticeable and difficult to see except by a dental health care professional.

- Moderate and severe forms of dental fluorosis—teeth have larger white spots and, in the rare, severe form, rough, pitted surfaces.

What causes dental fluorosis?

Dental fluorosis is caused by taking in too much fluoride over a long period when the teeth are forming under the gums. Only children aged eight years and younger are at risk because this is when permanent teeth are developing under the gums. The severity of the condition depends on the dose (how much), duration (how long), and timing (when consumed) of fluoride intake.

Increases in the occurrence of mostly mild dental fluorosis were recognized as more sources of fluoride became available to prevent tooth decay. These sources include drinking water with fluoride, fluoride toothpaste—especially if swallowed by young children—and dietary prescription supplements in tablets or drops (particularly if prescribed to children already drinking fluoridated water).

What accounts for most of the fluoride intake?

In the United States, water and processed beverages (soft drinks and fruit juices) can provide approximately 75% of a person's fluoride intake. Inadvertent swallowing of toothpaste and inappropriate use of other dental products containing fluoride can result in greater intake than desired. For this reason the Centers for Disease Control and Prevention (CDC) recommends parents supervise the use of fluoride toothpaste by children under the age of six years to encourage them to spit out excess toothpaste. Also, avoid the use of fluoride mouth rinses in children who are younger than six years old because the mouth rinse could be repeatedly swallowed.

In which communities can dental fluorosis be found?

Dental fluorosis occurs among some persons in all communities, even in those with a low natural concentration of fluoride in the drinking water.

What parents and caregivers can do to reduce the occurrence of dental fluorosis?

Know the fluoride concentration of your drinking water: You should know the fluoride concentration in your primary source of drinking water, especially if you have young children. This information should help with decisions about using other fluoride products, particularly fluoride tablets or drops, that your physician or dentist may prescribe for your young child. Fluoride tablets or drops should not be used at all if your drinking water has the recommended fluoride concentration of 0.7 milligrams per liter (mg/L) or higher.

If you live in a state that participates in CDC's "My Water's Fluoride," you can find out your water system's fluoridation status online. If you are on a public water system, you can call the water utility company and request a copy of the utility's most recent *Consumer Confidence Report*.

For very young children, less than two years old: Do not use fluoride toothpaste unless advised to do so by your doctor or dentist. You should clean your child's teeth as soon as the first tooth appears by brushing without toothpaste with a small, soft-bristled toothbrush and plain water.

For children aged 2–6 years, apply no more than a pea-sized amount of fluoride toothpaste to the brush and supervise their toothbrushing, encouraging the child to spit out the toothpaste rather than swallow it. Until about age six years, children have poor control of their swallowing reflex and frequently swallow most of the toothpaste placed on their brush.

Use an alternative source of water for children aged eight years and younger if your primary drinking water contains greater than 2 mg/L of fluoride. In some regions of the United States, public water systems, and private wells contain a natural fluoride concentration of more than 2 mg/L, and at this concentration children eight years and younger have a greater chance for developing dental fluorosis, including the moderate and severe forms. These children should have an alternative source of drinking water that contains fluoride at the recommended level.

Target mouth rinses to children at high risk for developing tooth decay: Because fluoride mouth rinses have resulted in only limited reductions in tooth decay among children, especially as their exposure to other sources of fluoride has increased, their use should be targeted to individuals and groups at high risk for decay.

Children younger than six years should not use a fluoride mouth rinse without parents first consulting a dentist or physician because there is a possibility for dental fluorosis if these rinses are repeatedly swallowed.

Fluoride supplements can be prescribed for children at high risk for tooth decay and whose primary source of drinking water has a low fluoride level. If the children are younger than six years, however, then the dentist or physician should weigh the risks for developing decay without supplements with the possibility of developing dental fluorosis. Other sources of fluoride, especially drinking water, should be considered when determining this balance. Parents and caregivers should be informed of both the benefits and risks of fluoride supplements.

Fluoride supplements can be prescribed for persons as appropriate or used in school-based programs. When practical, supplements should be prescribed as chewable tablets or lozenges to maximize the topical effects of fluoride.

Section 23.2

Infant Formula and Fluorosis

Excerpted from "Infant Formula Safety—Community Water Fluoridation," Centers for Disease Control and Prevention (CDC), January 7, 2011.

The proper amount of fluoride from infancy through old age helps prevent and control tooth decay. Community water fluoridation is a widely accepted practice for preventing and controlling tooth decay by adjusting the concentration of fluoride in the public water supply. Recent evidence suggests that mixing powdered or liquid infant formula concentrate with fluoridated water on a regular basis may increase the chance of a child developing the faint, white markings of very mild or mild enamel fluorosis.

You can use fluoridated water for preparing infant formula. However, if your child is exclusively consuming infant formula reconstituted with fluoridated water, there may be an increased chance for mild dental fluorosis. To lessen this chance, parents can use low-fluoride bottled water some of the time to mix infant formula; these bottled waters are labeled as de-ionized, purified, demineralized, or distilled.

What is the best source of nutrition for infants?

Breastfeeding is ideal for infants. The Center for Disease Control and Prevention (CDC) is committed to increasing breastfeeding throughout the United States and promoting optimal breastfeeding practices. Both babies and mothers gain many benefits from breastfeeding. Breast milk is easy to digest and contains antibodies that can protect infants from bacterial and viral infections. If breastfeeding is not possible, several types of formula are available for infant feeding.

Why is there a focus on infant formula as a source of fluoride?

Infants consume little other than breast milk or formula during the first 4–6 months of life, and continue to have a high intake of liquids during the entire first year. Therefore, proportional to body weight, fluoride intake may be higher for younger or smaller children than for older children, adolescents, or adults.

What types of infant formula may increase the chance of dental fluorosis?

There are three types of formula available in the United States for infant feeding. These are powdered formula which comes in bulk or single-serve packets, concentrated liquid, and ready-to-feed formula. Those types of formula that require mixing with water—powdered or liquid concentrates—can be a child's main source of fluoride intake (depending upon the fluoride content of the water source used) and may increase the chance of dental fluorosis.

Can I use optimally fluoridated tap water to mix infant formula?

Yes, you can use fluoridated water for preparing infant formula. However, if your child is exclusively consuming infant formula reconstituted with fluoridated water, there may be an increased chance for mild dental fluorosis. To lessen this chance, parents can use low-fluoride bottled water some of the time to mix infant formula; these bottled waters are labeled as de-ionized, purified, demineralized, or distilled.

How can I find out the level (concentration) of fluoride in my tap water?

The best source of information on fluoride levels in your water system is your local water utility. Other knowledgeable sources may be a local public health authority, dentist, dental hygienist, or physician. CDC's website "My Water's Fluoride" allows consumers in some states to learn the fluoridation status of their water system.

Will using only low fluoride water to mix formula eliminate my child's risk for dental fluorosis?

Using only water with low fluoride levels to mix formula will reduce, but will not eliminate, the risk for dental fluorosis. Children can take in fluoride from other sources during the time that teeth are developing (birth through age eight years). These sources include drinking water, foods and beverages processed with fluoridated water, and dental products, such as fluoride toothpaste, that can be swallowed by young children whose swallowing reflex is not fully developed.

Chapter 24

Preventing Tooth Decay in Children Six Years and Younger

Chapter Contents

Section 24.1

Fluoride Varnish

This section begins with "When Primary Care Providers Apply Fluoride Varnish," Agency for Healthcare Research and Quality (A HRQ), 2011; and concludes with "Fluoride Varnish: An Effective Tool for Preventing Dental Caries," © 2010 National Maternal and Child Oral Health Resource Center, Georgetown University (www.mchoralhealth.org). Reprinted with permission.

When Primary Care Providers Apply Fluoride Varnish

Tooth decay among children younger than five years, referred to as early childhood caries (ECC), is preventable. Yet, as many as 11% of 2-year-olds and 44% of 5-year-olds develop ECC, with children from low-income families bearing a disproportionate burden of the disease. According to a new study, application of topical fluoride varnish by non-dental pediatric primary care providers can reduce dental caries-related treatments among children. A North Carolina Medicaid program called "Into the Mouths of Babes" (IMB), initiated in 2000, had primary care providers apply fluoride varnish to children's teeth during office visits. Analysis of the State's Medicaid enrollment and claims data from 2000 to 2006 showed that the program reduced dental caries-related treatments among children with four or more IMB visits by 17% up to six years of age, compared with children with no IMB visits.

When Bhavna T. Pahel, PhD, and her University of North Carolina colleagues simulated data for initial IMB visits at 12 and 15 months of age, there was a cumulative 49% reduction in dental caries-related treatments at 17 months of age. However, there was an increase in treatments for children from 24 to 42 months of age. The authors hypothesize that this increase in dental caries-related treatments likely occurred due to greater detection of disease in teeth of children who received and benefitted from the program, longer time since fluoride application, and emergence of teeth not initially treated with fluoride. Therefore, the authors concluded that multiple applications of fluoride at the time of primary tooth emergence seem to be most beneficial. In total, the reduction in caries-related treatments from the IMB preventive dental services represents a substantial improvement in the oral health of Medicaid-enrolled children, who historically have had high rates of dental caries but poor access to care from dentists, comment the researchers.

The IMB Program was based on the perception that, although very young children are unlikely to get checkups at the dentist, they frequently make well-child visits to their pediatricians or other primary care providers. The study was supported in part by the Agency for Healthcare Research and Quality (T32 HS00032).

Fluoride Varnish Is an Effective Tool for Preventing Dental Caries

Because frequent exposure to small amounts of fluoride each day is the best way to reduce the risk for dental caries (tooth decay), it is recommended that individuals drink water with an optimal fluoride concentration and brush their teeth with fluoride toothpaste twice a day. Among those at high risk for dental caries, additional forms of fluoride may be necessary to reduce risk.[1]

Background

Fluoride-containing varnishes were developed to improve on the shortcomings of other topical fluoride vehicles (for example, mouthrinse, gels) by prolonging contact of fluoride with tooth enamel.[2]

The decision to professionally apply topical fluoride should be based on assessment of dental caries risk, and fluoride varnish should ideally be applied by a dental or medical professional as part of a comprehensive, continuously accessible, coordinated, and family-centered oral health care program.[3,4]

Fluoride varnish applied every six months is effective in preventing dental caries in the primary and permanent teeth of children and adolescents at moderate to high risk for dental caries. For those at high risk, receiving fluoride varnish every three months may provide an additional caries-prevention benefit.[5,6]

The prescription and application of highly concentrated fluoride, including fluoride varnish, is regulated by state professional practice acts for dentists, dental hygienists, physicians, nurses, pharmacists, and others.[7]

Effectiveness

The quality of evidence for the efficacy of high-concentration fluoride varnish in preventing dental caries in children at moderate to high risk for caries is high.[1]

To be most effective, fluoride varnish applications should occur before dental caries develop and therefore should be started in infancy.[8]

In a study of children ages 3–5 enrolled in Head Start, among the children with active dental caries who received fluoride varnish application, 81% of the active caries became inactive after nine months, compared with 38% in children who did not receive fluoride varnish application.[9]

In a caries prevention program at an urban pediatric clinic serving families with low incomes, children ages 6–27 months who received a caries-risk assessment, fluoride varnish application, oral hygiene instruction, referral for treatment (if needed), and periodic recall had a significantly lower incidence of caries than did a comparison group who did not receive these services.[10]

Among 376 Chinese and Latino infants and children (ages 6–44 months) from families with low incomes, those who received oral hygiene counseling as well as fluoride varnish application had a lower incidence of dental caries than their counterparts who received only counseling.[11]

Safety

When recommendations for dosages and frequency of fluoride varnish application are followed, no side effects are expected to occur.[12]

Risk of fluorosis from fluoride varnish is minimal.[13]

No adverse events or safety issues were reported among 376 Chinese and Latino infants and children (ages 6–44 months) from families with low incomes who received fluoride varnish application.[11]

Service Delivery and Access

Fluoride varnish, in comparison with gels or foams, is applied easily, sets quickly, and is less likely to be swallowed by young children.[2, 13] This is especially advantageous in young children, in children or adults with special health care needs, and in public health programs.[13]

Having oral health professionals as well as medical professionals (physicians, nurse practitioners) apply fluoride varnish creates a wider array of access points at which children and adolescents enrolled in Medicaid can receive preventive services.[14]

The use of fluoride varnish to assist in the prevention of dental caries in children is expanding in both public and private settings that incorporate oral health risk assessments and parental counseling. These settings include Head Start programs; Special Supplemental Nutrition Programs for Women, Infants, and Children (WIC) clinics; well-child clinics; medical offices; and other community programs.[15]

In a study of post-residency pediatricians, more than 90% said they should assess children's teeth for dental caries and educate families about preventive oral health. Pediatricians and dentists need to work together to improve the quality of preventive oral health care available to all young children.[16]

Reimbursement

After Wisconsin changed its Medicaid policy to allow medical professionals (rather than just oral health professionals) to be reimbursed for fluoride varnish application, the number of fluoride varnish application claims for children enrolled in Medicaid (ages 1–6) increased significantly. The greatest increase was among children ages 1–2.[14]

If reimbursed at an appropriate level, a high proportion of primary care pediatric and family physicians are willing to provide fluoride varnish application to children who are eligible for Medicaid.[17]

A preventive initiative that includes an oral evaluation and fluoride varnish application for children and oral hygiene instruction for their parents receiving public assistance and seen in a pediatric medical residency setting provides an additional access point for preventive services to children at high risk for dental caries.[18]

References

1. Centers for Disease Control and Prevention. 2001. Recommendations for using fluoride to prevent and control dental caries in the United States. *Morbidity and Mortality Weekly Reports 50(RR–14)*:1–42. http://www.cdc.gov/mmwr/preview/ mmwrhtml/rr5014a1.htm.

2. Beltrán-Aguilar ED, Goldstein JW, Lockwood, SA. 2000. Fluoride varnishes: A review of their clinical use, cariostatic mechanism, efficacy and safety. *Journal of the American Dental Association 131(5)*:589–596. http://jada.ada.org/cgi/content/ abstract/131/5/589.

3. American Academy of Pediatric Dentistry, Council on Clinical Affairs. 2006. Definition of a dental home. *Pediatric Dentistry 31(6)*:10. http://www.aapd.org/media/Policies_Guide lines/D_ DentalHome.pdf.

4. American Academy of Pediatric Dentistry, Liaison with Other Groups Committee. 2008. Guideline on fluoride therapy. *Pediatric Dentistry 31(6)*:128–131. http://www.aapd.org/media/ Policies_Guidelines/G_Fluoride therapy.pdf.

5. Marinho VC, Higgins JP, Logan S, Sheiham A. 2002. Fluoride varnishes for preventing dental caries in children and adolescents. *Cochrane Database of Systemic Reviews (1):*CD 002279. http://www.cochrane.org/reviews/en/ab002279.html.

6. American Dental Association, Council on Scientific Affairs. 2006. Professionally applied topical fluoride: Evidence-based clinical recommendations. *Journal of the American Dental Association 137(8)*:1151–1159. http://jada.ada.org/cgi/content/full/137/8/1151.

7. Food and Drug Administration. 2009. *Regulatory Procedures Manual.* http://www.fda.gov/ICECI/ComplianceManuals/Regulatory ProceduresManual/default.htm.

8. Kagihara LE, Niederhauser VP, Stark M. 2009. Assessment, management, and prevention of early childhood caries. *Journal of the American Academy of Nurse Practitioners 21(1)*:1–10. http://www.ingentaconnect.com/content/bsc/jaan/2009/00000021/00000001/art00001.

9. Autio-Gold JT, Courts F. 2001. Assessing the effect of fluoride varnish on early enamel carious lesions in the primary dentition. *Journal of the American Dental Association 132(9)*:1247–1253. http://jada.ada.org/cgi/content/full/132/9/1247.

10. Minah G, Lin C, Coors S, Rambob I, Tinanoff N, Grossman LK. 2008. Evaluation of an early childhood caries prevention program at an urban pediatric clinic. *Pediatric Dentistry 30(6)*:499–504. http://www.ingentaconnect.com/content/aapd/pd/2008/00000030/0000 0006/art00007.

11. Weintraub JA, Ramos-Gomez B, Jue SS, Hoover CI, Featherstone JDB, Gansky SA. 2006. Fluoride varnish efficacy in preventing early childhood caries. *Journal of Dental Research 85(2)*:172–176. http://jdr.sagepub.com/cgi/reprint/85/2/172.pdf.

12. Ekstrand J. 1980. Plasma fluoride concentration and urinary fluoride excretion in children following application of the fluoride-containing varnish Duraphat. *Caries Research 14(4)*: 185–189.

13. Ramaswami N. 2008. Fluoride varnish: A primary prevention tool for dental caries. *Journal of the Michigan Dental Association 90(1)*:44–47.

14. Okunseri C, Szabo A, Jackson S, Pajewski NM, Garcia RI. 2009. Increased children's access to fluoride varnish treatment

by involving medical care providers: Effect of a Medicaid policy change. *HSR: Health Services Research 44(4)*:1144–1156. http://www.hsr.org/hsr/abstract.jsp?aid=44115147736.

15. Association of State and Territorial Dental Directors, Fluorides Committee. 2007. *Fluoride Varnish: An Evidence-Based Approach—Research Brief*. Reno, NV: Association of State and Territorial Dental Directors, Fluorides Committee. http://www .astdd.org/docs/Sept2007FINALFl varnishpaper.pdf.

16. Lews C, Robertson AS, Phelps S. 2005. Unmet dental care needs among children with special health care needs: Implications for the medical home. *Pediatrics 116(3)*:426–431. http:// www.pediatrics.org/cgi/content/full/116/3/e426.

17. Slade GD, Rozier RG, Zeldin LP, Margolis PA. 2007. Training pediatric health care providers in prevention of dental decay. *BMC Health Services Research 7*:176. http://www.biomed central.com/1472-6963/7/176/abstract.

18. Grant JS, Roberts MW, Brown WD, Quinoñez RB. 2007. Integrating dental screening and fluoride varnish application into a pediatric residency outpatient program: Clinical and financial implications. *Journal of Pediatric Dentistry 31(3)*:175–178. http://pediatricdentistry.metapress.com/content/ y7501427n240u793.

Section 24.2

Xylitol Syrup Helps to Prevent Toddler Tooth Decay

"Xylitol Syrup Helps to Prevent Childhood Tooth Decay,"
National Institute of Dental and Craniofacial Research
(NIDCR), July 21, 2009.

In December 1869, an Ohio dentist named William Sample received the first patent on chewing gum. His recipe: rubber, sugar, licorice, and charcoal. Although Sample never actively pursued the patent, many subsequently wiled away a precious hour adding and subtracting ingredients to his crude, chewy concoction. Among them was Walter Dierner, an accountant in the 1920s for the Fleer Chewing Gum Company in Philadelphia. When the 23-year-old Dierner wasn't crunching numbers, he dabbled on the side with his homespun chewing gum recipes. One day Dierner got his latest recipe wrong and "ended up with something with bubbles." As Dierner recalled, his colleagues at Fleer recognized the novelty of "bubble gum" and launched plans to manufacture it. To show just how different bubble gum was from regular chewing gum, Dierner and company decided to give it a different look. The men dashed off to find a bottle of food coloring to do the trick, and by chance the only one to be found in the entire factory was pink. The rest is history.

So in 1963, when scientists discovered that the natural sweetener xylitol inhibits the adhesion of the caries-causing oral bacterium *Streptococcus mutans*, it seemed logical to include the ingredient in chewing gum. As great as the idea has been, it has had its limitations for small children. The problem—toddlers need a fair amount of xylitol to protect their primary teeth as they erupt, and manufacturers can only pack so much of the compound into a stick of gum. The toddlers would need to chew at least three sticks of gum per day to get the full decay-preventing benefit. That has left researchers grasping for a more practical alternative.

In the July 2009 issue of the *Archives of Pediatrics & Adolescent Medicine*, researchers partially funded through the National Institute of Dental and Craniofacial Research (NIDCR), may have found the answer. It is a soft capsule filled with eight milliliters of strawberry-flavored xylitol syrup. Parents can pull it apart and squeeze the syrup directly into their child's mouth. In a year-long randomized trial of 94 toddlers whose primary teeth were coming in, the researchers found that children who received two capsules a day could prevent up to 70% of decayed teeth. They found that the protection against decay was not increased with three capsules per day. The study was conducted in the Micronesian Marshall Islands, where the caries rate is two to three times that of the typical American mainland community. According to the authors, this marks the first time to their knowledge that xylitol has been shown to be "effective for the prevention of decay in primary teeth for toddlers."

Reference

Milgrom P, Ly KA, Tut OK, Mancl L, Roberts MC, Briand K, and Gancio MJ. Xylitol pediatric topical oral syrup to prevent dental caries, *Arch Pediatr Adolsc Med 2009:163*: 601-607.

Chapter 25

Preventing Tooth Decay in School-Age Children

Chapter Contents

Section 25.1

Sealants Seal Out Tooth Decay

This section includes "Dental Sealants Fact Sheet," Centers for Disease Control and Prevention (CDC), September 2, 2009, and Figure 25.1 which is excerpted from "Seal Out Tooth Decay: A Booklet for Parents," National Institute of Dental and Craniofacial Research (NIDCR), September 2009.

What are dental sealants?

Dental sealants are thin plastic coatings that are applied to the grooves on the chewing surfaces of the back teeth to protect them from tooth decay. Most tooth decay in children and teens occurs on these surfaces. Sealants protect the chewing surfaces from tooth decay by keeping germs and food particles out of these grooves.

Which teeth are suitable for sealants?

Permanent molars are the most likely to benefit from sealants. The first molars usually come into the mouth when a child is about six years old. Second molars appear at about age 12. It is best if the sealant is applied soon after the teeth have erupted, before they have a chance to decay.

How are sealants applied?

Applying sealants does not require drilling or removing tooth structure. The process is short and easy. After the tooth is cleaned, a special gel is placed on the chewing surface for a few seconds. The tooth is then washed off and dried. Then, the sealant is painted on the tooth. The dentist or dental hygienist also may shine a light on the tooth to help harden the sealant. It takes about a minute for the sealant to form a protective shield.

Are sealants visible?

Sealants can only be seen up close. Sealants can be clear, white, or slightly tinted, and usually are not seen when a child talks or smiles.

Will sealants make teeth feel different?

As with anything new that is placed in the mouth, a child may feel the sealant with the tongue. Sealants, however, are very thin and only fill the pits and grooves of molar teeth.

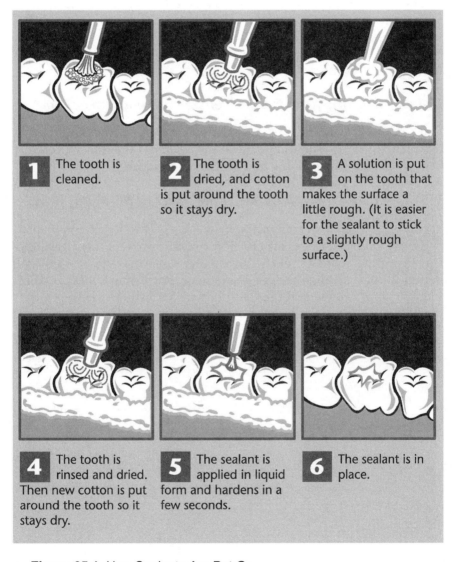

1 The tooth is cleaned.

2 The tooth is dried, and cotton is put around the tooth so it stays dry.

3 A solution is put on the tooth that makes the surface a little rough. (It is easier for the sealant to stick to a slightly rough surface.)

4 The tooth is rinsed and dried. Then new cotton is put around the tooth so it stays dry.

5 The sealant is applied in liquid form and hardens in a few seconds.

6 The sealant is in place.

Figure 25.1. How Sealants Are Put On

How long will sealants last?

A sealant can last for as long as 5–10 years. Sealants should be checked at your regular dental appointment and can be reapplied if they are no longer in place.

Will sealants replace fluoride for cavity protection?

No. Fluorides, such as those used in toothpaste, mouth rinse, and community water supplies also help to prevent decay, but in a different way. Sealants keep germs and food particles out of the grooves by covering them with a safe plastic coating. Sealants and fluorides work together to prevent tooth decay.

How do sealants fit into a preventive dentistry program?

Sealants are one part of a child's total preventive dental care. A complete preventive dental program also includes fluoride, twice-daily brushing, wise food choices, and regular dental care.

Why is sealing a tooth better than waiting for decay and filling the cavity?

Decay damages teeth permanently. Sealants protect them. Sealants can save time, money, and the discomfort sometimes associated with dental fillings. Fillings are not permanent. Each time a tooth is filled, more drilling is done and the tooth becomes a little weaker.

Section 25.2

Re-Think Drinks for School-Age Children

This section includes: "Drinks Destroy Teeth," © 2011 Indiana Dental Association (www.indental.org). All rights reserved. Reprinted with permission. And, excerpts from "Children's Food Environment State Indicator Report, 2011," Centers for Disease Control and Prevention (CDC).

Fizzy drinks make fuzzy teeth! Keeping teeth healthy for a lifetime means preventing tooth decay and erosion. Though fluoride in community drinking water dramatically reduces the amount of decay in all age groups, tooth erosion is a newer phenomenon and one that is preventable.

What is erosion?

Erosion is the chemical loss of enamel due to acid. Acid is found primarily in soft drinks, sports drinks, juices and acidic foods. Acid reflux, vomiting, and other illnesses that produce stomach acid in the mouth can also erode tooth enamel.

What is enamel?

Enamel is the protective outer layer of teeth. Throughout the day, your enamel undergoes a continuous dissolving and repairing cycle. Milk, fluoride, water, and fluoridated toothpastes can repair and build back the minerals essential to healthy teeth. Low pH beverages such as soft drinks, sports drinks, fruit juices, and wine dissolve enamel. Sour candies can also erode enamel.

How do fizzy drinks make fuzzy teeth?

When acid continuously attacks teeth, they cannot repair themselves and will gradually begin to turn fuzzy and dissolve. Dentists consider every sip of a low pH drink an acid attack. Even one bottle of soda or a single sports drink, if sipped over hours, can do extensive, irreversible damage to tooth enamel.

Table 25.1. Sugar and Acidity or pH of Common Drinks. The pH scale measures the acidity or alkalinity of a solution with pure water in the middle at neutral pH 7. The lower the pH, the stronger the acid.

Drink or Substance (12 oz. serving)	Acid pH	Tsp. Sugar
Water	7.0 (neutral)	0
Milk	6.7	1
Barq's Root Beer	4	11
Minute Maid Orange Juice	3.8	9
Propel Fitness Water	3.4	1
Red Bull Energy Drink	3.3	10
Sprite	3.3	10
Mountain Dew	3.3	12
Diet Coke	3.1	0
Sierra Mist	3.1	10
Full Throttle Energy Drink	3	11
Diet Pepsi	3	0
Gatorade	2.9	5
Sunkist Orange Soda	2.9	13
Dr. Pepper	2.9	10
Vault Energy Soda	2.9	12
Mountain Dew AMP[1]	2.8	11
SoBe Energy Citrus	2.6	12
Minute Maid Lemonade	2.6	10
Pepsi	2.5	11
Diet Schweppes Tonic Water	2.5	0
Coca-Cola Classic[2]	2.4	10
Battery Acid[3]	1	0

1. Now called AMP Energy.

2. In some geographical areas of the U.S. and Canada known simply as "Coca-Cola."

3. Battery acid is not a drink.

Test by Dr. John Ruby, University of Alabama, Birmingham School of Dentistry, 2007. Minnesota Dental Association: Sip All Day, Get Decay.

What is decay?

Decay is literally a soft spot in the enamel which penetrates the dentin, or a hole in the tooth. Decay is caused when the mouth's bacteria react to sugar. The chemical interaction between bacteria and sugar produces acid. The acid-producing bacteria eat the enamel until a hole is made in the tooth, also known as a cavity. Preventing cavities involves brushing, flossing and keeping sugar to a minimum. Fluoride hardens the outer layer of teeth, making it more difficult for bacteria to penetrate the enamel.

Tip: Always drink water when playing sports!

What role does saliva play?

Acid attacks do the most damage when you are very thirsty or have a dry mouth. Saliva, your mouth's natural defense shield, covers your teeth and provides some protection against acid attacks. When you're dehydrated, you lack saliva and your teeth are more vulnerable to acid attacks.

What can I do to prevent fuzzy teeth?

Stop the continuous acid and sugar attack on your teeth by limiting the quantity of soft drinks and sports drinks and instead choosing healthy drinks such as milk and water. Reduce the size of the drink and use a straw to draw the damaging liquid away from your teeth. Food consumed with acidic drinks can often help counteract acid attacks. Most important is to brush your teeth with fluoridated toothpaste before bed to reduce bacteria and to help harden your enamel. Wait at least one hour after drinking an acidic drink to brush your teeth to allow your saliva to begin the repair process. Drinking and swishing with water can also help.

Those with orthodontic appliances need to brush as soon as possible to remove food particles and plaque. They are at the greatest risk of decalcification and should limit soft drinks and sports drinks to occasional use.

Please note: Battery acid is listed in Table 25.1 only for purposes of comparison, and should never be confused for any reason as a beverage.

Children's Food Environment State Indicator Report, 2011

Sugar drinks are the largest source of added sugar and an important contributor of calories in the diets of children in the United States. Adolescent males consume, on average, around 300 calories from sugar

Table 25.2. Food Environment Indicators of Students by State, 2011

State	% HS Students Who Drank One or More Soda(s)/Day	% Middle and High Schools That Offer Sugar Drinks as Competitive Foods
US National	29.2	64.4*
Alabama	38.2	67.2
Alaska	20.1	53.2
Arizona	28.1	47.5
Arkansas	33.5	57.4
California		59.5
Colorado	24.6	69.8
Connecticut		16.7
Delaware	28.8	58.0
D.C.		
Florida	28.6	72.4
Georgia	29.7	
Hawaii	20.8	24.1
Idaho	18.3	66.4
Illinois	31.1	55.2
Indiana	29.7	71.9
Iowa		77.6
Kansas	30.7	80.3
Kentucky	35.7	48.6
Louisiana	36.6	
Maine		56.0
Maryland	21.3	56.2
Massachusetts	21.0	46.3
Michigan	27.6	69.9
Minnesota		65.9
Mississippi	40.2	56.2
Missouri	31.5	79.3

* Because national estimates are not available for these variables, the data presented in the "U.S. National" row is the median of the state estimates.

Table 25.2. *continued*

State	% HS Students Who Drank One or More Soda(s)/Day	% Middle and High Schools That Offer Sugar Drinks as Competitive Foods
Montana	25.7	76.3
Nebraska		74.0
Nevada	22.1	70.8
New Hampshire	22.1	59.5
New Jersey	19.9	44.4
New Mexico	30.4	
New York	24.5	66.8
North Carolina	32.5	65.0
North Dakota	26.3	63.3
Ohio		72.0
Oklahoma	38.1	76.1
Oregon		55.0
Pennsylvania	25.7	54.7
Rhode Island	21.2	48.8
South Carolina	33.2	71.9
South Dakota	28.8	76.3
Tennessee	41.3	36.3
Texas	32.8	56.0
Utah	14.5	81.0
Vermont	22.9	53.2
Virginia		64.4
Washington		68.0
West Virginia	34.5	43.6
Wisconsin	23.1	72.1
Wyoming	27.0	71.3

Data were not available for states that did not conduct a 2009 Youth Risk Behavior Surveillance (YRBS), or did not achieve a high enough overall response rate (greater than or equal to 60%) to receive weighted results; or for states that did not achieve a high enough overall response rate (greater than or equal to 70% on the 2008 School Health Profiles Survey) to receive weighted results.

drinks each day. High consumption of sugar drinks, which have few, if any, nutrients, has been associated with obesity.

The School Food Environment

The Institute of Medicine recommends that the sale of competitive foods in schools (food sold outside the United States Department of Agriculture [USDA] reimbursable school meal programs such as in vending machines, school stores, snack bars) be limited. Schools are uniquely positioned to facilitate and reinforce healthful eating behaviors by eliminating sugar drinks and high energy density foods (foods high in calories for their volume) from the selection of foods offered on the school campus.

Percentage of middle and high schools that offer sugar drinks as competitive foods: Although sodas are prohibited in an increasing number of schools, other sugar drinks that may not be commonly perceived as sources of added sugar and excess calories may be available, such as sports drinks and fruit flavored drinks that are not 100% juice. Schools should consider adopting policies that limit access to all sugar drinks in vending machines and schools stores.

Percentage of middle and high schools that offer less healthy foods as competitive foods: Because human appetite and satiation depend more on the volume of food consumed than on caloric content of the food, reducing the consumption of energy dense, low nutrient foods has been identified as a strategy to prevent weight gain. Foods of lower energy density and higher nutrient content such as fruits and vegetables in their natural forms, nonfat/low-fat dairy products, and whole grain products are healthful alternatives to high energy density foods such as candy, cakes, salty fried snacks, and ice cream.

Percentage of middle and high schools that allow advertising of less healthy foods: The Institute of Medicine has concluded that "food advertising to children affects their preferences, purchase behaviors, and consumption habits for different food and beverage categories, as well as for different product brands." In schools, advertising can take the form of posters and signage; logos or brand names on food and beverage coolers, cups, and plates or vending machines; food sales as fundraisers; corporate sponsorship of events; advertising in school publications; and corporate sponsored classroom curricula and scholarships. Such advertising may impact children's ability to make healthy choices in their diets.

Chapter 26

Dental Caries (Cavities) in Children

Dental Caries in Primary (Baby) Teeth

Overall dental caries in the baby teeth of children age 2–11 years declined from the early 1970s until the mid-1990s. From the mid-1990s until the most recent (1999–2004) National Health and Nutrition Examination Survey, this trend has reversed: a small but significant increase in primary decay was found. This trend reversal was more severe in younger children.

Prevalence

- 42% of children age 2–11 years have had dental caries in their primary teeth.

- Black and Hispanic children and those living in families with lower incomes have more decay.

Unmet needs

- 23% of children age 2–11 years have untreated dental caries.

- Black and Hispanic children and those living in families with lower incomes have more untreated decay.

This chapter includes "Dental Caries (Tooth Decay) in Children (Age 2 to 11)," National Institute of Dental and Craniofacial Research (NIDCR), March 25, 2011. Table 26.5 is excerpted from "Health, United States, 2010, Table 93," Centers for Disease Control and Prevention (CDC), 2010.

Severity

- Children age 2–11 years have an average of 1.6 decayed primary teeth and 3.6 decayed primary surfaces.

- Black and Hispanic subgroups and those with lower incomes have more severe decay in primary teeth.

- Black and Hispanic subgroups and those with lower incomes have more untreated primary teeth.

Dental Caries in Permanent (Adult) Teeth

Dental caries in children's permanent teeth declined from the early 1970s until the mid-1990s. Significant disparities are found in some population groups.

Table 26.1. Percent of Children with Caries in Primary Teeth Prevalence of caries in primary teeth (dft) among youths 2–11 years of age, by selected characteristics: United States, National Health and Nutrition Examination Survey, 1999–2004

Characteristic	Percent with caries in primary teeth
Age	
2 to 5 years	27.90
6 to 11 years	51.17
Sex	
Male	44.43
Female	39.80
Race and Ethnicity	
White, non-Hispanic	38.56
Black, non-Hispanic	43.34
Mexican American	55.40
Poverty Status (Income compared to Federal Poverty Level)	
Less than 100%	54.33
100% to 199%	48.75
Greater than 200%	32.30
Overall	42.17

Data source: The National Health and Nutrition Examination Survey (NHANES) has been an important source of information on oral health and dental care in the United States since the early 1970s.

Prevalence

- 21% of children 6 to 11 have had dental caries in their permanent teeth.

- Hispanic children and those living in families with lower incomes have more decay in their permanent teeth.

Unmet needs

- 8% of children age 6–11 years have untreated decay.

- Hispanic children and those living in families with lower incomes have more untreated decay.

Table 26.2. Percent of Children with Untreated Decay in Primary Teeth
Prevalence of untreated decay in primary teeth (dt) among youths 2–11 years of age, by selected characteristics: United States, National Health and Nutrition Examination Survey, 1999–2004

Characteristic	Percent with untreated decay in primary teeth (dt)
Age	
2 to 5 years	20.48
6 to 11 years	24.49
Sex	
Male	24.16
Female	21.66
Race and Ethnicity	
White, non-Hispanic	19.47
Black, non-Hispanic	27.58
Mexican American	33.09
Poverty Status (Income compared to Federal Poverty Level)	
Less than 100%	32.52
100% to 199%	28.40
Greater than 200%	15.01
Overall	22.94

Data Source: The National Health and Nutrition Examination Survey (NHANES) has been an important source of information on oral health and dental care in the United States since the early 1970s.

Severity

- Children age 6–11 years have about 0.45 decayed permanent teeth and 0.68 decayed permanent surfaces.

- Black and Hispanic subgroups and those with lower incomes have more severe decay in both permanent teeth and surfaces.

- Black and Hispanic subgroups and those with lower incomes have more untreated permanent teeth and surfaces.

Units of measure

Dental caries are measured by a dentist examining a child's teeth, and recording the ones with untreated decay and the ones with fillings. This provides three important numbers:

Table 26.3. Percent of Children with Decay in Permanent Teeth

Prevalence of tooth decay in permanent teeth (DFT) among youths 6–11 years of age, by selected characteristics: United States, National Health and Nutrition Examination Survey, 1999–2004

Characteristic	Percent with decay in permanent teeth
Age	
6 to 8 years	10.16
9 to 11 years	31.36
Sex	
Male	19.36
Female	22.87
Race and Ethnicity	
White, non-Hispanic	18.59
Black, non-Hispanic	19.03
Mexican American	30.76
Poverty Status (Income compared to Federal Poverty Level)	
Less than 100%	28.28
100% to 199%	24.09
Greater than 200%	16.31
Overall	21.06

Data Source: The National Health and Nutrition Examination Survey (NHANES) has been an important source of information on oral health and dental care in the United States since the early 1970s.

- ft (filled teeth): this is the number of decayed teeth that have been treated, which indicates access to dental care;

- dt (decayed teeth): this is the number decayed teeth that have not been treated, which measures unmet need; and

- dft (decayed and filled teeth): this is the sum of ft and dt, and is the measure of person's total lifetime tooth decay.

In addition to counting decayed and filled teeth, this same information can be gathered at the tooth surface level. Since every tooth has multiple surfaces, counting the decayed or filled surfaces provides a more accurate measure of the severity of decay. The following tables list both methods of measuring caries.

Table 26.4. Percent of Children with Untreated Decay in Permanent Teeth

Prevalence of untreated tooth decay in permanent teeth (DT) among youths 6–11 years of age, by selected characteristics: United States, National Health and Nutrition Examination Survey, 1999–2004

Characteristic	Percent with untreated decay in permanent teeth (DT)
Age	
6 to 8 years	4.05
9 to 11 years	11.05
Sex	
Male	7.45
Female	7.91
Race and Ethnicity	
White, non-Hispanic	5.56
Black, non-Hispanic	8.55
Mexican American	12.71
Poverty Status (Income compared to Federal Poverty Level)	
Less than 100%	11.76
100% to 199%	11.94
Greater than 200%	3.57
Overall	7.65

Data Source: The National Health and Nutrition Examination Survey (NHANES) has been an important source of information on oral health and dental care in the United States since the early 1970s.

Table 26.5. Dental Visits by Selected Characteristics: United States, 1997 and 2009

Data are based on household interviews of a sample of the civilian noninstitutionalized population.

Characteristic	Ages 2–17 years	
	1997	*2009*
Percent of persons with a dental visit in the past year[1]		
Total[2]	72.7	78.4
Sex		
Male	72.3	77.6
Female	73.0	79.3
Race		
White only	74.0	79.1
Black or African American only	68.8	76.7
American Indian or Alaska Native only	66.8	68.5
Asian only	69.9	76.2
Percent of poverty level[3]		
Below 100%	62.0	71.7
100%–199%	62.5	75.2
200%–399%	76.1	77.1
400% or more	85.7	87.8
Geographic region		
Northeast	77.5	82.6
Midwest	76.4	80.5
South	68.0	76.8
West	71.5	75.8

Notes:

[1] Respondents were asked, "About how long has it been since you last saw or talked to a dentist?"

[2] Includes all other races not shown separately and unknown disability status.

[3] Percent of poverty level is based on family income and family size and composition using U.S. Census Bureau poverty thresholds.

Chapter 27

Preventing Sports-Related Orofacial Injuries

Background

The tremendous popularity of organized youth sports and the high level of competitiveness have resulted in a significant number of dental and facial injuries. Over the past decade, approximately 46 million youths in the United States (U.S.) were involved in "some form of sports." It is estimated that 30 million children in the U.S. participate in organized sport programs. All sporting activities have an associated risk of orofacial injuries due to falls, collisions, contact with hard surfaces, and contact from sports-related equipment. Sports accidents reportedly account for 10–39% of all dental injuries in children. Children are most susceptible to sports-related oral injury between the ages of seven and 11 years. The administrators of youth, high school, and college football, lacrosse, and ice hockey have demonstrated that dental and facial injuries can be reduced significantly by introducing mandatory protective equipment. Popular sports such as baseball, basketball, soccer, softball, wrestling, volleyball, and gymnastics lag far behind in injury protection for girls and boys. Youths participating in leisure activities, such as skateboarding, inline or roller skating, and bicycling, also benefit from appropriate protective equipment.

Excerpted from "Policy on Prevention of Sports-related Orofacial Injuries," *Pediatric Dentistry, 33(6)*, 63–66, 2011. © 2011 American Academy of Pediatric Dentistry. Reprinted with permission via Copyright Clearance Center.

Studies of dental and orofacial athletic injuries are reported throughout the medical and dental literature. A review of literature published over the past 20 years showed that the injury rate varied greatly depending on the size of the sample, the sample's geographic location, the ages of the participants, and the specific sports involved in the study. Although the statistics vary, many studies reported that dental and orofacial injuries occurred regularly and concluded that participation in sports carries a considerable risk of injury.

Consequences of orofacial trauma for children and their families are substantial because of potential for pain, psychological effects, and economic implications. Children with untreated trauma to permanent teeth exhibit greater impacts on their daily living than those without any traumatic injury. The yearly costs of all injuries, including orofacial injuries, sustained by young athletes have been estimated to be as high as 1.8 billion dollars. The National Youth Sports Safety Foundation in 2005 estimated the cost to treat an avulsed permanent tooth and provide followup care is between $5000 and $20,000 over a lifetime. Traumatic dental injuries have additional indirect costs that include children's hours lost from school and parents' hours lost from work, consequences that disproportionately burden lower income, minority, and non-insured children.

The majority of sport-related dental and orofacial injuries affect the upper lip, maxilla, and maxillary incisors, with 50–90% of dental injuries involving the maxillary incisors. Use of a mouth guard can protect the upper incisors. However, studies have shown that even with a mouth guard in place, up to 25% of dentoalveolar injuries still can occur.

Identifying patients who participate in sports and recreational activities allows the healthcare provider to recommend and implement preventive protocols for individuals at risk for orofacial injuries. In 2000, a predictive index was developed to identify the risk factors involved in various sports. This index is based upon a defined set of risk factors that predict the chance of injury including demographic information (age, gender, dental occlusion), protective equipment (type/usage), velocity and intensity of the sport, level of activity and exposure time, level of coaching and type of sports organization, whether the player is a focus of attention in a contact or non-contact sport, history of previous sports-related injury, and the situation (for example, practice versus game). Behavioral risk factors (such as hyperactivity) also have been associated significantly with injuries affecting the face and/or teeth.

The frequency of dental trauma is significantly higher for children with increased overjet and inadequate lip coverage. A dental professional may be able to modify these risk factors. Initiating preventive orthodontic treatment in early- to middle-mixed dentition of patients with an overjet greater than three millimeters has the potential to reduce the severity of traumatic injuries to permanent incisors.

Although some sports-related traumatic injuries are unavoidable, most can be prevented. Helmets, facemasks, and mouth guards have been shown to reduce both the frequency and severity of dental and orofacial trauma. However, few sports have regulations that require their use. The National Federation of State High School Associations mandate mouth guards for only four sports: football, ice hockey, lacrosse, and field hockey. Several states have attempted to increase the number of sports which mandate mouth guard use, with various degrees of success and acceptance. Four New England states have been successful in increasing the number of sports requiring mouth guard use to include sports such as soccer, wrestling, and basketball.

Initially used by professional boxers, the mouth guard has been used as a protective device since the early 1900s. The mouth guard, also referred to as a gum shield or mouth protector, is defined as a "resilient device or appliance placed inside the mouth to reduce oral injuries, particularly to teeth and surrounding structures." The mouth guard was constructed to "protect the lips and intraoral tissues from bruising and laceration, to protect the teeth from crown fractures, root fractures, luxations, and avulsions, to protect the jaw from fracture and dislocations, and to provide support for edentulous space." The mouth guard works by "absorbing the energy imparted at the site of impact and by dissipating the remaining energy."

The American Society for Testing and Materials (ASTM) classifies mouth guards by three categories:

1. **Type I:** Custom-fabricated mouth guards are produced on a dental model of the patient's mouth by either the vacuum-forming or heat-pressure lamination technique. The ASTM recommends that for maximum protection, cushioning, and retention, the mouth guard should cover all teeth in one arch, customarily the maxillary arch, less the third molar. A mandibular mouth guard is recommended for individuals with a Class III malocclusion. The custom-fabricated type is superior in retention, protection, and comfort. When this type is not available, the mouth-formed mouth guard is preferable to the stock or preformed mouth guard.

2. **Type II:** Mouth-formed, also known as boil-and-bite, mouth guards are made from a thermoplastic material adapted to the mouth by finger, tongue, and biting pressure after immersing

the appliance in hot water. Available commercially at department and sporting-goods stores, these are the most commonly used among athletes but vary greatly in protection, retention, comfort, and cost.

3. **Type III:** Stock mouth guards are purchased over-the-counter. They are designed for use without any modification and must be held in place by clenching the teeth together to provide a protective benefit. Clenching a stock mouth guard in place can interfere with breathing and speaking, and for this reason, stock mouth guards are considered by many to be less protective. Despite these shortcomings, the stock mouth guard could be the only option possible for patients with particular clinical presentations (for example: use of orthodontic brackets and appliances, periods of rapidly changing occlusion during mixed dentition).

The Academy for Sports Dentistry (ASD) "recommends the use of a properly fitted mouth guard. It encourages the use of a custom fabricated mouth guard made over a dental cast and delivered under the supervision of a dentist. The ASD strongly supports and encourages a mandate for use of a properly fitted mouth guard in all collision and contact sports." During fabrication of the mouth guard, it is recommended to establish proper anterior occlusion of the maxillary and mandibular arches as this will prevent or reduce injury by better absorbing and distributing the force of impact. The practitioner also should consider the patient's vertical dimension of occlusion, personal comfort, and breathing ability. By providing cushioning between the maxilla and mandible, mouth guards also may reduce the incidence or severity of condylar displacement injuries as well as the potential for concussions.

Due to the continual shifting of teeth in orthodontic therapy, the exfoliation of primary teeth, and the eruption of permanent teeth, a custom-fabricated mouth guard may not fit the young athlete soon after the impression is obtained. Several block-out methods used in both the dental operatory and laboratory may incorporate space to accommodate for future tooth movement and dental development. By anticipating required space changes, a custom fabricated mouth guard may be made to endure several sports seasons.

Parents play an important role in the acquisition of a mouth guard for young athletes. In a 2004 national fee survey, custom mouth guards ranged from $60 to $285. In a study to determine the acceptance of the three types of mouth guards by 7- and 8-year old children playing soccer, only 24% of parents surveyed were willing to pay $25 for a custom mouth guard. Therefore, cost may be a barrier.

Attitudes of officials, coaches, parents, and players about wearing mouth guards influence their usage. Although coaches are perceived as the individuals with the greatest impact on whether or not players wear mouth guards, parents view themselves as equally responsible for maintaining mouth guard use. However, surveys of parents regarding the indications for mouth guard usage reveal a lack of complete understanding of the benefits of mouth guard use. Players' perceptions of mouth guard use and comfort largely determine their compliance and enthusiasm. Therefore, the dental profession needs to influence and educate all stakeholders about the risk of sports-related orofacial injuries and available preventive strategies. Routine dental visits can be an opportunity to initiate patient/parent education and make appropriate recommendations for use of a properly-fitted athletic mouth guard.

Policy Statement

The AAPD (American Academy of Pediatric Dentistry) recommends:

1. Dentists play an active role in educating the public in the use of protective equipment for the prevention of orofacial injuries during sporting and recreational activities.

2. Continuation of preventive practices instituted in youth, high school and college football, lacrosse, field hockey, and ice hockey.

3. For youth participating in organized baseball and softball activities, an ASTM-certified face protector be required (according to the playing rules of the sport).

4. Mandating the use of properly-fitted mouth guards in other organized sporting activities that carry risk of orofacial injury.

5. Prior to initiating practices for a sporting season, coaches/administrators of organized sports consult a dentist with expertise in orofacial injuries for recommendations for immediate management of sports-related injuries (for example avulsed teeth).

6. Continuation of research in development of a comfortable, efficacious, and cost-effective sports mouth guard to facilitate more widespread use of this proven protective device.

7. Dentists of all specialties, including pediatric and general dentists, provide education to parents and patients regarding prevention of orofacial injuries as part of the anticipatory guidance discussed during dental visits.

8. Dentists should prescribe, fabricate, or provide an appropriate referral for mouth guard protection for patients at increased risk for orofacial trauma.

9. That third party payers realized the benefits of mouth guards for the prevention and protection from orofacial sports-related injuries and, furthermore, encourages them to improve access to these services.

10. The ASD and the International Association of Dental Traumatology be consulted as valuable resources for the professions and public.

Chapter 28

Childhood Bruxism (Teeth Grinding or Clenching)

When you look in on your sleeping child, you want to hear the sounds of sweet dreams: easy breathing and perhaps an occasional sigh. But some parents hear the harsher sounds of gnashing and grinding teeth, called bruxism, which is common in kids.

About Bruxism

Bruxism is the medical term for the grinding of teeth or the clenching of jaws. Bruxism often occurs during deep sleep or while under stress. Two to three out of every ten kids will grind or clench, experts say, but most outgrow it.

Causes of Bruxism

Though studies have been done, no one knows why bruxism happens. But in some cases, kids may grind because the top and bottom teeth aren't aligned properly. Others do it as a response to pain, such as an earache or teething. Kids might grind their teeth as a way to ease the pain, just as they might rub a sore muscle. Many kids outgrow these fairly common causes for grinding.

"Bruxism (Teeth Grinding or Clenching)," November 2009, reprinted with permission from www.kidshealth.org. Copyright © 2009 The Nemours Foundation. This information was provided by KidsHealth, one of the largest resources online for medically reviewed health information written for parents, kids, and teens. For more articles like this one, visit www.KidsHealth.org, or www.TeensHealth.org.

Stress—usually nervous tension or anger—is another cause. For instance, a child might worry about a test at school or a change in routine (a new sibling or a new teacher). Even arguing with parents and siblings can cause enough stress to prompt teeth grinding or jaw clenching.

Some kids who are hyperactive also experience bruxism. And sometimes kids with other medical conditions (such as cerebral palsy) or on certain medications can develop bruxism.

Effects of Bruxism

Many cases of bruxism go undetected with no adverse effects, while others cause headaches or earaches. Usually, though, it's more bothersome to other family members because of the grinding sound.

In some circumstances, nighttime grinding and clenching can wear down tooth enamel, chip teeth, increase temperature sensitivity, and cause severe facial pain and jaw problems, such as temporomandibular joint disease (TMJ). Most kids who grind, however, do not have TMJ problems unless their grinding and clenching is chronic.

Diagnosing Bruxism

Lots of kids who grind their teeth aren't even aware of it, so it's often siblings or parents who identify the problem.

Some signs to watch for:

- grinding noises when your child is sleeping,

- complaints of a sore jaw or face in the morning,

- pain with chewing.

If you think your child is grinding his or her teeth, visit the dentist, who will examine the teeth for chipped enamel and unusual wear and tear, and spray air and water on the teeth to check for unusual sensitivity.

If damage is detected, the dentist may ask your child a few questions, such as:

- How do you feel before bed?

- Are you worried about anything at home or school?

- Are you angry with someone?

- What do you do before bed?

The exam will help the dentist determine whether the grinding is caused by anatomical (misaligned teeth) or psychological (stress) factors and come up with an effective treatment plan.

Treating Bruxism

Most kids outgrow bruxism, but a combination of parental observation and dental visits can help keep the problem in check until they do.

In cases where the grinding and clenching make a child's face and jaw sore or damage the teeth, dentists may prescribe a special night guard. Molded to a child's teeth, the night guard is similar to the protective mouthpieces worn by football players. Though a mouthpiece may take some getting used to, positive results happen quickly.

Helping Kids with Bruxism

Whether the cause is physical or psychological, kids might be able to control bruxism by relaxing before bedtime—for example, by taking a warm bath or shower, listening to a few minutes of soothing music, or reading a book.

For bruxism that's caused by stress, ask about what's upsetting your child and find a way to help. For example, a kid who is worried about being away from home for a first camping trip might need reassurance that mom or dad will be nearby if anything happens.

If the issue is more complicated, such as moving to a new town, discuss your child's concerns and try to ease any fears. If you're concerned, talk to your doctor.

In rare cases, basic stress relievers aren't enough to stop bruxism. If your child has trouble sleeping or is acting differently than usual, your dentist or doctor may suggest further evaluation. This can help determine the cause of the stress and an appropriate course of treatment.

How Long Does Bruxism Last?

Childhood bruxism is usually outgrown by adolescence. Most kids stop grinding when they lose their baby teeth. However, a few kids do continue to grind into adolescence. And if the bruxism is caused by stress, it will continue until the stress is relieved.

Preventing Bruxism

Because some bruxism is a child's natural reaction to growth and development, most cases can't be prevented. Stress-induced bruxism can be avoided, however, by talking with kids regularly about their feelings and helping them deal with stress. Take your child for routine dental visits to find and, if needed, treat bruxism.

Chapter 29

Oral Conditions in Children with Other Special Needs

Tooth eruption may be delayed, accelerated, or inconsistent in children with growth disturbances. Gums may appear red or bluish-purple before erupting teeth break through into the mouth. Eruption depends on genetics, growth of the jaw, muscular action, and other factors. Children with Down syndrome may show delays of up to two years. Review information about the variability in tooth eruption patterns and ask an oral health care provider any additional questions.

Malocclusion, a poor fit between the upper and lower teeth, and crowding of teeth occur frequently in people with developmental disabilities. Nearly 25% of the more than 80 craniofacial anomalies that can affect oral development are associated with intellectual disability. Muscle dysfunction contributes to malocclusion, particularly in people with cerebral palsy. Teeth that are crowded or out of alignment are more difficult to keep clean, contributing to periodontal disease and dental caries. Request a referral to an orthodontist or pediatric dentist for evaluation and specialized instruction in daily oral hygiene.

Tooth anomalies are variations in the number, size, and shape of teeth. People with Down syndrome, oral clefts, ectodermal dysplasias, or other conditions may experience congenitally missing, extra, or malformed teeth. Consult with an oral health care provider for dental treatment planning during a child's growing years.

"Oral Conditions in Children with Special Needs," National Institute of Dental and Craniofacial Research (NIDCR), September 2010.

Developmental defects appear as pits, lines, or discoloration in the teeth. Very high fever or certain medications can disturb tooth formation and defects may result. Many teeth with defects are prone to dental caries, are difficult to keep clean, and may compromise appearance. Make an appointment with an oral health care provider for evaluation of treatment options and advice on keeping teeth clean.

Trauma to the face and mouth occur more frequently in people who have intellectual disability, seizures, abnormal protective reflexes, or muscle incoordination. People receiving restorative dental care should be observed closely to prevent chewing on anesthetized areas. If a tooth is avulsed or broken, take the patient and the tooth to a dentist immediately. With the health care provider determine ways to prevent trauma and to know what to do when it occurs.

Bruxism, the habitual grinding of teeth, is a common occurrence in people with cerebral palsy or severe intellectual disability. In extreme cases, bruxism leads to tooth abrasion and flat biting surfaces. Ask a dentist for an evaluation; behavioral techniques or a bite guard may be recommended.

Dental caries, or tooth decay, may be linked to frequent vomiting or gastroesophageal reflux, less than normal amounts of saliva, medications containing sugar, or special diets that require prolonged bottle feeding or snacking. When oral hygiene is poor, the teeth are at increased risk for caries. Include frequent rinsing with plain water and use of a fluoride-containing toothpaste or mouth rinse as part of oral hygiene. Supervise children to avoid swallowing fluoride. Ask for a referral to an oral health care provider and/or gastroenterologist for prevention and treatment. Ask for sugarless medications when available.

Viral infections are usually due to the herpes simplex virus. Children rarely get herpetic gingivostomatitis or herpes labialis before six months of age. Herpetic gingivostomatitis is most common in young children, but may occur in adolescents and young adults. Viral infections can be painful and are usually accompanied by a fever. Counsel about the infectious nature of the lesions, the need for frequent fluids to prevent dehydration, and methods of symptomatic treatment.

Early, severe periodontal (gum) disease can occur in children with impaired immune systems or connective tissue disorders and inadequate oral hygiene. Simple gingivitis results from an accumulation of bacterial plaque and presents as red, swollen gums that bleed easily. Periodontitis is more severe and leads to tooth loss if not treated. Professional cleaning by an oral health care provider, systemic antibiotics, and instructions on home care may be needed to stop the infection. The parent/caregiver may need to help with daily toothbrushing and flossing and frequent appointments with an oral health care provider may be necessary.

Gingival overgrowth may be a side effect from medications such as calcium channel blockers, phenytoin sodium, and cyclosporine. Poor oral hygiene aggravates the condition and can lead to superimposed infections. Severe overgrowth can impair tooth eruption, chewing, and appearance. Ask an oral health care provider about prevention and treatment. A preventive regimen of antimicrobial rinses and frequent appointments may be needed. Consider alternative medications if possible.

Tips for Health Care Providers

- Take time to talk and listen to parents and caregivers.

- Tell parents and caregivers to seek a dental consultation no later than a child's first birthday.

- Seek advice on behavior management techniques; early intervention and familiarization with the dental team may take several visits.

- Evaluate and treat orthodontic problems early to minimize risk of more complicated problems later in life.

- Advise caregivers to avoid serving snacks at bedtime.

Part Four

Orthodontic, Endodontic, Periodontic, and Orofacial Procedures

Chapter 30

Orthodontia

Chapter Contents

Section 30.1

Orthodontia Overview

"All About Orthodontia," January 2011, reprinted with permission from www.kidshealth.org. Copyright © 2011 The Nemours Foundation. This information was provided by KidsHealth, one of the largest resources online for medically reviewed health information written for parents, kids, and teens. For more articles like this one, visit www.KidsHealth.org, or www .TeensHealth.org.

All about Orthodontia

Why Do People Need Braces?

Braces are a common and almost expected part of puberty (and many adults get braces, too). To better understand why braces and other orthodontic devices are needed, it helps to talk a bit about the teeth first.

As you made your way through childhood, your "baby" teeth fell out one by one, to be replaced by permanent, adult teeth. Although some people's adult teeth grow in at the right angle and with the right spacing, many people's teeth don't. Some teeth may grow in crooked or overlapping. In other people, some teeth may grow in rotated or twisted. Some people's mouths are too small, and this crowds the teeth and causes them to shift into crooked positions. And in some cases, a person's upper jaw and lower jaw aren't the same size. When the lower half of the jaw is too small, it makes the upper jaw hang over when the jaw is shut, resulting in a condition called an overbite. When the opposite happens (the lower half of the jaw is larger than the upper half), it's called an underbite.

All of these different types of disorders go by one medical name: malocclusion. This word comes from Latin and means "bad bite." In most cases, a "bad bite" isn't anyone's fault; crooked teeth, overbites, and underbites are often inherited traits, just like brown eyes or big feet are inherited traits. In some cases, things like dental disease, early loss of baby or adult teeth, some types of medical problems, an accident, or a habit like prolonged thumb sucking can cause the disorders.

Malocclusion can be a problem because it interferes with proper chewing—crooked teeth that aren't aligned properly don't work as well as straight ones. Because chewing is the first part of eating and digestion, it's important that teeth can do the job. Teeth that aren't aligned correctly can also be harder to brush and keep clean, which can lead to tooth decay, cavities, and gum disease. And finally, many people who have crooked teeth may feel self-conscious about how they look; braces can help them feel better about their smile and entire appearance.

If a dentist suspects that someone needs braces or other corrective devices, he or she will refer the patient to an orthodontist. Orthodontists are dentists who have special training in the diagnosis and treatment of misaligned teeth and jaws.

Most regular dentists can tell if teeth will be misaligned once a patient's adult teeth begin to come in—sometimes as early as age 6 or 7—and the orthodontist may recommend interceptive treatment therapy. (Interceptive treatment therapy involves the wearing of appliances to influence facial growth and help teeth grow in better, and helps prevent more serious problems from developing.) In many cases, the patient won't be referred to an orthodontist until closer to the teen years.

Diagnosis

Before giving someone braces, the orthodontist needs to diagnose what the problem is. This means making use of several different methods, including x-rays, photographs, impressions, and models.

The x-rays give the orthodontist a good idea of where the teeth are positioned and if any more teeth have yet to come through the gums. Special x-rays that are taken from 360 degrees around the head may also be ordered; this type of x-ray shows the relationships of the teeth to the jaws and the jaws to the head. The orthodontist may also take regular photographs of the patient's face to better understand these relationships.

And finally, the orthodontist may need an impression made of the patient's teeth. This is done by having the patient bite down on a soft material that is used later to form an exact model of the teeth.

Treatment

Once a diagnosis is made, the orthodontist can then decide on the right kind of treatment. In some cases, a removable retainer will be all that's necessary. In other rare cases (especially when there is an extreme overbite or underbite), an operation will be necessary. But in most cases, the answer is braces.

Braces straighten teeth because they do two very important things: stay in place for an extended amount of time, and exert steady pressure. It's this combination that allows braces to successfully change the position of teeth in a patient's mouth, through periodic adjustments by the orthodontist.

Different Types of Braces

An orthodontist can outfit patients with a few different kinds of braces. Some are made of lightweight metal and go around each tooth, while other metal ones are attached to the outside surfaces of the teeth with special glue.

Clear braces can be attached to the outside surfaces of the teeth, as can ceramic ones that are the same color as teeth. Some patients can get newer "mini-braces," which are much smaller, or "invisible braces," which are affixed to the inside surfaces of the teeth. In many cases, patients can choose which kind they want.

A recent addition to treatment options, braceless orthodontics, uses a series of clear removable appliances that are custom made and worn for specified amounts of time. These appliances exert pressure on the malpositioned teeth and move them gradually into their correct position.

How long each appliance in the series must be worn depends on the individual treatment plan the dentist or orthodontist creates. These appliances and the treatment plan are computer generated from the models of the teeth taken. Your dentist or orthodontist must decide if you are a candidate for this type of treatment since it is not right for everyone.

Correcting the position of the teeth often takes anywhere from six months to two or three years with any of the methods.

With braces, after the amount of time needed for correction has been established for the patient, the orthodontist must work on the other part of the treatment: making sure the braces exert steady pressure. To achieve this, the patient must come for regular visits, usually once a month or so. During the visits, the orthodontist attaches wires, springs, or rubber bands to the braces in order to create more tension and pressure on the teeth. Sometimes the rubber bands will connect certain teeth to one another to create a kind of opposing tension.

With some teens, the orthodontist may decide that extra tension is needed outside the mouth if braces alone aren't enough to straighten the teeth or shift the jaw. In such cases, a patient may need to wear head or neck gear with wires that attach inside the mouth and elastic that attaches the gear to the head. Many times, someone will only need to wear this type of gear while sleeping or in the evening, while at home.

It may take a while, but with the right combination and timing of wires, springs, rubber bands, and sometimes head gear, the teeth will slowly but surely move into their correct positions.

Some of the adjustments can make your mouth feel a bit sore or uncomfortable because the tension tends to make itself felt in more places than your teeth. Most of the time, taking ibuprofen or acetaminophen can help relieve the pain.

If you always have a lot of pain after your braces are adjusted, talk to your orthodontist about it; he or she may able to make the adjustments a bit differently.

Caring for Teeth with Braces

Your orthodontist will make sure that you know how to take special care of your teeth while your braces are on.

Braces, wires, springs, rubber bands, and other appliances can act like magnets for food and plaque, which can leave permanent stains on the teeth if not brushed away. Most orthodontists recommend brushing after meals with fluoride toothpaste and taking special care to remove food stuck in braces. Some orthodontists will also prescribe or recommend a fluoride mouthwash, which can get into places in a mouth with braces that a toothbrush can't.

Some people with braces find that they are more prone to canker sores (from the braces hitting the inside surface of the mouth). If this happens, an orthodontist may recommend an over-the-counter medicine that can be placed directly on the canker sore to help heal it. Wax can sometimes be applied to wires or braces that are causing irritation.

Faces after Braces

After what can seem like a long time to someone who has braces, the magic day finally comes: the orthodontist takes the braces off! After your teeth are cleaned thoroughly, the orthodontist may actually want to repeat the process of taking x-rays and impressions of the teeth. This allows the orthodontist to really check the work, and in the case of x-rays, see if wisdom teeth are now visible.

In some cases, an orthodontist may recommend that a patient have wisdom teeth removed if they do not appear to be coming in correctly after the braces have been removed. The reason? The wisdom teeth may cause the newly straightened teeth to shift and move in the mouth.

And speaking of teeth shifting and moving, a very important part of orthodontic treatment is retention, or keeping the teeth in their new place. The truth is that most teens, after wearing braces and going for adjustments for up to two years or longer, don't want anything to do with the orthodontist or having appliances in their mouths.

But even though the teeth have been successfully moved, they are still not completely stable—they need to settle in their corrected positions until the bones, gums, and muscles adapt to the change. This is usually accomplished with the use of retainers, which work by retaining the straight position of the teeth.

Some retainers are made of clear plastic and metal wires that cover the outside surface of the teeth, whereas others are made of rubber. Most retainers need to be worn all the time for the first six months, then usually only during sleeping. How long a retainer must be worn depends on the patient—one person might wear it for a few months, while another might have to wear it for several years.

Whatever the timeframe, retainers are very important; without them, the teeth could shift back into their old, crooked positions, making all the orthodontist's work and your years of patience useless!

The most important things to remember when you're feeling frustrated about having a face full of braces? That during every school photo where you can't be persuaded to open your mouth because of your braces, there are millions of other people experiencing the same thing.

And that no matter what, your braces will come off eventually—and you'll be left with a wonderful, straight smile.

Section 30.2

Invisible Braces

Braces for Adults and Teens

According to a Invisalign 2000 survey, 74% of American women and men believe that an attractive smile is important for getting their dream job, while 84% fell it is critical for their love lives.

Invisalign can give you the beautiful straight teeth you've always wanted. It works through a series of invisible, removable, and comfortable aligners that no one can tell you're wearing. You can smile during treatment as well as after.

What is Invisalign?

Invisalign can help you get the great smile you've always wanted because it is:

- Invisible, so no one can tell you're straightening your teeth. So now you can smile more during treatment as well as after.

- Removable, so you can eat and drink what you want while in treatment, plus brushing and flossing are no problem.

- Comfortable, because it has no metal to cause mouth abrasions during treatment. And no metal and wires usually means you spend less time in your doctor's office getting adjustments.

Invisalign also allows you to view your own virtual treatment plan when you start, so you can see how your straight teeth will look when your treatment is complete.

- Invisalign is the invisible way to straighten your teeth without braces.

- Invisalign aided by computer imagery uses a series of clear removable aligners to straighten your teeth without metal wires or brackets.

- Invisalign has been proven effective in clinical research.

How does Invisalign Work?

- You wear each set of aligners for about two weeks, removing them only to eat, drink, brush, and floss. Each set of aligners, move the teeth about 0.25 millimeters per aligner

- As you replace each aligner with the next in the series, your teeth will move—little by little, week by week—until they have straightened to the final position.

- You'll visit your dentist about once every 6 weeks to ensure that your treatment is progressing as planned.

- Total treatment time averages 9–15 months and the average number of aligners worn during treatment is between 18 and 30, but both will vary from case to case.

How Are Aligners Made?

- The aligners are made through a combination of your orthodontist's or dentist's expertise and 3-dimensional (3-D) computer imaging technology. You will be required to have full mouth vinyl polysiloxane impression, completed records and a panoramic x-ray, intra-oral photographs, and extra-oral photographs.

Table 30.1. A Comparison of Traditional Orthodontic Treatment and the Invisalign Technique

Factor	Traditional Orthodontics	Invisalign
Materials	Wires and brackets	Clear plastic trays "aligners"
Type of treatment	Broad range of orthodontic therapy	Most suitable for patients with certain orthodontic needs
Suitability	Suitable for many patients	Suited mainly for a vast majority of adults and for adolescents who have their permanent teeth.

Invisalign's distinct advantage to give you the great smile you have always wanted:

- Invisible, so no one can tell you are straightening your teeth. So now you can smile more during treatment as well as after.

- Removable, so you can eat and drink what you want while in treatment, plus brushing and flossing are no problem.

- Comfortable, because it has no metal to cause mouth abrasions during treatment. And no metal and wires means you spend less time in your doctor's office getting adjustments.

- Oral hygiene is improved.

- Invisalign allows you to view your own virtual treatment plan when you start, so you can see how your straight teeth will look when you treatment is complete.

- May reduce the risk of cavities and gum disease when compared to wire braces that trap food and plaque.

- Visit dentist only once every six weeks.

- Is usually faster than conventional braces.

- No metal braces.

- In most cases the aligners are doing multiple tooth movements simultaneously. Commonly, in conventional bracketing, some movements get ignored until another movement is completed by the current mechanics

- Work usually completed in 15 months conventional braces takes on the average of two years

Disadvantages of Invisalign:

- They are "not designed to treat patients with mixed dentition, changing a bite and/or growing palates, and therefore are not appropriate for children."

- All restorative work must be completed before or after the treatment.

- Designed to treat patients with less complex orthodontic needs.

- It is difficult to change this system after treatment has begun because this system is so exacting.

- The system is dependent on the patient wearing the retainers.

- May temporarily affect your speech.

- They are to be worn full time, day or night, except while eating and brushing or flossing.

- Teeth may be sore with a slight ache from the pressure especially for the first few days with each new aligner.

- After the work is completed you may have to wear a retainer at night.

- Need for good patient compliance.

- Cash up front is needed in order to assure that you will wear the aligners.

Costs

Invisalign typically costs $3,000 to $9,000.

American Association of Orthodontists states, "It is a very good additional tool....but there are many oral problems it cannot handle and it certainly does not replace braces." They work best if you already have "a good bite, small rotation, small gap, or a minor problem." "They will not work with biting or crowding problems and are not meant to be used with children."

Dentistry has moved beyond just treating the teeth and oral cavity. They can now give patients beautiful faces and alleviate a multitude of medical problems.

Braces for Adults

Options Available

Metal braces, made of high-grade stainless steel and attached to the front of teeth, are the most common. Some patients may complain about discomfort from metal brackets rubbing against the skin. If you experience any pain or discomfort, ask your dentist or orthodontist for some dental wax to place over the brackets.

Clear ceramic braces are worn on the front of the teeth just like traditional steel braces. Unlike metal braces, they blend with the color of the teeth for a much less noticeable appearance. They may look better but also may break more easily than metal braces.

Invisible braces are a series of clear, customized, removable appliances called aligners. Not only are these braces invisible, but they also are removable so they won't trap food and plaque between your teeth like metal braces. You'll wear each aligner for about two weeks and only remove it for eating, brushing, and flossing. This may be an option for individuals with mild spacing problems

The latest reports indicate that 25% of all individuals or one million adults wear braces. Benefits of braces for adults include the following:

- Reduce decay and gum disease due to crowding
- Relieve headaches and earaches
- Improve speaking, biting, or chewing problems
- Prevent or improve temporomandibular disorders (TMD) troubles

Disadvantage of braces in adulthood is that they take longer than teenagers. The average adult wears braces for 18 months to three years. Braces are custom-made appliances that use gentle pressure to straighten teeth and bite, this process can cause discomfort. The cost can range between $4,000–$9,000. However, Invisalign can reduce the length of time of wearing braces to 18 months or less and with less discomfort.

Remember that while wearing braces keep your teeth and brackets clean to reduce the risk of cavities. Avoid hard foods such as candy, raw carrots, corn on the cob, pretzels, nuts, popcorn, and crushed ice because they will damage or dislodge braces. Avoid sticky foods to decrease your risk of cavities.

How do I adjust to life with braces?

You probably will experience some discomfort or difficulty speaking or eating at first. While wearing braces, keep your teeth and brackets clean. If you wear cemented, non-removable braces, food and plaque can get trapped between teeth and gums. To reduce your risk of cavities, follow a regimen of brushing, flossing and rinsing, and reduce your consumption of sweets and carbohydrates. Plaque and sugar combine to make acid, which can cause decalcification (white spots) on teeth and tooth decay if left behind.

Which foods should I avoid?

It's a good idea not to eat foods that can damage or dislodge braces. Hard foods such as candy, raw carrots, corn on the cob, pretzels, nuts, popcorn, and crushed ice are off limits. Sticky foods to avoid include caramel, taffy, and gum. These foods can get stuck between teeth and gums or bend wires and knock bands or brackets loose. If this results in damage to braces, treatment may be extended.

Do I need to see my dentist during orthodontic treatment?

Yes. Remember that going to the orthodontist is not a substitute for regular dental checkups. If you're going to invest time and financial resources in a healthy smile, be prepared to go the distance to achieve results. That means you should consult your dentist for a schedule that's appropriate for you.

No matter your age, it is never too late to improve your dental health and beautify your smile Since braces are being worn by more adults.

Conventional Braces

Continuing research shows that health problems as varied as headaches and breathing problems may be related to abnormal alignments of the bones of the face and jaw. For example, a person with a long, narrow face is more likely to have problems breathing through his/her nose.

The key to successful diagnosis and treatment is early intervention should begin as early as possible. Many parents wait until children are in their teens before considering braces. But once a child reaches the age of 13, jaw development slows and there is limited room for growth.

When a child is treated between the ages of five and eleven, a dentist can redirect the child's growth and reduce the length of time that a child wears braces along with also alleviating problems such as headaches, jaw pain, earache, mouth breathing, and sleep apnea.

Braces are made of metal or plastic, braces include brackets attached to the teeth and wires that connect them. Pressure to move the teeth is created by adjusting the wires regularly.

The length of time a person wears braces depends on age, the severity of the problem, and the condition of the mouth. However, the average child wears braces for 18–30 months. After the braces are removed, a removable retainer must be worn for several months to hold the teeth in their proper position until they're more secure.

Wearing braces usually begins around age ten although braces can be worn at any age. A good thing is your smile is something you can change. Early orthodontic intervention, where appropriate, can make treatment more predictable. It can also help to alleviate that ugly duckling teeth phase much earlier, which can be helpful to a child's self-image as well.

When Braces Leave Scratches on Teeth

When a child has been wearing braces, it can be a shock for parents when they come off. Braces can leave scratches on teeth. Chinese researchers at Beijing Medical University found that brushing with a fluoride toothpaste promoted mineral deposits on teeth, and that the scratches were gone in a few weeks. Longer brushing time with three times a day regularity promoted fastest improvement.

Section 30.3

The Reality of Retainers

You've probably seen a kid in the cafeteria take out his retainer before eating lunch. Carefully, he places it in a plastic container to make sure that it's safe while he eats. You can tell that this small plastic and metal mouthpiece is important to him. You might wonder why. Let's find out.

What's a Retainer?

A retainer is a piece of plastic and metal that is custom-made for each individual kid who needs one. It fits the top of the teeth and mouth. No two retainers are alike, even though many look similar.

Retainers are really common. In fact, most people (kids and adults) who have braces have to wear a retainer for at least a little while after getting their braces taken off. Other people wear them to close gaps in their teeth, to help with speech problems, or to solve certain medical problems.

Why Do I Need to Wear a Retainer?

You might need a retainer for a few reasons. The most common reason is to help your teeth stay set in their new positions after wearing braces. It's important to wear your retainer because as your body grows, your teeth do some shifting. The retainer helps to control this shifting, which occurs naturally.

After your braces are removed, your orthodontist (a special dentist who helps straighten teeth and correct jaw problems) will fit you for a retainer and tell you how long to wear it and when. For example, you might have to wear it all day for three months but then only at night after that. Some kids may wear their retainer only at night right from the start, but they may have to wear it for more than a year. The retainer keeps the teeth in line and you won't even notice it while you're sleeping.

Other kids may wear retainers to close a space between their teeth or just to move one tooth. In these cases, braces aren't needed because retainers can do the job. Often, retainers will be worn for several years to close a space, for example, and then keep the gap closed by holding the teeth in place.

When you wear a retainer for any reason, certain teeth may feel pressure and might even feel sore for the first few days. If you experience this, don't worry—it's completely normal.

Retainers can help many mouth problems besides shifting teeth. Sometimes they're used to help a medical problem. For example, you may have a tongue thrust (a condition where your tongue sneaks through your teeth when you talk). Some retainers, known as a crib or tongue cage retainers, are designed with small metal bars that hang down from the roof of your mouth. These retainers keep your tongue from going forward in between your teeth when you speak. Your tongue is trained to go to the roof of your mouth instead of through your teeth. The length of time kids wear a tongue cage varies depending on the kid.

Another use for retainers is to help people with temporomandibular disorder (TMD). This disorder is usually a result of a bite problem (the teeth don't meet together properly when the jaws are closed) called malocclusion (say: mal-uh-kloo-zhun) or bruxism (say: bruk-sih-zum), which is grinding your teeth while you sleep. Grinding stretches the muscles and joints in your mouth and jaws and sometimes can cause jaw pain or headaches. Retainers can help you by preventing your mouth from closing completely at night, which keeps you from grinding your teeth.

Getting Fitted for and Wearing a Retainer

This is the easy part. Your orthodontist will fit you for the retainer using a material known as alginate (say: al-juh-nate). It's a chewy, chalky kind of thick liquid that makes a mold of your teeth when you sink them into it. The fitting process is fast, painless, and doesn't even taste bad—and you can choose from different flavors.

Your finished retainer can be designed to express your style and likes. Sometimes you can have a picture such as Batman, Christmas trees, or Halloween bats on the plastic part of the retainer. Once you've been fitted for the retainer, you usually have to wait less than a week to get the real thing.

You may think your retainer feels weird at first. That's normal. But see your orthodontist for an adjustment if the retainer causes pain, or cuts or rubs against your gums.

At first, you'll need to get used to talking with it in your mouth. Talking slowly at first is a good way to practice and eventually, you won't even notice it's there. Dentists advise reading aloud for several minutes each day. You may also notice an increased saliva flow (more spit in your mouth) in the first few days of wearing your new retainer, which is normal.

Caring for Your Retainer

Retainers live in your mouth along with bacteria, plaque, and left-over food particles. You should clean your retainer every day, but make sure to check with your orthodontist about how your type of retainer should be cleaned (some kinds shouldn't be cleaned with toothpaste). You can also soak it in mouthwash or a denture-cleaning agent to freshen it up and kill germs.

Because the plastic of your retainer can crack if it gets too dry, you should always soak it when it isn't in your mouth. Plastic can warp easily, so don't put it in hot water or leave it near a heat source—like on your radiator, for example. Finally, do not bend the wires. Flipping the retainer around in your mouth will cause the wires to bend.

One important way to take care of your retainer is not to lose it. They are expensive and your mom or dad might have to pay for lost or damaged retainers. Worse yet, they might ask you to help pay for a new one. So look before you dump your lunch tray and try to keep it in the same spot at home when you're not wearing it. In other words, retain your retainer!

Chapter 31

Endodontic Conditions and Treatment

Chapter Contents

Section 31.1

What Is Endodontic Surgery?

Why would I need endodontic surgery?

- Surgery can help save your tooth in a variety of situations.

- Surgery may be used in diagnosis. If you have persistent symptoms but no problems appear on your x-ray, your tooth may have a tiny fracture or canal that could not be detected during nonsurgical treatment. In such a case, surgery allows your endodontist to examine the entire root of your tooth, find the problem, and provide treatment.

- Sometimes calcium deposits make a canal too narrow for the instruments used in nonsurgical root canal treatment to reach the end of the root. If your tooth has this calcification, your endodontist may perform endodontic surgery to clean and seal the remainder of the canal.

- Usually, a tooth that has undergone a root canal can last the rest of your life and never need further endodontic treatment. However, in a few cases, a tooth may not heal or become infected. A tooth may become painful or diseased months or even years after successful treatment. If this is true for you, surgery may help save your tooth.

- Surgery may also be performed to treat damaged root surfaces or surrounding bone.

Although there are many surgical procedures that can be performed to save a tooth, the most common is called apicoectomy or root-end resection. When inflammation or infection persists in the bony area around the end of your tooth after a root canal procedure, your endodontist may have to perform an apicoectomy.

What is an apicoectomy?

In this procedure, the endodontist opens the gum tissue near the tooth to see the underlying bone and to remove any inflamed or infected tissue. The very end of the root is also removed. A small filling may be placed in the root to seal the end of the root canal, and a few stitches or sutures are placed in the gingiva to help the tissue heal properly. Over a period of months, the bone heals around the end of the root.

Are there other types of endodontic surgery?

Other surgeries endodontists might perform include dividing a tooth in half, repairing an injured root, or even removing one or more roots. Your endodontist will be happy to discuss the specific type of surgery your tooth requires.

In certain cases, a procedure called intentional replantation may be performed. In this procedure, a tooth is extracted, treated with an endodontic procedure while it is out of the mouth, and then replaced in its socket. These procedures are designed to help you save your tooth.

Will the procedure hurt?

Local anesthetics make the procedure comfortable. Of course, you may feel some discomfort or experience slight swelling while the incision heals. This is normal for any surgical procedure. Your endodontist will recommend appropriate pain medication to alleviate your discomfort.

Your endodontist will give you specific postoperative instructions to follow. If you have questions after your procedure, or if you have pain that does not respond to medication, call your endodontist.

Can I drive myself home?

Often you can, but you should ask your endodontist before your appointment so that you can make transportation arrangements if necessary.

When can I return to my normal activities?

Most patients return to work or other routine activities the next day. Your endodontist will be happy to discuss your expected recovery time with you.

Does insurance cover endodontic surgery?

Each insurance plan is different. Check with your employer or insurance company prior to treatment.

How do I know the surgery will be successful?

Your dentist or endodontist is suggesting endodontic surgery because he or she believes it is the best option for saving your own natural tooth. Of course, there are no guarantees with any surgical procedure. Your endodontist will discuss your chances for success so that you can make an informed decision.

What are the alternatives to endodontic surgery?

Often, the only alternative to surgery is extraction of the tooth. The extracted tooth must then be replaced with an implant, bridge, or removable partial denture to restore chewing function and to prevent adjacent teeth from shifting. Because these alternatives require surgery or dental procedures on adjacent healthy teeth, endodontic surgery is usually the most biologic and cost-effective option for maintaining your oral health.

No matter how effective modern artificial tooth replacements are— and they can be very effective—nothing is as good as a natural tooth. You've already made an investment in saving your tooth. The pay-off for choosing endodontic surgery could be a healthy, functioning natural tooth for the rest of your life.

Section 31.2

Root Canals

What is endodontic treatment?

Endo is the Greek word for inside and *odont* is Greek for tooth. Endodontic treatment treats the inside of the tooth.

To understand endodontic treatment, it helps to know something about the anatomy of the tooth. Inside the tooth, under the white enamel and a hard layer called the dentin, is a soft tissue called the pulp. The pulp contains blood vessels, nerves, and connective tissue, and creates the surrounding hard tissues of the tooth during development.

The pulp extends from the crown of the tooth to the tip of the roots where it connects to the tissues surrounding the root. The pulp is important during a tooth's growth and development. However, once a tooth is fully mature it can survive without the pulp, because the tooth continues to be nourished by the tissues surrounding it.

Why would I need an endodontic procedure?

Endodontic treatment is necessary when the pulp, the soft tissue inside the root canal, becomes inflamed or infected. The inflammation or infection can have a variety of causes: deep decay, repeated dental procedures on the tooth, or a crack or chip in the tooth. In addition, an injury to a tooth may cause pulp damage even if the tooth has no visible chips or cracks. If pulp inflammation or infection is left untreated, it can cause pain or lead to an abscess.

What are the signs of needing endodontic treatment?

Signs to look for include pain, prolonged sensitivity to heat or cold, tenderness to touch and chewing, discoloration of the tooth, and swelling, drainage and tenderness in the lymph nodes as well as nearby bone and gingival tissues. Sometimes, however, there are no symptoms.

How does endodontic treatment save the tooth?

The endodontist removes the inflamed or infected pulp, carefully cleans and shapes the inside of the canal, a channel inside the root, then fills and seals the space. Afterwards, you will return to your dentist, who will place a crown or other restoration on the tooth to protect and restore it to full function. After restoration, the tooth continues to function like any other tooth.

Will I feel pain during or after the procedure?

Many endodontic procedures are performed to relieve the pain of toothaches caused by pulp inflammation or infection. With modern techniques and anesthetics, most patients report that they are comfortable during the procedure.

For the first few days after treatment, your tooth may feel sensitive, especially if there was pain or infection before the procedure. This discomfort can be relieved with over-the-counter or prescription medications. Follow your endodontist's instructions carefully.

Your tooth may continue to feel slightly different from your other teeth for some time after your endodontic treatment is completed. However, if you have severe pain, or pressure or pain that lasts more than a few days, call your endodontist.

Endodontic Procedure

Endodontic treatment can often be performed in one or two visits and involves the following steps:

1. The endodontist examines and x-rays the tooth, then administers local anesthetic. After the tooth is numb, the endodontist places a small protective sheet called a dental dam over the area to isolate the tooth and keep it clean and free of saliva during the procedure.

2. The endodontist makes an opening in the crown of the tooth. Very small instruments are used to clean the pulp from the pulp chamber and root canals and to shape the space for filling.

3. After the space is cleaned and shaped, the endodontist fills the root canals with a biocompatible material, usually a rubber-like material called gutta-percha. The gutta-percha is placed with an adhesive cement to ensure complete sealing of the root canals. In most cases, a temporary filling is placed to close

the opening. The temporary filling will be removed by your dentist before the tooth is restored.

4. After the final visit with your endodontist, you must return to your dentist to have a crown or other restoration placed on the tooth to protect and restore it to full function.

If the tooth lacks sufficient structure to hold the restoration in place, your dentist or endodontist may place a post inside the tooth. Ask your dentist or endodontist for more details about the specific restoration planned for your tooth.

How much will the procedure cost?

The cost varies depending on how complex the problem is and which tooth is affected. Molars are more difficult to treat, the fee is usually more. Most dental insurance policies provide some coverage for endodontic treatment.

Generally, endodontic treatment and restoration of the natural tooth are less expensive than the alternative of having the tooth extracted. An extracted tooth must be replaced with a bridge or implant to restore chewing function and prevent adjacent teeth from shifting. These procedures tend to cost more than endodontic treatment and appropriate restoration. With root canal treatment you save your natural teeth and money.

Will the tooth need any special care or additional treatment after endodontic treatment?

You should not chew or bite on the treated tooth until you have had it restored by your dentist. The unrestored tooth is susceptible to fracture, so you should see your dentist for a full restoration as soon as possible. Otherwise, you need only practice good oral hygiene, including brushing, flossing, and regular checkups and cleanings.

Most endodontically treated teeth last as long as other natural teeth. In a few cases, a tooth that has undergone endodontic treatment does not heal or the pain continues. Occasionally, the tooth may become painful or diseased months or even years after successful treatment. Often when this occurs, redoing the endodontic procedure can save the tooth.

What causes an endodontically treated tooth to need additional treatment?

New trauma, deep decay, or a loose, cracked or broken filling can cause new infection in your tooth. In some cases, the endodontist may discover additional very narrow or curved canals that could not be treated during the initial procedure.

Can all teeth be treated endodontically?

Most teeth can be treated. Occasionally, a tooth can't be saved because the root canals are not accessible, the root is severely fractured, the tooth doesn't have adequate bone support, or the tooth cannot be restored. However, advances in endodontics are making it possible to save teeth that even a few years ago would have been lost. When endodontic treatment is not effective, endodontic surgery may be able to save the tooth.

Section 31.3

Endodontic Retreatment

Why do I need another endodontic procedure?

As occasionally happens with any dental or medical procedure, a tooth may not heal as expected after initial treatment for a variety of reasons:

- Narrow or curved canals were not treated during the initial procedure.

- Complicated canal anatomy went undetected in the first procedure.

- The placement of the crown or other restoration was delayed following the endodontic treatment.

- The restoration did not prevent salivary contamination to the inside of the tooth.

In other cases, a new problem can jeopardize a tooth that was successfully treated. For example:

- New decay can expose the root canal filling material to bacteria, causing a new infection in the tooth.

- A loose, cracked, or broken crown or filling can expose the tooth to new infection.

- A tooth sustains a fracture.

What will happen during retreatment?

First, the endodontist will discuss your treatment options. If you and your endodontist choose retreatment, the endodontist will reopen your tooth to gain access to the root canal filling material. In many cases, complex restorative materials—crown, post and core material—must be disassembled and removed to permit access to the root canals.

After removing the canal filling, the endodontist can clean the canals and carefully examine the inside of your tooth using magnification and illumination, searching for any additional canals or unusual anatomy that requires treatment.

After cleaning the canals, the endodontist will fill and seal the canals and place a temporary filling in the tooth. If the canals are unusually narrow or blocked, your endodontist may recommend endodontic surgery. This surgery involves making an incision to allow the other end of the root to be sealed.

After your endodontist completes retreatment, you will need to return to your dentist as soon as possible to have a new crown or other restoration placed on the tooth to protect and restore it to its full function.

Is retreatment the best choice for me?

Whenever possible, it is best to save your natural tooth. Retreated teeth can function well for years, even for a lifetime.

Advances in technology are constantly changing the way root canal treatment is performed, so your endodontist may use new techniques that were not available when you had your first procedure. Your endodontist may be able to resolve your problem with retreatment.

As with any dental or medical procedure, there are no guarantees. Your endodontist will discuss your options and the chances of success before beginning retreatment.

How much will the procedure cost?

The cost varies depending on how complicated the procedure will be. The procedure will probably be more complex than your first root canal treatment, because your restoration and filling material may need to be removed to accomplish the new procedure. In addition, your endodontist may need to spend extra time searching for unusual canal anatomy. Therefore, you can generally expect retreatment to cost more than the initial endodontic treatment.

While dental insurance may cover part or all of the cost for retreatment, some policies limit coverage to a single procedure on a tooth in a given period of time. Check with your employer or insurance company prior to retreatment to be sure of your coverage.

What are the alternatives to retreatment?

If nonsurgical retreatment is not an option, then endodontic surgery should be considered. This surgery involves making an incision to allow access to the tip of the root. Endodontic surgery may also be recommended in conjunction with retreatment or as an alternative. Your endodontist will discuss your options and recommend appropriate treatment.

What are the alternatives to endodontic retreatment and/ or endodontic surgery?

The only other alternative is extraction of the tooth. The extracted tooth must then be replaced with an implant, bridge, or removable partial denture to restore chewing function and to prevent adjacent teeth from shifting. Because these options require extensive surgery or dental procedures on adjacent healthy teeth, they can be far more costly and time consuming than retreatment and restoration of the natural tooth.

No matter how effective tooth replacements are—nothing is as good as your own natural tooth. You've already made an investment in saving your tooth. The payoff for choosing retreatment could be a healthy, functioning natural tooth for many years to come.

Chapter 32

Periodontal (Gum) Disease

Chapter Contents

Section 32.1

Facts about Periodontal Disease

Excerpted from "Periodontal (Gum) Disease: Causes, Symptoms, and Treatments," National Institute of Dental and Craniofacial Research (NIDCR), NIH Publication 10–1142, July 2011.

What Causes Gum Disease?

Our mouths are full of bacteria. These bacteria, along with mucus and other particles, constantly form a sticky, colorless plaque on teeth. Brushing and flossing help get rid of plaque. Plaque that is not removed can harden and form tartar that brushing doesn't clean. Only a professional cleaning by a dentist or dental hygienist can remove tartar.

Gingivitis

The longer plaque and tartar are on teeth, the more harmful they become. The bacteria cause inflammation of the gums that is called gingivitis. In gingivitis, the gums become red, swollen, and can bleed easily. Gingivitis is a mild form of gum disease that can usually be reversed with daily brushing and flossing, and regular cleaning by a dentist or dental hygienist. This form of gum disease does not include any loss of bone and tissue that hold teeth in place.

Periodontitis

When gingivitis is not treated, it can advance to periodontitis (which means inflammation around the tooth.) In periodontitis, gums pull away from the teeth and form spaces (called pockets) that become infected. The body's immune system fights the bacteria as the plaque spreads and grows below the gum line. Bacterial toxins and the body's natural response to infection start to break down the bone and connective tissue that hold teeth in place. If not treated, the bones, gums, and tissue that support the teeth are destroyed. The teeth may eventually become loose and have to be removed.

Risk Factors

- **Smoking:** Need another reason to quit smoking? Smoking is one of the most significant risk factors associated with the development of gum disease. Additionally, smoking can lower the chances for successful treatment.

- **Hormonal changes in girls and women:** These changes can make gums more sensitive and make it easier for gingivitis to develop.

- **Diabetes:** People with diabetes are at higher risk for developing infections, including gum disease.

- **Other illnesses:** Diseases like cancer or acquired immunodeficiency syndrome (AIDS) and their treatments can also negatively affect the health of gums.

- **Medications:** There are hundreds of prescription and over-the-counter medications that can reduce the flow of saliva, which has a protective effect on the mouth. Without enough saliva, the mouth is vulnerable to infections such as gum disease. And some medications can cause abnormal overgrowth of the gum tissue; this can make it difficult to keep gums clean.

- **Genetic susceptibility:** Some people are more prone to severe gum disease than others.

Who Gets Gum Disease?

People usually do not show signs of gum disease until they are in their 30s or 40s. Men are more likely to have gum disease than women. Although teenagers rarely develop periodontitis, they can develop gingivitis, the milder form of gum disease. Most commonly, gum disease develops when plaque is allowed to build up along and under the gum line.

How Do I Know if I Have Gum Disease?

Symptoms of gum disease include the following:

- Bad breath that will not go away
- Red or swollen gums
- Tender or bleeding gums
- Painful chewing

- Loose teeth
- Sensitive teeth
- Receding gums or longer appearing teeth

Any of these symptoms may be a sign of a serious problem, which should be checked by a dentist. At your dental visit the dentist or hygienist should do the following:

- Ask about your medical history to identify underlying conditions or risk factors (such as smoking) that may contribute to gum disease.
- Examine your gums and note any signs of inflammation.
- Use a tiny ruler called a probe to check for and measure any pockets. In a healthy mouth, the depth of these pockets is usually between 1–3 millimeters. This test for pocket depth is usually painless.

The dentist or hygienist may also do the following:

- Take an x-ray to see whether there is any bone loss.
- Refer you to a periodontist. Periodontists are experts in the diagnosis and treatment of gum disease and may provide you with treatment options that are not offered by your dentist.

Section 32.2

Types of Gum Disease

Periodontal (gum) diseases, including gingivitis and periodontitis, are serious infections that, left untreated, can lead to tooth loss. The word periodontal literally means "around the tooth." Periodontal disease is a chronic bacterial infection that affects the gums and bone supporting the teeth. Periodontal disease can affect one tooth or many teeth. It begins when the bacteria in plaque (the sticky, colorless film that constantly forms on your teeth) causes the gums to become inflamed.

Gingivitis

Gingivitis is the mildest form of periodontal disease. It causes the gums to become red, swollen, and bleed easily. There is usually little or no discomfort at this stage. Gingivitis is often caused by inadequate oral hygiene. Gingivitis is reversible with professional treatment and good oral home care.

Periodontitis

Untreated gingivitis can advance to periodontitis. With time, plaque can spread and grow below the gum line. Toxins produced by the bacteria in plaque irritate the gums. The toxins stimulate a chronic inflammatory response in which the body in essence turns on itself, and the tissues and bone that support the teeth are broken down and destroyed. Gums separate from the teeth, forming pockets (spaces between the teeth and gums) that become infected. As the disease progresses, the pockets deepen and more gum tissue and bone are destroyed. Often, this destructive process has very mild symptoms. Eventually, teeth can become loose and may have to be removed.

There are many forms of periodontitis. The most common ones include the following.

- **Aggressive periodontitis** occurs in patients who are otherwise clinically healthy. Common features include rapid attachment loss and bone destruction and familial aggregation.

- **Chronic periodontitis** results in inflammation within the supporting tissues of the teeth, progressive attachment and bone loss. This is the most frequently occurring form of periodontitis and is characterized by pocket formation and/or recession of the gingiva. It is prevalent in adults, but can occur at any age. Progression of attachment loss usually occurs slowly, but periods of rapid progression can occur.

- **Periodontitis as a manifestation of systemic diseases** often begins at a young age. Systemic conditions such as heart disease, respiratory disease, and diabetes are associated with this form of periodontitis.

- **Necrotizing periodontal disease** is an infection characterized by necrosis of gingival tissues, periodontal ligament, and alveolar bone. These lesions are most commonly observed in individuals with systemic conditions such as human immunodeficiency virus (HIV) infection, malnutrition, and immunosuppression.

Section 32.3

Older Adults Greatly Affected by Gum Disease

Oral Health and Older Adults

People are living longer and healthier lives. And, older adults also are more likely to keep their teeth for a lifetime than they were a decade ago. However, studies indicate that older people have the highest rates of periodontal disease and need to do more to maintain good oral health.

Whatever your age, it's important to keep your mouth clean, healthy, and feeling good. And it's important to know the state of your periodontal health.

- At least half of non-institutionalized people over age 55 have periodontitis.

- Almost one out of four people age 65 and older have lost all of their teeth.

- Receding gum tissue affects the majority of older people.

- Periodontal disease and tooth decay are the leading causes of tooth loss in older adults.

What you may not realize is that oral health is not just important for maintaining a nice-looking smile and being able to eat corn on the cob. Good oral health is essential to quality of life. Consider a few of the reasons:

- Every tooth in your mouth plays an important role in speaking, chewing, and in maintaining proper alignment of other teeth.

- A major cause of failure in joint replacements is infection, which can travel to the site of the replacement from the mouth in people with periodontal disease.

- People with dentures or loose and missing teeth often have restricted diets since biting into fresh fruits and vegetables is often not only difficult, but also painful. This likely means they don't get proper nutrition.

- Most men and women age 65 and older report that a smile is very important to a person's appearance.

- And, maybe most importantly, recent research has advanced the idea that periodontal disease is linked to a number of major health concerns such as heart disease, stroke, respiratory disease, and diabetes.

While your likelihood of developing periodontal disease increases with age, the good news is that research suggests that these higher rates may be related to risk factors other than age. So, periodontal disease is not an inevitable aspect of aging. Risk factors that may make older people more susceptible include general health status, diminished immune status, medications, depression, worsening memory, diminished salivary flow, functional impairments, and change in financial status.

Medications and Oral Side Effects

Older adults are likely to take medications that can impact oral health and affect dental treatment. Hundreds of common medications—including antihistamines, diuretics, pain killers, high blood pressure medications, and antidepressants—can cause side effects such as dry mouth, soft tissue changes, taste changes, and gingival overgrowth.

Dry mouth leaves the mouth without enough saliva to wash away food and neutralize plaque, leaving you more susceptible to tooth decay and periodontal disease. In addition, dry mouth can cause sore throat, problems with speaking, difficulty swallowing, and hoarseness. Your dentist or periodontist can recommend various methods to restore moisture, including sugarless gum, oral rinses, or artificial saliva products.

Be sure to tell your periodontist and other dental professionals about any medications that you are taking, including herbal remedies and over-the-counter medications.

Special Concerns for Older Women

Women who are menopausal or post-menopausal may experience changes in their mouths. Recent studies suggest that estrogen deficiency could place post-menopausal women at higher risk for severe periodontal disease and tooth loss. In addition, hormonal changes in older women may result in discomfort in the mouth, including dry mouth, pain and burning sensations in the gum tissue, and altered taste, especially salty, peppery, or sour.

In addition, menopausal gingivostomatitis affects a small percentage of women. Gums that look dry or shiny, bleed easily, and range from abnormally pale to deep red mark this condition. Most women find that estrogen supplements help to relieve these symptoms.

Bone loss is associated with both periodontal disease and osteoporosis. Osteoporosis could lead to tooth loss because the density of the bone that supports the teeth may be decreased. More research is being done to determine if and how a relationship between osteoporosis and periodontal disease exists. Women considering hormone replacement therapy (HRT) to help fight osteoporosis should note that this may help protect their teeth as well as other parts of the body.

Dental Implants

More and more older people are selecting dental implants over dentures as a replacement option for lost teeth. Whether you have lost one or all of your teeth, dental implants allow you to have teeth that look and feel just like your own.

Older adults have similar success rate with implants compared with younger people. As long as you're in good health and your periodontist can restore healthy gums and adequate bone to support the implant, you're never too old to receive a dental implant.

A dental implant is an artificial tooth root placed into your jaw to hold a replacement tooth or bridge in place. While high-tech in nature, dental implants are actually more tooth-saving than traditional bridgework, since implants do not rely on neighboring teeth for support.

In addition, dental implants are intimately connected with the gum tissues and underlying bone in the mouth. Therefore, they prevent the bone loss and gum recession that often accompanies bridgework and dentures and preserve the integrity of facial features. When teeth are missing, the bone which previously supported these teeth begins to deteriorate. This can result in dramatic changes in your appearance, such as increased wrinkles around the mouth and lips that cave in and lose their natural shape.

Since periodontists are the dental experts who specialize in precisely these areas, they are ideal members of your dental implant team. Not only do periodontists have experience working with other dental professionals, they also have the special knowledge, training, and facilities that you need to have teeth that look and feel just like your own. Talk with your periodontist to find out if dental implants are an option for you.

Denture Care

Denture wearers need to avoid plaque buildup that can irritate the tissues under the dentures. Thoroughly clean dentures daily and remove dentures at night to avoid bacteria growth. If you wear dentures, you need to continue to see a dental professional regularly. Because mouths continually change, dentures need to be checked for proper fit to avoid irritation, increased bone loss, and infections. A change in the fit of partial dentures could indicate periodontal disease.

Perfecting Your Smile

Cosmetic periodontal procedures are not just for people in their 20s and 30s. You can have the smile you desire at any age.

A study by the American Dental Association and Oral-B in 1998 found that nearly half of survey respondents age 65 and older selected a smile as the first thing they notice about people. Almost 80% in this age group also reported that a smile is very important to a person's appearance.

Preventing Periodontal Disease

Even if you've managed to avoid periodontal disease until now, it is especially important to practice a meticulous oral care routine as you age. Receding gum tissue affects a large percentage of older people. This condition exposes the roots of teeth and makes them more vulnerable to decay and periodontal infection.

To keep your teeth for a lifetime, you must remove the plaque from your teeth and gums every day with proper brushing and flossing. Regular dental visits are also important. Daily cleaning will help keep calculus formation to a minimum, but it won't completely prevent it. A professional cleaning at least twice a year is necessary to remove calculus from places your toothbrush and floss may have missed.

If you have dexterity problems or a physical disability, you may find it difficult to use your toothbrush or dental floss. Your dentist or periodontist can suggest options such as an electric toothbrush or floss holder or a toothbrush with a larger handle.

Treating Periodontal Disease

In the earlier stages of periodontal disease, most of the treatment involves scaling and root planing, which means removing plaque and calculus in the pockets around the tooth and smoothing the root surfaces. In most cases of early periodontal disease, scaling and root planing and proper daily home care are all that are required for a satisfactory result. More advanced cases may require surgical treatment.

Once you've been treated for periodontal disease, periodontal maintenance procedures or supportive periodontal therapy enables you to gain control of the disease and increase your chances of keeping your natural teeth. In addition to a dental examination, a thorough periodontal evaluation is performed. Harmful bacterial plaque and calculus are then removed from above and below the gum line. If necessary, root planing may be used to smooth root surfaces that are infected. In addition, your periodontist or other dental professional will review your at-home oral hygiene routine and may suggest modifications tailored for your condition.

Section 32.4

Treatment of Gum Disease

Excerpted from "Periodontal (Gum) Disease: Causes, Symptoms, and Treatments," National Institute of Dental and Craniofacial Research (NIDCR), NIH Publication 10–1142, July 2011.

How Is Gum Disease Treated?

The main goal of treatment is to control the infection. The number and types of treatment will vary, depending on the extent of the gum disease. Any type of treatment requires that the patient keep up good daily care at home. The doctor may also suggest changing certain behaviors, such as quitting smoking, as a way to improve treatment outcome.

Deep Cleaning (Scaling and Root Planing)

The dentist, periodontist, or dental hygienist removes the plaque through a deep-cleaning method called scaling and root planing.

Scaling means scraping off the tartar from above and below the gum line. Root planing gets rid of rough spots on the tooth root where the germs gather, and helps remove bacteria that contribute to the disease. In some cases, a laser may be used to remove plaque and tartar. This procedure can result in less bleeding, swelling, and discomfort compared to traditional deep cleaning methods.

Surgical Treatments

Flap surgery: Surgery might be necessary if inflammation and deep pockets remain following treatment with deep cleaning and medications. A dentist or periodontist may perform flap surgery to remove tartar deposits in deep pockets or to reduce the periodontal pocket and make it easier for the patient, dentist, and hygienist to keep the area clean. This common surgery involves lifting back the gums and removing the tartar. The gums are then sutured back in place so that the tissue fits snugly around the tooth again. After surgery the gums will heal and fit more tightly around the tooth. This sometimes results in the teeth appearing longer.

Bone and tissue grafts: In addition to flap surgery, your periodontist or dentist may suggest procedures to help regenerate any bone or gum tissues lost to periodontitis. Bone grafting, in which natural or synthetic bone is placed in the area of bone loss, can help promote bone growth. A technique that can be used with bone grafting is called guided tissue regeneration. In this procedure, a small piece of mesh-like material is inserted between the bone and gum tissue. This keeps the gum tissue from growing into the area where the bone should be, allowing the bone and connective tissue to regrow. Growth factors—proteins that can help your body naturally regrow bone—may also be used. In cases where gum tissue has been lost, your dentist or periodontist may suggest a soft tissue graft, in which synthetic material or tissue taken from another area of your mouth is used to cover exposed tooth roots.

Since each case is different, it is not possible to predict with certainty which grafts will be successful over the long term. Treatment results depend on many things, including how far the disease has progressed, how well the patient keeps up with oral care at home, and certain risk factors, such as smoking, which may lower the chances of success. Ask your periodontist what the level of success might be in your particular case.

Second Opinion

When considering any extensive dental or medical treatment options, you should think about getting a second opinion. To find a dentist or periodontist for a second opinion, call your local dental society. They can provide you with names of practitioners in your area. Also, dental schools may sometimes be able to offer a second opinion. Call the dental school in your area to find out whether it offers this service.

How Can I Keep My Teeth and Gums Healthy?

- Brush your teeth twice a day (with a fluoride toothpaste).

- Floss regularly to remove plaque from between teeth. Or use a device such as a special brush or wooden or plastic pick recommended by a dental professional.

- Visit the dentist routinely for a check-up and professional cleaning.

- Don't smoke.

Can Gum Disease Cause Health Problems beyond the Mouth?

In some studies, researchers have observed that people with gum disease (when compared to people without gum disease) were more likely to develop heart disease or have difficulty controlling blood sugar. Other studies showed that women with gum disease were more likely than those with healthy gums to deliver preterm, low birthweight babies. But so far, it is not been determined whether gum disease is the cause of these conditions.

There may be other reasons people with gum disease sometimes develop additional health problems. For example, something else may be causing both the gum disease and other condition, or it could be a coincidence that gum disease and other health problems are present together.

More research is needed to clarify whether gum disease actually causes health problems beyond the mouth, and whether treating gum disease can keep other health conditions from developing. In the meantime, it's a fact that controlling gum disease can save your teeth—a very good reason to take care of your teeth and gums.

Clinical Trials

Clinical trials are research studies of new and promising ways to prevent, diagnose, or treat disease. If you want to take part in a clinical trial about periodontal disease, visit http://clinicaltrials.gov. In the box under "Search Clinical Trials," type in: periodontal diseases. This will give you a list of clinical trials on gum disease for which you might be eligible.

Section 32.5

Medications for Periodontal Treatment

Excerpted from "Periodontal (Gum) Disease: Causes, Symptoms, and Treatments," National Institute of Dental and Craniofacial Research (NIDCR), NIH Publication 10–1142, July 2011.

Medications may be used with treatment that includes scaling and root planing, but they cannot always take the place of surgery. Depending on how far the disease has progressed, the dentist or periodontist may still suggest surgical treatment. Long-term studies are needed to find out if using medications reduces the need for surgery and whether they are effective over a long period of time. Here are some medications that are currently used:

Table 32.1. Medications Used for Treatment of Gum Disease

Medication	What is it?	Why is it used	How is it used?
Prescription antimicrobial mouthrinse	A prescription mouthrinse containing an antimicrobial called chlorhexidine	To control bacteria when treating gingivitis and after gum surgery	It's used like a regular mouthwash.
Antiseptic chip	A tiny piece of gelatin filled with the medicine chlorhexidine	To control bacteria and reduce the size of periodontal pockets	After root planing, it's placed in the pockets where the medicine is slowly released over time.
Antibiotic gel	A gel that contains the antibiotic doxycycline	To control bacteria and reduce the size of periodontal pockets	The periodontist puts it in the pockets after scaling and root planing. The antibiotic is released slowly over a period of about seven days.

Table 32.1. *continued*

Medication	What is it?	Why is it used	How is it used?
Antibiotic microspheres	Tiny, round particles that contain the antibiotic minocycline	To control bacteria and reduce the size of periodontal pockets	The periodontist puts the microspheres into the pockets after scaling and root planing. The particles release minocycline slowly over time.
Enzyme suppressant	A low dose of the medication doxycycline that keeps destructive enzymes in check	To hold back the body's enzyme response—If not controlled, certain enzymes can break down gum tissue	This medication is in pill form. It is used in combination with scaling and root planing.
Oral antibiotics	Antibiotic tablets or capsules	For short term treatment of an acute or locally persistent periodontal infection	These come as tablets or capsules and are taken by mouth.

Chapter 33

Dental Implants

Chapter Contents

Section 33.1

Dental Implants Result in Minimal Bone Loss

Dental implants are frequently used as a replacement for missing teeth in order to restore the patient's tooth function and appearance. Previous research demonstrates that the placement of a dental implant disrupts the host tissue in the area of the implant, so practitioners often focus their treatment planning to carefully maintain the patient's bone and gum tissue surrounding the implant. A study published in the *Journal of Periodontology* found that the majority of bone remodeling occurred in the time between the implant placement and final prosthesis placement.

Subsequently, little mean bone change was observed in the five years following the implant placement, independent of type of restoration or implant length. The study, conducted at the University of Texas Health Science Center at San Antonio, evaluated 596 dental implants placed in 192 patients over the age of 18. Patients were screened for adequate oral hygiene and bone volume. Exclusion criteria included heavy smoking, chewing tobacco use, drug abuse, and untreated periodontal disease, amongst others.

Study author Dr. David Cochran, DDS, PhD, Chair of the Department of Periodontics at the University of Texas Health Science Center at San Antonio, and President of the American Academy of Periodontology (AAP), believes that this study provides additional support for the use of dental implants to replace missing teeth. "As a periodontist, I am committed to saving my patients' natural dentition whenever possible. However, the results of this study help further indicate that a dental implant is an effective and dependable tooth replacement option. Since the patient's host tissue surrounding the dental implant largely remains unchanged in the five years following placement, the dental team can now focus on periodic assessment and treatment of other areas in the mouth as needed, and know that the implant is doing its job as a viable substitute solution."

Section 33.2

Replacement Teeth That Look and Feel Like Your Own

A dental implant is an artificial tooth root that a periodontist places into your jaw to hold a replacement tooth or bridge. Dental implants are an ideal option for people in good general oral health who have lost a tooth or teeth due to periodontal disease, an injury, or some other reason. While high-tech in nature, dental implants are actually more tooth-saving than traditional bridgework, since implants do not rely on neighboring teeth for support.

Dental implants are so natural-looking and feeling, you may forget you ever lost a tooth. You know that your confidence about your teeth affects how you feel about yourself, both personally and professionally. Perhaps you hide your smile because of spaces from missing teeth. Maybe your dentures don't feel secure. Perhaps you have difficulty chewing. If you are missing one or more teeth and would like to smile, speak, and eat again with comfort and confidence, there is good news. Dental implants are teeth that can look and feel just like your own. Under proper conditions, such as placement by a periodontist and diligent patient maintenance, implants can last a lifetime. Long-term studies continue to show improving success rates for implants.

What Dental Implants Can Do

- Replace one or more teeth without affecting bordering teeth.

- Support a bridge and eliminate the need for a removable partial denture.

- Provide support for a denture, making it more secure and comfortable.

315

Types of Implants in Use Today

- **Endosteal (in the bone):** This is the most commonly used type of implant. The various types include screws, cylinders, or blades surgically placed into the jawbone. Each implant holds one or more prosthetic teeth. This type of implant is generally used as an alternative for patients with bridges or removable dentures.

- **Subperiosteal (on the bone):** These are placed on top of the jaw with the metal framework's posts protruding through the gum to hold the prosthesis. These types of implants are used for patients who are unable to wear conventional dentures and who have minimal bone height.

Advantages of Dental Implants over Dentures or a Bridge

Every way you look at it, dental implants are a better solution to the problem of missing teeth.

- **Esthetic:** Dental implants look and feel like your own teeth. Since dental implants integrate into the structure of your bone, they prevent the bone loss and gum recession that often accompany bridgework and dentures. No one will ever know that you have a replacement tooth.

- **Tooth-saving:** Dental implants don't sacrifice the quality of your adjacent teeth like a bridge does because neighboring teeth are not altered to support the implant. More of your own teeth are left untouched, a significant long-term benefit to your oral health.

- **Confidence:** Dental implants will allow you to once again speak and eat with comfort and confidence. They are secure and offer freedom from the irksome clicks and wobbles of dentures. They'll allow you to say goodbye to worries about misplaced dentures and messy pastes and glues.

- **Reliable:** The success rate of dental implants is highly predictable. They are considered an excellent option for tooth replacement.

Are You a Candidate for Dental Implants?

The ideal candidate for a dental implant is in good general and oral health. Adequate bone in your jaw is needed to support the implant, and the best candidates have healthy gum tissues that are free of periodontal disease.

Dental implants are intimately connected with the gum tissues and underlying bone in the mouth. Since periodontists are the dental experts who specialize in precisely these areas, they are ideal members of your dental implant team. Not only do periodontists have experience working with other dental professionals, they also have the special knowledge, training and facilities that you need to have teeth that look and feel just like your own. Your dentist and periodontist will work together to make your dreams come true.

What Is Treatment Like?

This procedure is a team effort between you, your dentist, and your periodontist. Your periodontist and dentist will consult with you to determine where and how your implant should be placed. Depending on your specific condition and the type of implant chosen, your periodontist will create a treatment plan tailored to meet your needs

- **Replacing a single tooth:** If you are missing a single tooth, one implant and a crown can replace it. A dental implant replaces both the lost natural tooth and its root.

- **Replacing several teeth:** If you are missing several teeth, implant-supported bridges can replace them. Dental implants will replace both your lost natural teeth and some of the roots.

- **Replacing all of your teeth:** If you are missing all of your teeth, an implant-supported full bridge or full denture can replace them. Dental implants will replace both your lost natural teeth and some of the roots.

- **Sinus augmentation:** A key to implant success is the quantity and quality of the bone where the implant is to be placed. The upper back jaw has traditionally been one of the most difficult areas to successfully place dental implants due to insufficient bone quantity and quality and the close proximity to the sinus. Sinus augmentation can help correct this problem by raising the sinus floor and developing bone for the placement of dental implants.

- **Ridge modification:** Deformities in the upper or lower jaw can leave you with inadequate bone in which to place dental implants. To correct the problem, the gum is lifted away from the ridge to expose the bony defect. The defect is then filled with bone or bone substitute to build up the ridge. Ridge modification has been shown to greatly improve appearance and increase your chances for successful implants that can last for years to come.

What Can I Expect after Treatment?

As you know, your own teeth require conscientious at-home oral care and regular dental visits. Dental implants are like your own teeth and will require the same care. In order to keep your implant clean and plaque-free, brushing and flossing still apply.

After treatment, your periodontist will work closely with you and your dentist to develop the best care plan for you. Periodic follow-up visits will be scheduled to monitor your implant, teeth and gums to make sure they are healthy.

Section 33.3

Dental Implant Placement Options

A dental implant is an artificial tooth root that a periodontist places into your jaw to hold a replacement tooth or bridge. Dental implants are an ideal option for people in good general oral health who have lost a tooth or teeth due to periodontal disease, an injury, or some other reason. Dental implants are so natural-looking and feeling, you may forget you ever lost a tooth.

Under proper conditions, such as placement by a periodontist and diligent patient maintenance, implants can last a lifetime. Dental implants are intimately connected with the gum tissues and underlying bone in the mouth. Since periodontists are the dental experts who specialize in precisely these areas, they are ideal members of your dental implant team. Not only do periodontists have experience working with other dental professionals, they also have the special knowledge, training and facilities that you need to have teeth that look and feel just like your own.

Your periodontist and dentist will consult with you to determine where and how your implant should be placed. Depending on your specific condition and the type of implant chosen, your periodontist will create a treatment plan tailored to meet your needs.

Replacing a Single Tooth

If you are missing a single tooth, one implant and a crown can replace it. A dental implant replaces both the lost natural tooth and its root.

What are the advantages of a single-tooth implant over a bridge?

A dental implant provides several advantages over other tooth replacement options. In addition to looking and functioning like a natural tooth, a dental implant replaces a single tooth without sacrificing the health of neighboring teeth. The other common treatment for the loss of a single tooth, a tooth-supported fixed bridge, requires that adjacent teeth be ground down to support the cemented bridge.

Because a dental implant will replace your tooth root, the bone is better preserved. With a bridge, some of the bone that previously surrounded the tooth begins to resorb (deteriorate). Dental implants integrate with your jawbone, helping to keep the bone healthy and intact.

In the long term, a single implant can be more esthetic and easier to keep clean than a bridge. Gums can recede around a bridge, leaving a visible defect when the metal base or collar of the bridge becomes exposed. Resorbed bone beneath the bridge can lead to an unattractive smile. And, the cement holding the bridge in place can wash out, allowing bacteria to decay the teeth that anchor the bridge.

How will the implant be placed?

First, the implant, which looks like a screw or cylinder, is placed into your jaw. Over the next two to six months, the implant and the bone are allowed to bond together to form an anchor for your artificial tooth. During this time, a temporary tooth replacement option can be worn over the implant site.

Often, a second step of the procedure is necessary to uncover the implant and attach an extension. This small metal post, called an abutment, completes the foundation on which your new tooth will be placed. Your gums will be allowed to heal for a couple of weeks following this procedure.

There are some implant systems (one-stage) that do not require this second step. These systems use an implant which already has the extension piece attached. Your periodontist will advise you on which system is best for you.

Finally, a replacement tooth called a crown will be created for you by your dentist and attached to the abutment. After a short time, you will experience restored confidence in your smile and your ability to chew and speak. Dental implants are so natural-looking and feeling, you may forget you ever lost a tooth.

Replacing Several Teeth

If you are missing several teeth, implant-supported bridges can replace them. Dental implants will replace both your lost natural teeth and some of the roots.

What are the advantages of implant-supported bridges over fixed bridges or removable partial dentures?

Dental implants provide several advantages over other teeth replacement options. In addition to looking and functioning like natural teeth, implant-supported bridges replace teeth without support from adjacent natural teeth. Other common treatments for the loss of several teeth, such as fixed bridges or removable partial dentures, are dependent on support from adjacent teeth.

In addition, because implant-supported bridges will replace some of your tooth roots, your bone is better preserved. With a fixed bridge or removable partial denture, the bone that previously surrounded the tooth root may begin to resorb (deteriorate). Dental implants integrate with your jawbone, helping to keep the bone healthy and intact.

In the long term, implants are esthetic, functional, and comfortable. Gums and bone can recede around a fixed bridge or removable partial denture, leaving a visible defect. Resorbed bone beneath bridges or removable partial dentures can lead to a collapsed, unattractive smile. The cement holding bridges in place can wash out, allowing bacteria to decay teeth that anchor the bridge. In addition, removable partial dentures can move around in the mouth and reduce your ability to eat certain foods.

Replacing All of Your Teeth

If you are missing all of your teeth, an implant-supported full bridge or full denture can replace them. Dental implants will replace both your lost natural teeth and some of the roots.

How will the implants be placed?

First, implants, which look like screws or cylinders, are placed into your jaw. Then, over the next two to six months, the implants and the bone are allowed to bond together to form anchors for your artificial teeth. During this time, a temporary teeth replacement option can be worn over the implant sites.

Often, a second step of the procedure is necessary to uncover the implants and attach extensions. These small metal posts, called abutments, along with various connecting devices that allow multiple crowns to attach to the implants, complete the foundation on which your new teeth will be placed. Your gums will be allowed to heal for a couple of weeks following this procedure.

There are some implant systems (one-stage) that do not require this second step. These systems use an implant which already has the extension piece attached. Your periodontist will advise you on which system is best for you.

Depending upon the number of implants placed, the connecting device that will hold your new teeth can be tightened down on the implant, or it may be a clipped to a bar or a round ball anchor to which a denture snaps on and off.

Finally, full bridges or full dentures will be created for you and attached to your implants or the connecting device. After a short time, you will experience restored confidence in your smile and your ability to chew and speak.

Sinus Augmentation

A key to implant success is the quantity and quality of the bone where the implant is to be placed. The upper back jaw has traditionally been one of the most difficult areas to successfully place dental implants due to insufficient bone quantity and quality and the close proximity to the sinus. If you've lost bone in that area due to reasons such as periodontal disease or tooth loss, you may be left without enough bone to place implants.

Sinus augmentation can help correct this problem by raising the sinus floor and developing bone for the placement of dental implants. Several techniques can be used to raise the sinus and allow for new bone to form. In one common technique, an incision is made to expose the bone. Then a small circle is cut into the bone. This bony piece is lifted into the sinus cavity, much like a trap door, and the space underneath is filled with bone graft material. Your periodontist can explain your options for graft materials, which can regenerate lost bone and tissue.

Finally, the incision is closed and healing is allowed to take place. Depending on your individual needs, the bone usually will be allowed to develop for about four to 12 months before implants can be placed.

After the implants are placed, an additional healing period is required. In some cases, the implant can be placed at the same time the sinus is augmented.

Sinus augmentation has been shown to greatly increase your chances for successful implants that can last for years to come. Many patients experience minimal discomfort during this procedure.

Ridge Modification

Deformities in the upper or lower jaw can leave you with inadequate bone in which to place dental implants. This defect may have been caused by periodontal disease, wearing dentures, developmental defects, injury or trauma. Not only does this deformity cause problems in placing the implant, it can also cause an unattractive indentation in the jaw line near the missing teeth that may be difficult to clean and maintain.

To correct the problem, the gum is lifted away from the ridge to expose the bony defect. The defect is then filled with bone or bone substitute to build up the ridge. Your periodontist can tell you about your options for graft materials, which can help to regenerate lost bone and tissue.

Finally, the incision is closed and healing is allowed to take place. Depending on your individual needs, the bone usually will be allowed to develop for about four to 12 months before implants can be placed. In some cases, the implant can be placed at the same time the ridge is modified.

Ridge modification has been shown to greatly improve appearance and increase your chances for successful implants that can last for years to come. Ridge modification can enhance your restorative success both esthetically and functionally.

Chapter 34

Facial Trauma

Facial trauma is any injury of the face and upper jaw bone (maxilla).

Causes, Incidence, and Risk Factors

Blunt or penetrating trauma can cause injury to the area of the face that includes the upper jaw, lower jaw, cheek, nose, or forehead. Common causes of injury to the face include:

- automobile accidents,
- penetrating injuries, and
- violence.

Symptoms

- Changes in sensation and feeling over the face
- Deformed or uneven face or facial bones
- Difficulty breathing through the nose due to swelling and bleeding
- Double vision
- Missing teeth
- Swelling around the eyes that may cause vision problems

This chapter includes: "Facial Trauma," © 2012 A.D.A.M., Inc. Reprinted with permission. And, text excerpted from, "Dentists, Oral and Maxillofacial Surgeon: Job Description and Summary," NIH Office of Science Education Lifeworks, 2012.

Signs and Tests

The doctor will perform a physical exam, which may show:

- bleeding from the nose, eyes, or mouth, or nasal blockage;
- breaks in the skin (lacerations);
- bruising around the eyes or widening of the distance between the eyes, which may mean injury to the bones between the eye sockets.

The following may suggest bone fractures:

- Abnormal sensations on the cheek and irregularities that can be felt
- An upper jaw that moves when the head is still

A computed tomography (CT) scan of the head may be done.

Treatment

Patients who cannot function normally or who have significant deformity will need surgery. The goal of treatment is to:

- control bleeding,
- create a clear airway,
- fix broken bone segments with titanium plates and screws,
- leave the fewest scars possible,
- rule out other injuries,
- treat the fracture.

Treatment should be immediate, as long as the person is stable and there are no neck fractures or life-threatening injuries.

Expectations (Prognosis)

Patients generally do very well with proper treatment. You will probably look different than you did before your injury. You may need to have more surgery 6–12 months later.

Complications

General complications include, but are not limited to these:

- Bleeding

- Uneven face

- Infection

- Brain and nervous system problems

- Numbness or weakness

- Loss of vision or double vision

Calling Your Health Care Provider

Go to the emergency room or call the local emergency number (such as 911) if you have a severe injury to your face.

Prevention

Wear seat belts and use protective head gear when appropriate. Avoid violent confrontations with other people.

Oral and Maxillofacial Surgeons

Oral and maxillofacial surgeons do all kinds of surgery involving the mouth, teeth, jaws, and face. They reconstruct faces shattered by car accidents and gunshots, remove tumors and cancerous lesions, correct bites by surgically repositioning the jaws, place dental implants, repair cleft palates, perform all kinds of facial cosmetic surgery, and extract impacted wisdom teeth.

Oral and maxillofacial surgeons care for patients who experience such conditions as problem wisdom teeth, facial pain, and misaligned jaws. They treat accident victims suffering facial injuries, offer reconstructive and dental implant surgery, and care for patients with tumors and cysts of the jaws, and functional and esthetic conditions of the maxillofacial areas. With specialized knowledge in pain control and advanced training in anesthesia, the oral and maxillofacial surgeon is able to provide quality care with maximum patient comfort and safety in the office setting.

According to the American Board of Oral and Maxillofacial Surgery, board certified oral and maxillofacial surgeons provide the following services: "Oral and maxillofacial surgeons remove impacted, damaged, and non-restorable teeth. They also provide sophisticated, safe, and effective anesthesia services in their office including intravenous (IV) sedation and general anesthesia."

Dental implants: Oral and maxillofacial surgeons, in close collaboration with restorative dentists, help plan and then place implants used to replace missing teeth. They can also reconstruct bone in places needing bone for implant placement and modify gingival (gum) tissue surrounding implants when necessary to make teeth placed on implants look even more natural.

Facial trauma: Oral and maxillofacial surgeons care for facial injuries by repairing routine and complex facial skin lacerations (cuts), setting fractured jaw and facial bones, reconnecting severed nerves and ducts, and treating other injuries. These procedures include care of oral tissues, the jaws, cheek and nasal bones, the forehead, and eye sockets.

Pathologic conditions: Oral and maxillofacial surgeons manage patients with benign and malignant cysts and tumors of the oral and facial regions. Severe infections of the oral cavity, salivary glands, jaws, and neck are also treated.

Reconstructive and cosmetic surgery: Oral and maxillofacial surgeons correct jaw, facial bone, and facial soft tissue problems left as the result of previous trauma or removal of pathology. This surgery to restore form and function often includes moving skin, bone, nerves, and other tissues from other parts of the body to reconstruct the jaws and face. These same skills are also used when oral and maxillofacial surgeons perform cosmetic procedures for improvement of problems due to unwanted facial features or aging.

Facial pain including temporomandibular joint disorders: Oral and maxillofacial surgeons possess skills in the diagnosis and treatment of facial pain disorders including those due to temporomandibular joint (TMJ) problems.

Correction of dentofacial (bite) deformities and birth defects: Oral and maxillofacial surgeons, usually in conjunction with an orthodontist, surgically reconstruct and realign the upper and lower jaws into proper dental and facial relationships to provide improved biting function and facial appearance. They also surgically correct birth defects of the face and skull including cleft lip and palate.

Chapter 35

Corrective Jaw Surgery

Many oral and dental problems can be treated with orthodontic braces, tooth extractions, and similar measures. However, there are situations where this is not enough. In many of these cases, corrective jaw surgery may be the best solution.

Why Perform Corrective Jaw Surgery?

Corrective jaw surgery is different than most other dental procedures in that the shape of the jaw itself is changed, rather than just the positions of teeth. It is usually performed when there is a significant abnormality of the size and shape of the jaw. This can involve the upper jaw, lower jaw, or both, and may be isolated or part of a more complex facial deformity.

In some people, the jaw does not develop adequately during infancy or childhood (hypoplastic jaw), or in severe cases, may not form at all. One of the jaws can grow much larger than the other jaw, or one of the jaws can grow asymmetrically. In other cases, an injury can seriously damage or change the shape of the jaw and require reconstruction.

Abnormalities of the jaw can cause serious problems. Mismatch or asymmetry of the jaws may cause abnormal tooth wear, tooth loss, or pain with chewing. An overly short jaw can crowd the mouth and throat causing the airway to close during sleep and prevent normal breathing

"Corrective Jaw Surgery," by David A. Cooke, MD, FACP. © 2012 Omnigraphics, Inc.

(sleep apnea). Additionally, some jaw deformities can seriously affect the shape and appearance of a person's face.

Oral and maxillofacial surgeons usually perform corrective jaw surgeries. However, most procedures are collaborative efforts that also involve a dentist and an orthodontist. Altering the jaw can have major impacts on the mouth and teeth, and several different kinds of treatment may be needed in combination with the surgery.

Corrective jaw surgeries may be done in stages, and can take several years to be complete. Orthodontic braces are almost always necessary as part of a corrective jaw procedure. Otherwise, the teeth will not fit together properly after surgery. Most often, the orthodontics are done prior to the surgery, to prepare the teeth for the new shape of the jaw. Once the surgery has been performed, the teeth will fit perfectly their new positions.

Corrective jaw surgery is usually performed under general anesthesia, but may be performed in a hospital or an outpatient surgical center, depending upon the patient and the procedure. Most corrective jaw surgeries are performed through incisions inside the mouth and do not usually scar the face. However, some procedures do require incisions outside the mouth that can lead to visible scars.

Types of Corrective Jaw Surgery

There are many different kinds of jaw surgeries, each appropriate to different types of jaw and facial deformities. However, most of these procedures are variations on one of three basic types of surgery:

- **Upper jaw advancement (LeFort I osteotomy):** This surgery is used to correct an abnormality of the upper jaw, typically when it is too short relative to the lower jaw, or tilted at an angle. The upper jaw (maxilla) and palate are cut free from the rest of the skull and reattached in a new position using screws, plates, or bone grafts. This changes the shape of the face, and may improve bite, airway size, and appearance quite dramatically.

- **Mandibular shortening (mandibular osteotomy):** There are many varieties of this surgery, all of which involve cutting through the bones of the lower jaw, then resetting them in new positions. Depending upon the specific case, the jaw may also be split at the center of the chin and reoriented. Screws, plates, or bone grafts are used to fix the lower jaw into a new shape. This procedure is usually performed for a protruding lower jaw (prognathism) which can have significant effects on bite and appearance, depending on the severity.

- **Mandibular lengthening:** As with mandibular shortening, there are many variants of this kind of surgery. Generally speaking, the forward part of the lower jaw is cut free from the rear part, and the bone is reattached in a new position that lengthens the jaw. The jaw may also be split vertically at the chin to allow proper angling of the sides of the jaw. Plates, screws, and bone grafts may be used to hold the cut bones in place. There are also procedures that pull sections of the mandible apart and encourage new bone to form between them (distraction osteogenesis). Mandibular lengthening is usually performed to correct an overly short lower jaw (retrognathism), or disproportion between the upper and lower jaws. This can cause a striking improvement in appearance in people with so-called "weak chin."

Considerations for Corrective Jaw Surgery

If you are considering corrective jaw surgery, try to choose a surgeon who has performed many procedures of the type you are planning to undergo. Be sure to ask questions about your different surgical options, as well as any alternatives to surgery. Getting a second opinion from another surgeon is usually a good idea, and may help you feel more secure that you understand the choices and risks involved.

Pain and bruising are to be expected after corrective jaw surgery, although they are temporary and can usually be managed easily with medications. During the recovery period, it may be necessary to modify your diet and avoid heavy activity for a period of time. Initial recovery from these surgeries occurs within a few weeks, but full healing may take up to a year. Your surgeon can give you more detailed information on what you can expect for a given procedure.

Studies indicate that corrective jaw surgeries, in general, are quite safe. However, complications definitely can occur. In some cases, the bones may not heal together properly after surgery, or the bones can partially reabsorb. There can also be problems with the metal hardware used to hold the bones in place. The alveolar nerves, which provide sensation to the teeth and inside of the mouth, can be damaged during surgery. In procedures where bone grafting is performed, bone is often removed from the pelvis, and there can be problems from where the bone is taken. Excessive bleeding and infection are rare, but potentially serious.

Corrective jaw surgery often changes the appearance of the face, and in some cases can be quite dramatic. This usually improves appearance, but the change can have significant psychological effects on the patient. After corrective jaw surgery, seeing a different face in the mirror can affect a person's sense of identity. Most people adjust well to their changes, but some require psychological care after surgery.

Summary

Corrective jaw surgery can be highly useful in treating some jaw deformities and bite abnormalities that are too extensive to repair with other dental or orthodontic techniques. It can also be very effective for correcting some types of sleep apnea, and can have dramatic cosmetic benefits. A decision about corrective jaw surgery should never be taken lightly and requires careful consideration of the risks and benefits.

Part Five

Oral Diseases and Disorders

Chapter 36

Bad Breath (Halitosis)

Four Sources of Bad Breath

The Mouth

The mouth includes the teeth, the gums, and the top surface (dorsum) of the tongue, especially the very back of the tongue. Since this type of bad breath is the most common, its diagnosis and treatment will be covered extensively.

The term for odors from the mouth is fetor oris (not halitosis). Fetor means "a strong offensive smell" and is a generic term. Oris means "from the mouth." Fetor oris is a strong offensive smell originating specifically from the mouth. Fetor oris is the most common type of bad breath and accounts for about 80% of all cases. If you are young and generally healthy, the chances are good that your problem falls into this category.

The structures in the mouth that can harbor bad breath are:

- the teeth,
- the gums, and
- the tongue (especially the back of the tongue).

The Upper Respiratory Tract

The upper respiratory tract includes the nasal cavities, sinuses, throat, tonsils, and the larynx (voice box). The term for bad breath from the upper respiratory tract is ozostomia. Ozostomia is the second most common type of bad breath, and is most commonly associated with post-nasal drip, but can be associated with infections of the various organs in the upper respiratory tracts as well including sinusitis, sore throat, and laryngitis.

The Lungs or Stomach

Bad breath originating from the lungs is either a temporary phenomenon caused by consuming certain foods or drugs, or it is a chronic problem caused by disease processes.

Stomatodysodia is the term for bad breath caused by outright disease processes in the lungs, such as various infections, emphysema, bronchitis, or lung cancer.

Halitosis is the term for bad breath that results from:

- physiologic processes elsewhere in the body and carried to the lungs by the bloodstream; or,

- odors originating in the stomach and carried to the mouth by vomiting.

Bacteria and How They Produce Bad Breath—The Role of Anaerobic Bacteria in Fetor Oris

Eighty percent of all bad breath originates from bacterial overgrowth within, or upon structures in the mouth. If you are young, healthy, and do not suffer chronic sinusitis, tonsillitis, or laryngitis, chances are good that this section is the most relevant to your problem.

When someone has bad breath caused by structures in the mouth, the chemicals you actually smell are sulfur compounds created by anaerobic bacteria. Anaerobic bacteria grow in the absence of oxygen and they most easily colonize areas where there is some mechanism to limit exposure to oxygen. As a class, the chemicals these anaerobes produce are called volatile sulfur compounds (VSC), and they include such beauties as hydrogen sulfide (rotten egg smell), methyl mercaptan (smells like rotten cabbage, and is the chemical added to natural gas to give it a recognizable odor), and dimethyl sulfide (smells like decayed vegetables). There are over 400 types of bacteria found in the average mouth. Several dozen of these can cause bad breath when allowed to flourish. They metabolize proteins such as dead tissue cells, blood, and mucous. Proteins are made from building blocks called amino acids, and the digestion of these amino acids supply the bacteria with energy. Some of the amino acids contain sulfur, and these sulfur compounds are converted to VSC as a waste product.

A healthy mouth contains many different kinds of bacteria. In any given part of the mouth, they establish a sort of balance between the competing species of bacteria depending on the conditions there. A healthy mouth does not smell bad because the conditions in all parts of it encourage a balance of bacteria that does not cause odors. We call a healthy balance of bacteria a normal flora, or a normal floral pattern. There is a very wide range of floral patterns which are healthy. Everyone has a slightly different floral pattern. But when conditions in any area of the mouth change due to disease or other factors such as dehydration or the presence of fermentable substances such as blood, dead cells, and shreds of food, the balance of bacterial species shifts, allowing the overgrowth of anaerobic bacteria at the expense of the rest of the normal floral organisms. Thus odors begin to emanate from that area due to the production of VSC.

Chronic and Temporary Oral Conditions That Cause Fetor Oris

Before discussing the actual structures of the mouth that must be treated in order to cure fetor oris, it is necessary to understand that there are several chronic or temporary conditions that can shift the balance of microbial flora toward an overgrowth of the bacteria which produce VSC:

Xerostomia

Xerostomia is the technical term for dry mouth. Dry mouth dehydrates and concentrates the layers of salivary protein and mucous which coats the structures of the mouth. This concentration of mucous, saliva, and food detritus makes for overgrowth of all sorts of different bacteria in different parts of the mouth. In some areas of a dry mouth, anaerobic bacteria overgrow and produce serious amounts of volatile sulfur compounds. Other areas favor the overgrowth of aerobes which produce their own volatile waste products which can smell and taste nearly as bad as the VCS produced by the anaerobes. The most common type of bad breath caused by dry mouth is morning breath, which is a result of breathing through the mouth while sleeping. Some people tend to develop chronic dry mouth due to conditions such as Sjögren syndrome. Elderly people are also prone to dry mouth due partly to the ageing process, but mostly to the numerous drugs they consume which tend to cause dry mouth. Dry mouth is a separate problem with its own diagnostic and treatment protocols.

Drugs

Certain drugs tend to cause dry mouth and thus are a prime cause of chronic bad breath. These include both prescription and non-prescription drugs as well as both legal and illegal drugs.

Prescription and over-the-counter drugs that cause dry mouth include, but are not limited to:

- antihistamines (the older types such as Benadryl),
- antidepressants (older types such as Elavil and Flexeril),
- anticholinergics (often used as decongestants as well as surgical drying agents such as atropine and scopolamine),
- anorexiants (diet pills),
- antihypertensives (blood pressure meds),
- antipsychotics (psychiatric drugs),
- antiparkinson agents,
- diuretics (water pills),
- sedatives (sleeping pills).

Some drugs actually cause halitosis (odors not originating in the mouth, but resulting from metabolic processes elsewhere in the body). Recovery room and operating room personnel can all attest to the incredibly bad breath (originating from the lungs) exhaled by patients recovering from general anesthetic agents after operations. Phenergan is an antihistamine used as a sedative and to control nausea and vomiting in patients recovering from the DTs (delirium tremens caused by chronic alcohol addiction). Patients on this drug have a halitosis which can permeate entire hospital wards. Note that this type of bad breath is temporary, and only happens during sedation. It is not permanent since once the drug has left the bloodstream, the odor stops.

Illegal recreational drugs may also cause chronic dry mouth and thus are a source of bad breath. Illegal drugs have the added liability of lifestyle issues which interact with the dry mouth and make the bad breath much worse. Addicts and other recreational users often neglect their oral hygiene and use huge amounts of sugar leading to massive tooth decay. In addition, poor oral hygiene combined with poor nutrition causes gum disease. Both of these conditions are major causes of bad breath. The drugs most likely to cause problems in this category are the metabolic stimulants: cocaine, crack, ecstasy, and methamphetamines.

Heroin and marijuana are not metabolic stimulants; however, they predispose users to high sugar use and poor oral hygiene, and thus are associated with bad breath due to tooth decay and periodontal disease.

Chapter 37

Burning Mouth Syndrome

Burning mouth syndrome (BMS) is a painful, frustrating condition often described as a scalding sensation in the tongue, lips, palate, or throughout the mouth. Although BMS can affect anyone, it occurs most commonly in middle-aged or older women.

BMS often occurs with a range of medical and dental conditions, from nutritional deficiencies and menopause to dry mouth and allergies. But their connection is unclear, and the exact cause of burning mouth syndrome cannot always be identified with certainty.

Signs and Symptoms

Moderate to severe burning in the mouth is the main symptom of BMS and can persist for months or years. For many people, the burning sensation begins in late morning, builds to a peak by evening, and often subsides at night. Some feel constant pain; for others, pain comes and goes. Anxiety and depression are common in people with burning mouth syndrome and may result from their chronic pain.

Other symptoms of BMS include:

- tingling or numbness on the tip of the tongue or in the mouth,

- bitter or metallic changes in taste, and

- dry or sore mouth.

"Burning Mouth Syndrome," National Institute of Dental and Craniofacial Research (NIDCR), NIH Publication No. 11-6288, May 2011.

339

Causes

There are a number of possible causes of burning mouth syndrome, including:

- damage to nerves that control pain and taste;

- hormonal changes;

- dry mouth, which can be caused by many medicines and disorders such as Sjögren syndrome or diabetes;

- nutritional deficiencies;

- oral candidiasis, a fungal infection in the mouth;

- acid reflux;

- poorly-fitting dentures or allergies to denture materials; and

- anxiety and depression.

In some people, burning mouth syndrome may have more than one cause. But for many, the exact cause of their symptoms cannot be found.

Diagnosis

A review of your medical history, a thorough oral examination, and a general medical examination may help identify the source of your burning mouth. Tests may include:

- blood work to look for infection, nutritional deficiencies, and disorders associated with BMS such as diabetes or thyroid problems;

- oral swab to check for oral candidiasis;

- allergy testing for denture materials, certain foods, or other substances that may be causing your symptoms.

Treatment

Treatment should be tailored to your individual needs. Depending on the cause of your BMS symptoms, possible treatments may include:

- adjusting or replacing irritating dentures;

- treating existing disorders such as diabetes, Sjögren syndrome, or a thyroid problem to improve burning mouth symptoms;

- recommending supplements for nutritional deficiencies;

- switching medicine, where possible, if a drug you are taking is causing your burning mouth;

- prescribing medications to relieve dry mouth, treat oral candidiasis, help control pain from nerve damage, or relieve anxiety and depression.

When no underlying cause can be found, treatment is aimed at the symptoms to try to reduce the pain associated with burning mouth syndrome.

Helpful Tips

You can also try these self-care tips to help ease the pain of burning mouth syndrome.

- Sip water frequently.

- Suck on ice chips.

- Avoid irritating substances like hot, spicy foods; mouthwashes that contain alcohol; and products high in acid, like citrus fruits and juices.

- Chew sugarless gum.

- Brush your teeth or dentures with baking soda and water.

- Avoid alcohol and tobacco products.

Talk with your dentist and doctor about other possible steps you can take to minimize the problems associated with burning mouth syndrome.

Chapter 38

Cleft Palate

Chapter Contents

Section 38.1

Understanding Craniofacial Defects

Excerpted from "July: National Cleft and Craniofacial
Awareness and Prevention Month," Centers for Disease Control
and Prevention (CDC), July 11, 2011.

Craniofacial defects—such as orofacial clefts, craniosynostosis, and microtia, and anotia—have a significant public health impact.

Craniofacial defects are conditions present at birth that affect the structure and function of a baby's head and face. Two of the most common craniofacial defects are orofacial clefts which occur when the lip and mouth do not form properly, and craniosynostosis which happens when the bones in the baby's skull fuse too early. Microtia is when the external portion of the ear does not form properly, and anotia occurs when the external portion of the ear is missing. Treatments and services for children with craniofacial defects can vary depending on the severity of the defect; the presence of associated syndromes or other birth defects, or both; as well as, the child's age and other medical or developmental needs. Children with certain craniofacial defects can have a greater risk for physical, learning, developmental, or social challenges, or a mix of these. Craniofacial defects have significant effects on families and the health care system:

- Each year, about 4,400 infants in the United States are born with a cleft lip with or without a cleft palate, and about 2,700 infants are born with a cleft palate alone.

- About four infants per 10,000 live-births in the metropolitan Atlanta, Georgia, area are born with craniosynostosis.

- Recent studies have found that direct medical and health care use and average costs per child were a lot higher for children with orofacial clefts than for children of the same age without these conditions.

Recently, Centers for Disease Control and Prevention (CDC) researchers and National Birth Defects Prevention Study (NBDPS) partners have reported important findings about some risk factors for craniofacial defects:

- **Diabetes:** Women who have diabetes before they get pregnant have been shown to be more at risk of having a baby with anotia or microtia or a cleft lip with or without cleft palate.

- **Smoking:** Women who smoke anytime during the month before they get pregnant through the end of the third month of pregnancy have been shown to be more likely to have a baby with a cleft lip with or without cleft palate.

- **Maternal thyroid disease:** Women with thyroid disease or who are treated for thyroid disease while they are pregnant have been shown to be at higher risk of having an infant with craniosynostosis.

- **Certain medications:** Women who report using clomiphene citrate (a fertility medication) just before or early in pregnancy have been shown to be more likely to have a baby with craniosynostosis.

Section 38.2

Choosing a Cleft Palate or Craniofacial Team

Throughout the United States there are many qualified health professionals caring for children with cleft lip and palate as well as other craniofacial anomalies. However, because these children frequently require a variety of services which need to be provided in a coordinated manner over a period of years, you may want to search for an interdisciplinary team of specialists. The principal role of the interdisciplinary team is to provide integrated case management for your child and to assure the quality and continuity of care and long-term follow-up. Here are some points to consider when selecting a team:

The Number of Different Specialists Who Participate on the Team

The more specialists participating on the team, the more likely every aspect of treatment can be considered during the team evaluation. The specific staff will be determined by the availability of qualified personnel and by the types of patients served by the team. When the team cannot provide all the services required by its patients, team members are responsible for making appropriate referrals, and for communicating with those to whom patients are referred. This arrangement will allow treatment plans to be coordinated and carried out in an efficient manner.

Although not all patients will need each type of specialist, the team may include:

- an audiologist (who assesses hearing);

- a surgeon (such as a plastic surgeon, an oral/maxillofacial surgeon, a craniofacial surgeon, or a neurosurgeon);

- a pediatric dentist or other dental specialist (for example: a prosthodontist who makes prosthetic devices for the mouth);

346

- an orthodontist (who straightens the teeth and aligns the jaws);

- a geneticist (who screens patients for craniofacial syndromes and helps parents and adult patients understand the chances of having more children with these conditions);

- a nurse (who helps with feeding problems and provides ongoing supervision of the child's health);

- an otolaryngologist (an ear, nose, and throat doctor, or ENT);

- a pediatrician (to monitor overall health and development);

- a psychologist, social worker, or other mental health specialist (to support the family and assess any adjustment problems);

- a speech-language pathologist (who assesses not only speech but also feeding problems); and

- other necessary specialists who treat specific aspects of complex craniofacial anomalies.

When these specialists work together and with the family as an interdisciplinary team, treatment goals can be individualized for each child, and parents and health care providers can make the best choices for treatment by consulting with each other. Because growth is a significant factor in the ultimate outcome of treatment, the child must be assessed thoroughly and regularly by the team until young adulthood.

The *Parameters for Evaluation and Treatment of Patients with Cleft Lip / Palate or Other Craniofacial Anomalies* document summarizes the current guidelines for team care endorsed by the American Cleft Palate-Craniofacial Association. By adhering to these guidelines, teams are promoting the best possible outcome for children born with clefts or other craniofacial birth defects.

Qualifications of the Individual Members on the Team

All the professionals on the team should be fully trained and appropriately certified and licensed. This issue may impact your insurance coverage, as well as the quality of care the team can deliver.

Experience of the Team

Each team must take responsibility for assuring that team members not only possess appropriate and current credentials but also have requisite experience in evaluation and treatment of patients with cleft lip/palate and other craniofacial anomalies. You should ask how often the team meets and approximately how many patients are seen at each meeting. You may also want to try to determine how long this group of professionals has been meeting as a team, and also how much experience the various individual professionals have had.

Location of the Team

The distance of the team from your home may not be an important consideration in choosing a team. In general, the team will be seeing your child only periodically throughout his or her growing years. Usually routine treatment such as general dental care, orthodontics, speech therapy, and pediatric care will be provided by professionals in your own community who will be in regular contact with professionals on the team. Your travel to a team will usually be limited to several trips a year or even once a year.

Affiliation of the Team and Its Members

You may want to ask if the team is listed with the American Cleft Palate-Craniofacial Association (ACPA) and how many of the individual members of the team are also members of ACPA. Staying current with recent developments in the field is one sign of a conscientious and concerned health care professional. You may also want to determine whether the team has any relationship to an established hospital or to a medical school or university. Facilities for diagnostic studies and treatment are often better with such an affiliation.

Communication with the Team

Your child may require care over a period of years, so you want to make sure you are comfortable communicating and working with the members of the team. Treatment recommendations should be communicated to you in writing as well as in face-to-face discussion. The team should assist you in locating parent-patient support groups and any other sources for services that are either not provided by the team itself or are better provided at the community level.

Section 38.3

Frequently Asked Questions about Cleft Lip and Cleft Palate

A to Z: What's First?

If there's a baby in your world, congratulations! If the baby is affected by cleft issues, there are a few things to think about, a few things to do, and a few pieces of information that may be helpful to you as you and baby begin your life together:

- **Take a deep breath:** Both before and after their arrival, babies can be exhausting. Learning that your family's newest addition may bring some unexpected experiences along with his or her arrival can take a bit of adjustment. Catch your breath, encourage family members and friends to do the same, and remember that medical communities and hospitals all over the world offer great care for cleft issues.

- **Identify treatment teams in your area:** You may call, email, or link online to the Geographical Listing of Cleft and Craniofacial Teams to find a cleft palate-craniofacial treatment team in your region.

- **Request booklets and brochures for parents of newborns:** E-mail Cleft Palate Foundation, or call, 800-242-5338. Provide your name, phone number, mailing address, and e-mail address.

What is cleft lip and cleft palate?

A cleft lip is an opening in the lip. A cleft palate is an opening in the roof of the mouth. Clefts result from incomplete development of the lip or palate while the baby is forming before birth. Babies' lips and palates develop separately during the first three months of pregnancy. In most cases, the left and right parts of the lip come together, or fuse, creating the two vertical lines on the normal upper lip. In a similar way, the left and right parts of the palate come together to create a normal palate. The front-to-back line that can usually be seen along the roof of a normal mouth indicates where fusion occurred.

Why didn't our baby's mouth fully develop?

We don't know the answer to this question, but it was not because you did something wrong. Sometimes clefts run in families, and in many cases, they rely on genetic predisposition. Some clefts occur in combination with other problems and are associated with a syndrome. It was not your fault. Scientists have learned that there are many possible causes for clefts. Research is under way to discover more about these causes.

How many babies are born with clefts?

Cleft lip and/or palate make up the most common birth defect in the United States. Approximately one out of every 594 newborns, or over 6,800 children, per year in the U.S. is affected by cleft lip and/or palate.

What can be done to help our baby?

A cleft lip can usually be repaired in the first few months of life. A cleft palate can usually be repaired some months later. The exact timing of these repairs depends on the baby's health and considerations of his or her future development, as determined by the doctor who performs the surgery.

Can our baby be fed properly?

Some babies with clefts have very few or no problems feeding, while others have more difficulty. Use of special bottles and careful positioning of the baby are sometimes helpful modifications. Your pediatrician will give you proper guidance.

Will our baby's teeth grow properly?

If the cleft affects only the lip, the teeth will probably not be affected. If the cleft affects the gums where the teeth grow, your baby will probably need the care of dental specialists.

Will our baby have trouble learning to talk?

If the cleft affects only the lip, speech problems are unlikely. However, many children with cleft palate need the help of a speech pathologist, and some may need an additional operation to improve their speech. The goal is to help the child develop normal speech as soon as possible.

Will our baby be mentally retarded?

There is no relationship between mental retardation and cleft lip and palate. However, if the cleft is part of a cluster of other problems (a syndrome), learning ability is sometimes affected.

How can we pay for the treatment our baby will need?

Health insurance will pay for all or part of the necessary care. Additional financial assistance may be available from an agency in your state which is supported by your tax dollars. Your family physician can direct you to the proper agency.

How do other parents feel when their child is born with a cleft?

It is natural for parents to feel upset at this time. Feelings of concern, anxiety, and grief are not unusual. Your family physician and the hospital staff members will guide you to a team of specialists who can provide you and your baby with the help you will need.

How can we tell our relatives and friends about the baby's cleft?

Most new parents feel that this is a difficult task. Although you may feel uncomfortable, it is important that you tell relatives and friends as soon as possible. Try to be as direct and honest as you can. Your baby is much more than his or her cleft, and everyone needs to remember that. If the people closest to you can visit while the mother and baby are still in the hospital, this is often helpful. You may want to use this chapter to answer their questions.

I've read the word hare lip what does it mean?

The word hare refers to a rabbit, which has a natural indentation in the center of its lip. The term is rarely used by professionals, because it is inaccurate and insensitive. Cleft lip is the correct description of the condition.

How can I get more information?

The Cleft Palate Foundation (CPF) has a number of publications for parents of children with clefts, including booklets on infant feeding, on the child from birth to four years, on the school-aged child, and on genetics. Modern care of a child born with a cleft lip or cleft palate is best managed by a team of medical, dental, speech, and other specialists. Ask your doctor to refer you to a cleft palate team in your community or state, or call 800-242-5338 to help locate one.

Section 38.4

Breastfeeding Children with Cleft Palate

"What about Breastfeeding?" © 2009 Cleft Palate Foundation
(www.cleftline.org). All rights reserved. Reprinted with permission.

What You Should Know

Le Leche League International advises that, "except in rare cases, a baby with a cleft palate cannot get all the milk he needs by breastfeeding alone. An opening in the palate makes it impossible for the baby to seal off his mouth and make the suction typically used to keep the breast (or bottle) in place and pull the nipple to the back of his mouth. Over time, lactation consultants have found that feeding exclusively at the breast is a difficult goal for all but a few babies with uncorrected cleft palates." Source: *Breastfeeding a Baby with a Cleft Lip or Cleft Palate*, La Leche League International, November 2004.

What You Can Do

Learning that breastfeeding is an unlikely option can be a source of disappointment and sadness for some families. Give yourself time and space to grieve this loss. But remember, you can still share many benefits of breastfeeding with your child:

- Express breast milk with a pump, but feed your baby with one of the bottle-feeding methods described in both the video and booklet, *Feeding Your Baby* by Cleft Palate Foundation (CPF).

- During feedings, make sure that you both enjoy eye-to-eye and skin-to-skin contact whenever possible.

- Once your baby has become successful feeding on a bottle, your baby may be put to the breast for non-nutritive sucking. Non-nutritive sucking at the breast can be a satisfying experience for both moms and babies.

- Non-nutritive sucking exercises and stimulates important muscles in your baby's mouth and tongue, and can facilitate the bonding experience. It may also help stimulate milk production for those moms who continue to pump breast milk.

What You Need

A hospital-grade breast pump: Your lactation consultant, hospital pharmacy, or local medical supply business are good places to ask for sales and rental information for these machines.

Cleft palate nurser: Your treatment team will include a feeding specialist who will help you determine which cleft palate nurser or other feeding system works best for you and your baby.

Support system: Ask a spouse, partner, other family member, or friend to help care for you and your baby while you are learning how to use the breast pump and feed your baby.

Time: Learning to feed a baby with a cleft can be challenging. Learning to feed a baby with a cleft while learning to use a breast pump can be overwhelming. Allow your support system to help you make time to relax and explore how the pump best works for you.

Know When to Say When

Once you're home, experiment with a hospital-grade breast pump for a few days, use your support system, and take time to learn to express milk and feed your baby. If you decide that the pumping process isn't becoming easier or doesn't fit with the demands of work and/or other children, you may be ready to let it go. You can be pleased that you explored the possibility as fully as you could. Make the decision to move on to feeding with formula with the same love and care as breastfeeding.

Section 38.5

Questions about Scars from Cleft Palate Surgeries

Why is my child's scar red?

All new scars are red, more so in some people than in others. When the body first begins to heal a wound, it produces a lot of scar tissue. In order to nourish this healing process, the body creates many tiny blood vessels to bring in a temporary supply of extra blood, causing a red color. Scars in children typically get progressively red for perhaps three months. During this time the scar will often be raised off the skin and fairly stiff to the touch. Reaching a peak after several months, the scar gradually fades, softens, and flattens.

What will the scar look like?

Eventually, the scar should become a soft flat white line.

When will the scar go away?

Once there is a scar, it is there forever. However, when the scar matures it should be much less noticeable than when it was new. Some people heal with less obvious scars than others, so that the scar may be very fine or, at the other extreme, very wide. Most people's scars are fairly thin but not hairline. Normally, scars take 12 to 18 months to fully mature.

Will applications of vitamin E to the scar help?

Many people believe that there are special healing qualities to vitamin E, aloe vera, or cocoa butter. In fact, there is no consistent evidence that these will truly improve the long-term appearance of the scar. Since a normal scar will spontaneously improve, some people mistakenly think that the improvement is due to the vitamin E they are applying. Although we do not recommend the use of vitamin E, there is no evidence that it will do any harm. Therefore, aside from the very small risk of a skin allergy to vitamin E, there is no known ill effect that will result if you wish to use it. However, it should be avoided during the first two weeks after surgery.

What can I do to make it look better?

Since the scar will be getting better by itself, mostly you just need to wait. However, many doctors believe that applying sun screen for three or four months after surgery is beneficial because some people can develop permanent excess color in a scar as a result of early sun exposure.

My child's operation was two years ago. What can be done to make the scar less visible?

Once the scar has matured (become soft and white), it should not be expected to undergo further spontaneous changes. However, sometimes the scar is not as refined as might be possible. In this situation, your surgeon may recommend cutting out and re-closing a portion of the scar in an attempt to make it thinner or more level with the surrounding skin. Another treatment that might be recommended is dermabrasion, a process of sanding down the scar surface, again in an effort to make it more level with the surrounding skin.

What is a keloid?

A keloid is a tumor of scar tissue that can develop when the body continues to make scar tissue for many months or even years, rather than maturing normally and becoming white and flat. A keloid is a scar that is permanently red, hard, and raised. Fortunately, these are fairly rare. Your surgeon can tell you more about keloids.

Section 38.6

Information for
Adults with Clefts

Getting Along with Others

Attitudes toward Adults with Visible Difference

As an adult with a cleft you have lived all your life with the residual scars of the cleft surgery. The extent of facial scarring from a repaired cleft varies from person to person. The impact of having a visible difference is also very individual.

Perhaps you have been able to accept your visible differences. Facial scars have faded into the background of awareness and do not play a pivotal role when interacting with friends, colleagues, or other individuals with whom you have long-term relationships. Nevertheless, you may still experience irritation or a twinge of self-consciousness when someone asks about your scar, or when you notice that someone is looking a bit too long. Why is this?

If you have ever taken time to really study the appearance of others, you have probably realized that people come in many different sizes, shapes, and degrees of attractiveness. Yet as variable as appearance is, most people can walk into a room without drawing attention to themselves. However, this may not be the case for a person with visible scarring or asymmetry of facial features. If you have a visible difference, it is more difficult to fade into the crowd.

Looking different carries with it a particular social burden. There are social conventions for most interpersonal interactions. That is, people know how to behave, what to say, or what not to say in a social interaction. However, people feel quite self-conscious when they are in conversation for the first time with someone who looks different. They are uncertain about where to look or whether they should ignore the difference or acknowledge it by asking a question.

You may have already learned there are ways to help other people become more comfortable with your facial difference. While it may feel unfair, often in initial encounters the responsibility for establishing a comfortable relationship with another person will fall to you. When you are introduced to a new person, you may be able to ease the situation by looking directly at the other person, meeting his or her eyes, and smiling. At other times, a confident but brief explanation of your facial difference may be in order. Still other situations call for a humorous response. What is important is that you have several techniques you can use to help put the other person at ease and thus help you both to move on to other areas of conversation.

In order to handle social interactions comfortably and confidently, you must feel good about yourself. For some adults, the memories of teasing and social exclusion they experienced during their school years make it very difficult for them to feel socially confident. Some adults continue to be embarrassed about their appearance or feel angry because they were born with a cleft. If you have feelings which you believe interfere with your ability to get along with other people, be successful at work, or interact comfortably in romantic relationships, you are not alone. Joining a support group may provide you with the opportunity to interact with individuals who have had similar experiences. Professional counseling, often available through your local cleft/craniofacial team, may also be of benefit to you. In addition to support groups and professional counseling, further management of remaining physical and aesthetic problems related to the cleft may help.

Facial Appearance: Surgical Considerations in the Adult

Patient Input and Surgeon Selection

There is a major difference between adults considering reconstructive surgery for repair of a cleft problem and children undergoing cleft surgery; the adult can actively participate in the surgical goals. Most adults who are considering reconstructive surgery are able to express fairly clear desires and expectations. It is important for the surgeon to address these concerns before any surgery is done.

As a patient, you must be comfortable with the amount of time spent with your surgeon discussing your concerns before surgery. The success of the operation may depend upon how much you and your surgeon agree. It cannot be overemphasized that what is important is what you consider important. You should know that some surgeons may be uncomfortable with your particular goals and desires. If that happens, you should continue to seek consultations with other surgeons with the understanding that no reputable surgeon will agree to do something that he/she cannot accomplish or does not believe is right.

Since many aspects of cleft treatment are based on the surgeon's personal experience rather than hard scientific fact, you should expect a variety of opinions and treatment suggestions among surgeons. Although this may be confusing, it does not mean that any individual surgical plan is right or wrong. The variety of opinions should be viewed as an opportunity for you to find a surgeon who understands you and who is willing to proceed with a mutually agreeable plan.

Functional versus Aesthetic

It is not unusual for functional problems related to the cleft to remain into adulthood. These may include speech problems, hearing problems, fistulas (small holes in the palate), dental problems, or breathing problems due to nasal obstruction, to name only a few. You and your surgeon should agree about which, if any, of these problems should be dealt with first so that your long-term health and function will be the best it can be. If there is more than one functional problem, you are in the best position to decide how much each problem interferes with your daily activities. Of course, this may be different for different people due to personal desires or job demands.

If there is more than one problem, it is important that you and your surgeon develop a list of all the problems that are present and consider them individually and as a whole. This may allow more than one problem to be treated surgically while under the same anesthetic or during the same operation. Some of these problems may require the involvement of a variety of surgical, dental, or other specialists. This type of coordinated care is best delivered by a team of specialists who can address all problems that may be present after the initial repair of a cleft lip or palate.

Concerns about facial appearance after initial or primary cleft repair are more personal than the functional (for example: speech, chewing, swallowing) problems just discussed. Scarring, lip irregularities, and nasal deformities are probably the most common reasons you may seek later or secondary surgical correction. It is important that you understand before the surgery exactly what is and is not possible. It is also important to understand what the surgeon anticipates the recovery period to be and what, if any, limitations you will experience after the surgery is done.

Because insurance often does not cover the cost of aesthetic procedures, it is important that you have a clear understanding of exactly what your financial obligation will be before the procedure is done. Most surgeons who do secondary surgery feel that this type of surgery is reconstructive (to restore function) and not merely cosmetic (to improve appearance), because its purpose is to try to reconstruct the structures affected by the cleft. Increasingly, though, insurance companies are taking the position that these types of procedures are performed for cosmetic reasons only, and they are refusing to pay for some or all of the costs.

In summary, the needs and desires of adults with clefts are as varied as each person. Before any procedure, you should ask questions and explain your desires and expectations to your surgeon and, perhaps, other members of the cleft palate team. After discussions with your surgeon, you should understand the goals and limitations of surgery. Last, but certainly not least, you should understand the necessary financial arrangements associated with any proposed procedure.

Creating an Attractive Smile

Goals and Procedures

The overall goal of treatment for cleft lip and palate is to achieve the best possible facial appearance and function. An attractive, functional smile depends upon many things, including jaws that are positioned well and in harmony with the rest of the face, a bite that is comfortable and stable, and teeth that are healthy and attractive. The function and harmonious appearance of the lip and nose are also critical in achieving this goal.

When considering ways of improving facial appearance by surgery, there are several important things to remember. A cleft involves all soft and hard tissue layers, not just the skin. Although a scar on the lip may be the most obvious thing to you, more extensive treatment than scar revision may be necessary to achieve the best possible improvement.

Your lip and nose are supported by the underlying skeleton (bone and cartilage) and teeth. If these supporting structures are not properly formed or are not in the correct position, your lip and nose will not appear balanced, regardless of how noticeable the scar may be. Clefts result in defects in the bone which may interrupt or alter dental development. Missing or malformed teeth in the area of the cleft are likely. The cleft itself disrupts the continuity of the upper jaw, often leading to instability of the two bony segments on either side of the cleft. The bony segments may be out of line with one another. In addition, the growth of the upper jaw is often disturbed by either scarring from previous surgeries or other unknown factors. As a result, the upper jaw (maxilla) may be smaller, narrower, and positioned farther back than is usual relative to the lower jaw (mandible), causing the upper teeth to be inside the lower teeth. In addition, the teeth in the area of the cleft may erupt out of position.

Fortunately, these problems can be corrected to make an attractive and functional smile. The procedures are best done in a series of steps which may take years to fully complete. Therefore, they are done best when planned by a coordinated team of specialists. As stated earlier, this is usually accomplished through an interdisciplinary cleft palate team.

Orthodontic appliances move the teeth into the best position within their respective jaws. Extraction of certain teeth may be necessary in order to reposition the teeth and may sometimes result in the bite temporarily worsening. Ultimately, however, this leads to the best possible facial and dental form and function. If surgical widening of your upper jaw is needed, an orthodontic expansion device may be fixed to several teeth.

Your facial bones form the foundation of your face, and the bony dental ridges support your teeth. These bones need to be properly positioned before a good bite can be achieved. A variety of surgical procedures can be performed to widen or reposition the upper jaw. The lower jaw and chin can also be repositioned if necessary. These procedures must be planned jointly by the orthodontist and surgeon to insure that an acceptable bite and facial harmony will result. Orthodontic appliances are usually placed first, and surgery is only undertaken after adequate orthodontic preparation. An exception to this may be if bone grafting in the upper jaw is planned.

Bone grafting in the tooth-bearing dental (alveolar) ridge is an operation performed to stabilize the bony segments of the upper jaw and provide better support for permanent teeth. Usually this is done in childhood or early adolescence, but it may also be necessary in adults to achieve the best possible result.

Bone is removed from one part of the body and placed in the jaw to fill in the missing bone in the gum or dental ridge. While some surgeons use artificial materials in place of the body's own bone, most surgeons believe natural bone gives a better result. The bone can be taken (harvested) from a variety of places, including your hip, head, rib, or leg. You should discuss the choice of bone graft donor site with your surgeon.

You may also benefit from a bone graft to highlight your cheek bones or nose. If you and your surgeon agree these procedures may be helpful, they can usually be done at the same time. When jaw bones are moved, it is necessary to hold them in position until they heal solidly.

Traditionally, it was necessary to wire the patient's teeth together after surgery for up to six weeks to assist the healing process. (If your teeth are wired together, it is necessary to have a liquid diet, since normal chewing is not possible.) Increasingly, surgeons are using metal plates and screws to hold repositioned jaw segments and bone grafts in position during healing. This is known as "rigid internal fixation." Even if your teeth are not wired together, chewing is discouraged to prevent movement of healing bones. In this case, it will be necessary to have a soft diet for approximately eight weeks after surgery.

Following surgery, continued orthodontic treatment may be necessary to move the teeth into their final position. The usual length of treatment from start to finish (both orthodontics and jaw surgery) is eighteen to twenty-four months. If preoperative orthodontic treatment was performed, additional adjustments following surgery may be made to assure that all teeth come together in the best possible way.

An important consideration in planning the final dental result is whether teeth are either missing or malformed. If a tooth is missing, a decision must be made either to close the space it would have occupied by moving teeth into that space or to leave the space open and replace the tooth with a prosthetic (artificial) tooth. Many different prosthetic replacements are available, such as removable partial dentures, fixed bridges, bonded bridges, and implants. Factors influencing the decision about which might be best include the quality of the existing bite, the degree of crowding among the teeth, the location of the missing tooth, and the amount of bone support at that site. Plans also must be made to restore any malformed teeth. If a tooth is small or misshapen and needs to be restored to a larger size, adequate space must be reserved for the final size. If you have any of these problems, a dentist who makes dentures and other dental appliances (prosthodontist) or an experienced general dentist together with the dentist who moves teeth (orthodontist) should arrive at the best possible plan together and discuss with you the various choices available prior to treatment.

The final phase of making an attractive smile involves attention to the scar on the lip and the shape of the lip. It is important to keep in mind, as has been emphasized previously, that your lip will not look its best unless it is adequately supported by the skeletal and dental structures underneath the lip. Ideally, lip revision surgery should follow restoration or reconstruction of the teeth and jaws.

Sometimes speech is changed after jaw surgery. Your tongue will need to get used to the different space. In fact, the new jaw position may make it easier to produce better speech sounds. There will be a period of time right after surgery when you will naturally adapt to the new jaw positions. Even so, it may be helpful to see a speech-language pathologist for evaluation and treatment. Although the jaw surgery might be helpful for some aspects of speech, like making certain sounds more precisely, the surgery could change the nasality in your speech. That is, when the upper jaw is moved forward, this may affect your soft palate and change your ability to seal off your nose from your mouth during speech. Your surgeon and speech-language pathologist should discuss these possibilities with you before jaw surgery.

In summary, several stages of treatment including surgery, orthodontics, and prosthodontics are often necessary to achieve the most pleasing and functional smile possible. The key to the success of these varied steps is coordinated planning. Good results can be achieved with careful planning before any treatment is started.

The Adult Patient

Speaking Clearly

Although certain facial and jaw structures may continue to grow and develop into the late teens, and sometimes beyond, your speech structures have probably been adult size for several years. It is true that all body tissues including those of the mouth and throat mature and change to some degree all our lives, but in general, the size and shape of the structures involved in speech are finalized by approximately 13 to 16 years of age.

Let's assume you are at least 20 years old and, most likely, no longer making annual visits to your interdisciplinary team. In fact, you may have assumed that all that can be done has already been done, and you are getting on with your life. But you may still have some questions about your speech. If you do, it is important to try to answer them.

Am I satisfied with my speech now?

This is a very important question, and only you know the answer. Perhaps you are quite satisfied, and that is good. But perhaps you are not. You may not know precisely what concerns you about your speech—only that you are not totally satisfied. Your speech is part of your self-image, and your opinion is important.

What were my expectations for my speech some years ago?

This question is somewhat related to the first, because current satisfaction is most likely the result of what you expected your speech to be like as an adult. Was your expectation perfect speech? Normal speech? Acceptable speech? Able to get along speech? Acceptable speech is the minimum goal that your medical, dental, and speech-language professionals had for you from the start. They all wanted your speech to be the best it could be. Perhaps your speech has always been very good, and you have not really thought much about it. But for many, the expectation of what they hoped for has fallen somewhat short. You should feel comfortable expressing that feeling of dissatisfaction. Speech improvement may still be possible.

What impression does my speech make in comparison with other speakers?

You probably remember some negative comments made by others about your speech, or you may recall your speech-language pathologist reminding you to watch or monitor your articulation or nasality during conversational speech. In many respects, this is the bottom line concern of speech-language pathologists—to carryover what you could do in therapy sessions to all speaking situations. Perhaps you remember being told by your team that improved speech required some physical procedure like a speech prosthesis or surgery. Perhaps you, or your parents, were not interested at that time. You may be interested now. Your recent concern and interest may have been sparked by a comment you heard from a listener. Perhaps you feel you did not get that certain job because your speech was not good enough, or maybe your current job requires effective communication skills and you want your speech to be better. You may have options now of which you were not previously aware.

Is my speech understandable to others?

Ideally, your speech is almost totally understandable to others, a quality known as speech intelligibility. The expectation for your speech as an adult is that it should be either readily intelligible all the time or, at a minimum, that there are only occasional words that are not intelligible. If frequent words and phrases are not understood by your listeners, the reasons why should be evaluated further. Even some speakers who are readily intelligible continue to have concerns with other aspects of speech as follow.

Is my speech too nasal? Too denasal?

You may believe, or you may have heard, that you sound like you are talking through your nose, or you sound like you are all stuffed up or have a cold. These descriptions refer to the balance of sound between the nose and the mouth during speech. This balance normally changes when we speak depending on the speech sounds being produced. It is not normal when the balance does not change properly. Too much nasality is common with children or adults with cleft palate. This part of speech depends on the function of your speech structures. You may recall hearing as a child, if you received speech therapy, how important it was to seal off, close off, or separate the nasal cavity from the mouth and throat to produce good speech. You use your soft palate and throat walls to accomplish this closure. This is called velopharyngeal closure, and it is an important requirement for normal vowels and for almost all consonant sounds.

If you have had your soft palate repaired, it may still be too short to contact the back wall of your throat, or it may be that your throat walls do not move sufficiently. This is called velopharyngeal insufficiency (VPI), and it causes too much sound to pass through your nose when you speak.

You may have had surgery, such as a pharyngeal flap or a pharyngoplasty, or you may have had a speech prosthesis made for you that was intended to improve velopharyngeal closure for speech. Even if you have had one of these treatments, too much nasality may still concern you.

You may believe that the opposite is true of your speech; that is, you may have too little nasality (denasality). Although a complete closure between the nose and the mouth is required for most consonants, the nasal consonants are the exception. In the English language, there are three nasal consonants (/m/ as in *make*, /n/ as in *new*, and /ng/ as in *ring*). When these sounds are produced, the soft palate needs to stay down and leave an opening into the nasal cavity. If your nose is obstructed by crooked or enlarged structures within it, the nasal consonants will sound denasal and you may sound "stuffed up" like you have a cold. This is usually treated by surgically opening up the nasal passages.

You may also sound denasal if you have persistent congestion or allergies. Nasal congestion is temporary for most of us, and we return to normal speech when the congestion subsides. But for some, persistent nasal congestion prevents the free flow of sound and air into the nose, making it impossible for the denasal quality to go away. You may need to consult an allergist for treatment if allergies are the problem.

It is also possible to have too much and too little nasality at the same time. Careful evaluation by professionals with experience in cleft care should result in identification of the cause of the problem and recommendations for treatment. Finally, there may be a mild degree of nasality in your speech, but you and others consider it to be within acceptable limits. Unless you or those you interact with are concerned, mild nasality is not really a problem at all.

Is the way I make individual consonants different from others?

Perhaps your concern is the accuracy or preciseness of your consonant sounds. This is called articulation. For persons with cleft lip and palate, there is no reason to believe that all consonant sounds cannot be made in the correct place in the mouth. Many of the hazards to precise articulation were removed when your final dental work (dental bridge, crowns, jaw surgery) was done. Hopefully, the original surgery to repair the hard and soft palate and any other surgery to improve velopharyngeal closure gave you an adequate mechanism for acceptable speech, but perhaps not. You may still be concerned about the preciseness of your articulation—making better /s/ and /z/ sounds or /sh/ and /ch/ sounds. Also, you may still be concerned about the audible escape of air from your nose (audible nasal air emission) that sometimes occurs when you produce words containing sounds like /p/ or /b/ and /ch/ and /j/.

Is my voice okay?

Voice is the part of speech that is produced by your larynx or "voice box." Your voice may sound too high or too low in pitch, too soft or too loud, or too hoarse or raspy. Having a cleft lip and palate does not involve the larynx directly, but sometimes the way we use the voice box to compensate or adjust for velopharyngeal problems may affect the quality of voice. Perhaps you have experienced laryngitis when you have yelled, screamed, or cheered too much. This usually goes away after a couple of days. But misuse or abuse of the voice structures over time can cause some persistent problems. It may be this aspect of your speech that concerns you.

Any one or a combination of the above aspects of speech can be responsible for your dissatisfaction and concern. Speech that is socially and vocationally acceptable is a very reasonable expectation and goal for you. You may have heard professionals refer to your speech as acceptable, but you may, or may not, agree with that judgment. What is acceptable speech for some may not be for others. Perfect speech or normal speech mayor may not be realistic for you, and you have the right to disagree. Your opinion is important.

But you need to understand that there may be limitations to your current speech structures. Your choices for treatment that can make your speech better may or may not be similarly limited. Whether you decide to have treatment will depend on how much the problem bothers you and whether it interferes with others understanding and relating to you.

What is required to improve certain aspects of my speech?

Speech treatment or therapy may be all you need to help you. Following an evaluation by a qualified speech-language pathologist, it may be concluded that your present speech structures will allow you to change your speech with the help of some professional instruction. On the other hand, it may be concluded that in order to improve your speech, physical treatment is definitely needed. For example, after a complete evaluation, it may be found that you are doing the best you can with your current structures, but your soft palate is too short to accomplish velopharyngeal closure for acceptable speech. There may be a variety of physical treatments that can help—perhaps a surgical procedure or a speech prosthesis. Perhaps your hearing affects your speech performance. Careful and complete evaluation is the key to determine what is needed.

Where can I get help?

A professional speech and hearing evaluation can tell you whether your speech and hearing mechanisms are working properly, what aspects of speech are involved, and what the treatment options might be. Some speech-language pathologists work in the public schools and, in many states, provide evaluative and treatment services for persons up to 21 years of age. Other resources for speech, language, and hearing evaluation are through community-based speech and hearing clinics, university speech and hearing clinics, hospital rehabilitation centers, and private practitioners. Don't forget that your interdisciplinary cleft palate team is a very important resource for you at any time. Most cleft palate teams evaluate and provide treatment for adults with clefts even if the team is located in a children's hospital. The medical, dental, speech/language, and hearing professionals who make up your team will be able to evaluate and provide treatment or recommend treatment resources for you. It is never too late to change if you want to change. You can obtain a list of cleft teams in your geographic area by contacting the Cleft Palate Foundation at 800-24-CLEFT (800-242-5338).

Ear, Nose, and Throat Health

Children with clefts of the palate almost always experience problems with middle ear infections during the first few years of life. A few continue to experience difficulty with hearing and ear infections as adults.

If you have persistent ear problems during adulthood, you need the attention of an ear, nose, and throat specialist. Signs of possible problems include hearing loss in one or both ears, drainage from the ears, or ear aches that keep coming back or that never really go away. You may have a hearing loss caused by damage to the delicate middle ear bones or the ear drum, preventing sound vibrations from reaching the nerves that sense sound. This type of damage can often be repaired surgically.

Ear drainage or recurrent earaches may be due to a minor but persistent infection in the bone surrounding the middle ear. Surgery may be required to remove the infection and prevent irreversible damage and hearing loss. If hearing loss cannot be corrected by medical or surgical treatment, a hearing aid can help compensate for lost hearing.

In some persons who have had "nasal" speech for a long period of time, small growths (nodules) can develop on the vocal folds and give the voice a hoarse quality. Usually, voice improvement can be achieved by treating the cause of the nasality. Speech therapy may be helpful in some cases. Surgical removal of vocal fold nodules is necessary only as a last resort.

Unlike the ears, the nose, sinuses, and throat, usually are not prone to infection in persons with cleft palate. If the degree of nasal leakage allows liquid and food material to pass into the nasal cavity when you swallow; however, sinusitis can develop. This is generally not a problem and can be resolved with appropriate treatment to improve effective separation of the nose from the mouth (velopharyngeal closure) during swallowing. However, if symptoms persist, a thorough nasal examination including special x-rays may be desirable, and sinus surgery may be required.

Some adults with cleft palate may have problems breathing during sleep. Many adults who have had operations to improve speech (pharyngeal flap or pharyngoplasty, for example) snore loudly during sleep. While snoring may not be a problem for the affected individual, it might bother a sleep partner. A few adults may stop breathing altogether (sleep apnea) during sleep for more than a few seconds, and this can be a serious, even life-threatening, problem. If your sleep partner has noticed that you seem to stop breathing while sleeping, or if you have restless sleep with excessive daytime drowsiness, you may have sleep apnea. Your local cleft team can help if you are concerned about sleep problems.

Chapter 39

Dentinogenesis Imperfecta

What is dentinogenesis imperfecta?

Dentinogenesis imperfecta (DGI) is a disorder of tooth development. This condition causes the teeth to be discolored (most often a blue-gray or yellow-brown color) and translucent. Teeth are also weaker than normal, making them prone to rapid wear, breakage, and loss. These problems can affect both primary (baby) teeth and permanent teeth.

Researchers have described three types of dentinogenesis imperfecta with similar dental abnormalities. Type I occurs in people who have osteogenesis imperfecta, a genetic condition in which bones are brittle and easily broken. Dentinogenesis imperfecta type II and type III usually occur in people without other inherited disorders. A few older individuals with type II have had progressive high-frequency hearing loss in addition to dental abnormalities, but it is not known whether this hearing loss is related to dentinogenesis imperfecta.

Some researchers believe that dentinogenesis imperfecta type II and type III, along with a condition called dentin dysplasia type II, are actually forms of a single disorder. The signs and symptoms of dentin dysplasia type II are very similar to those of dentinogenesis imperfecta. However, dentin dysplasia type II affects the primary teeth much more than the permanent teeth.

Text in this chapter is excerpted from "Dentinogenesis Imperfecta," and "DSPP," from Genetics Home Reference, January 2012.

How common is dentinogenesis imperfecta?

Dentinogenesis imperfecta affects an estimated one in 6,000 to 8,000 people.

What genes are related to dentinogenesis imperfecta?

Mutations in the DSPP gene have been identified in people with dentinogenesis imperfecta type II and type III. Mutations in this gene are also responsible for dentin dysplasia type II. Dentinogenesis imperfecta type I occurs as part of osteogenesis imperfecta, which is caused by mutations in one of several other genes (most often the collagen, type I, alpha 1 [COL1A1] or collagen, type I, alpha 2 [COL1A2] genes).

The d*entin sialophosphoprotein* (DSPP) gene provides instructions for making two proteins that are essential for normal tooth development. These proteins are involved in the formation of dentin, which is a bone-like substance that makes up the protective middle layer of each tooth. DSPP gene mutations alter the proteins made from the gene, leading to the production of abnormally soft dentin. Teeth with defective dentin are discolored, weak, and more likely to decay and break. It is unclear whether DSPP gene mutations are related to the hearing loss found in a few older individuals with dentinogenesis imperfecta type II.

How do people inherit dentinogenesis imperfecta?

This condition is inherited in an autosomal dominant pattern, which means one copy of the altered gene in each cell is sufficient to cause the disorder. In most cases, an affected person has one parent with the condition.

DSPP Gene

What is the normal function of the DSPP gene?

The DSPP gene provides instructions for making a protein called dentin sialophosphoprotein. Soon after it is produced, this protein is cut into two smaller proteins: dentin sialoprotein and dentin phosphoprotein. These proteins are components of dentin, which is a bone-like substance that makes up the protective middle layer of each tooth. A third smaller protein produced from dentin sialophosphoprotein, called dentin glycoprotein, was identified in pigs but has not been found in humans.

Although the exact functions of the DSPP-derived proteins are unknown, these proteins appear to be essential for normal tooth development. Dentin phosphoprotein is thought to be involved in the normal hardening of collagen, the most abundant protein in dentin. Specifically, dentin phosphoprotein may play a role in the deposition of mineral crystals among collagen fibers (mineralization).

The DSPP gene is also active in the inner ear, although it is unclear whether it plays a role in normal hearing.

How are changes in the DSPP gene related to health conditions?

More than 20 mutations in the DSPP gene have been identified in people with dentinogenesis imperfecta. These genetic changes are responsible for two forms of this disorder, type II and type III. Mutations in this gene also cause dentin dysplasia type II, a disorder with signs and symptoms very similar to those of dentinogenesis imperfecta. However, dentin dysplasia type II affects the primary (baby) teeth much more than the permanent teeth. Some researchers believe that this type of dentin dysplasia and dentinogenesis imperfecta types II and III are actually forms of a single disorder.

About half of DSPP gene mutations affect dentin sialoprotein, altering its transport in cells. The remaining mutations affect dentin phosphoprotein, interfering with its normal production and/or secretion. As a result of these abnormalities of DSPP-related proteins, teeth have abnormally soft dentin. Teeth with defective dentin are discolored, weak, and prone to breakage and decay.

Although the DSPP gene is active in the inner ear, it is unclear whether DSPP gene mutations are related to the hearing loss found in a few older individuals with dentinogenesis imperfecta type II.

Chapter 40

Dry Mouth Disorders

Chapter Contents

Section 40.1

Causes and Treatment of Dry Mouth (Xerostomia)

Excerpted from "Dry Mouth? Don't Delay Treatment,"
U.S. Food and Drug Administration (FDA), May 9, 2011.

Almost everyone's mouth is dry sometimes. But if you feel like you have cotton in your mouth constantly, it may be time for treatment. Dry mouth, known medically as xerostomia, occurs when you don't have enough saliva, or spit, in your mouth. Feeling stressed can trigger dry mouth temporarily. But a persistently dry mouth may signal an underlying disease or condition, so it's important to see your doctor, says the Food and Drug Administration (FDA), which regulates products that relieve dry mouth. And because dry mouth can lead to tooth decay, you should see your dentist, too, says John V. Kelsey, DDS, of FDA's Division of Dermatology and Dental Products.

Dry mouth may make it difficult to speak, chew, and swallow, and may alter the taste of your food. It can also cause a sore throat, hoarseness, and bad breath. Dry mouth can affect people of any age, but older people are especially vulnerable. "It's not a normal consequence of aging," says Kelsey. "Older people may take multiple medications that can cause dry mouth." According to the *Surgeon General's Report on Oral Health in America*, dry mouth is a side effect of more than 400 prescription and over-the-counter drugs, such as antidepressants, antihistamines, muscle relaxants, and high blood pressure medicines.

Other causes of dry mouth include:

- cancer treatments, such as chemotherapy and radiation of the head or neck;

- hormone changes, such as those that occur during pregnancy or menopause;

- health problems, such as human immunodeficiency virus/acquired immunodeficiency syndrome (HIV/AIDS), diabetes, and Sjögren syndrome, a disease in which a person's immune system attacks the body's tissues, including moisture-producing glands;

- snoring or breathing open-mouthed.

The Role of Saliva

Saliva is produced by three major glands in the mouth (salivary glands) and plays a key role in:

- chewing, swallowing, and digesting food;
- preventing infection in the mouth by controlling bacteria; and
- preventing tooth decay.

"Saliva is mostly water, but it also contains enzymes and lubricants," says Kelsey. "The enzymes help digest food and the lubricants make speaking, chewing, and swallowing more comfortable." Saliva helps control bacteria, which cling to the surface of teeth. They feed on sugar in the food we eat and break down and use (metabolize) the sugar to grow. "A by-product of the metabolized sugar is acid, which starts to eat away at a tooth's surface," says Kelsey. Saliva neutralizes the acid and helps wash away food particles. If there is not enough saliva, cavities may occur.

Dry Mouth Treatments

Your doctor or dentist may recommend oral rinses and moisturizers, or prescribe an artificial saliva. Also called saliva substitutes, these products are regulated by FDA as medical devices. "Unlike drugs, artificial saliva [products] have no chemical action," says Susan Runner, DDS, chief of FDA's dental devices branch. "Their action is mechanical. They moisten and lubricate the mouth but do not stimulate the salivary glands to make saliva."

While not a cure, artificial saliva can provide short-term relief of the symptoms of dry mouth. "They can also help minimize discomfort after an oral procedure," says Runner.

Artificial saliva comes in a variety of forms, including rinses, sprays, swabs, gels, and tablets that dissolve in the mouth. Some are available by prescription only; others can be bought over-the-counter. FDA has also approved several prescription drugs to relieve dry mouth caused by certain medical treatments or conditions, such as Sjögren syndrome and radiation for head or neck cancer.

Advice for Consumers

If you have persistent dry mouth:

- Talk to your doctor, who may change your medications or adjust the doses.

- Talk to your dentist and provide a list of the medicines you take as well as any medical conditions or treatments you've had. The American Dental Association recommends seeing your dentist at least twice a year.

Tips for Relieving Dry Mouth

- Sip water or sugarless drinks, or suck on ice chips.

- Avoid irritants, such as alcohol, tobacco, and caffeine. Remember that caffeine is found in many sodas as well as in coffee and tea.

- Chew sugar-free gum or suck on sugar-free candy.

- Avoid salty or spicy foods, which may irritate the mouth.

- Use a humidifier in your bedroom at night.

- Consider using saliva substitutes.

Section 40.2

Salivary Gland Disorders

"Salivary Diagnostics," National Institutes of Health (NIH),
February 14, 2011.

Saliva is the watery fluid that moistens our mouths, helping us
eat, speak, and maintain good oral health. Saliva consists of a clear,
protein-rich fluid secreted by the salivary glands and trace amounts of
various biochemicals present in blood serum that filter into the mouth.
As certain health conditions arise, such as human immunodeficiency
virus (HIV) infection and cancer, proteins and substances linked to
these diseases can pass from the serum into the saliva. Increased
concentrations of these compounds over time make saliva a potentially
promising diagnostic fluid with several advantages over blood. Saliva
is easy to collect, requires no painful needle sticks, and can be tested
in many non-traditional settings because of the portability and lower
cost of salivary test kits.

Technologies that will enable saliva to be used as a window into the
body are being explored for their ability to detect disease and monitor
our health. Efforts are underway to develop miniaturized lab-on-a-
chip technology, where diagnostic tests and tools are made to be rapid,
automated, and portable. Combined with saliva sample collection or
cell collection (by gentle brushing of the skin surface), this technology
could eliminate the need for blood sampling or mouth tissue biopsy,
in many cases.

Yesterday

Getting a diagnosis used to mean making a trip to the doctor's office
or to a hospital. The examination often required providing a blood or
tissue sample. Collection of these samples involved insertion of needles
into blood vessels or cutting away a small area of the tissue (a biopsy).

Most tests detected full-blown disease. Few were sensitive enough
to detect subtle biochemical changes that might indicate a developing
health condition. No test analyzed saliva or was available for easy use
in the home.

Today

Currently available salivary diagnostic tests include various hormonal, HIV, and alcohol tests. Each test requires a small amount of saliva and produces rapid and highly accurate results.

In 2010, NIH funded two exciting new studies entitled, "Salivary biomarkers for early oral cancer detection," and "Salivary proteomic and genomic biomarkers for primary Sjögren syndrome."

Scientists have identified the genes and proteins that are expressed in the salivary glands. With these vast catalogues as their guide, they will define the patterns and certain conditions under which these genes and proteins are expressed in the salivary glands and how these parts function as a fully integrated biological system.

Tomorrow

Salivary diagnostic tests will provide immediate results to patients. The portable tests will initially approximate the size of a personal digital assistant (PDA). The fully integrated diagnostic systems will have the potential to measure from one to possibly hundreds of compounds in saliva within a matter of minutes.

An emergency medical technician will, with a patient's consent, collect a small saliva sample, load it into the fully automated test, and have an extensive saliva panel readout ready by the time the ambulance brings the patient to the emergency room. The readout will contain a profile of various proteins in the patient's mouth that are associated with various systemic diseases or conditions.

As miniaturization of the technology advances, it may become possible to attach a tiny device to a patient's tooth, allowing personalized monitoring of medication levels and the detection of biomarkers for specific disease states.

Section 40.3

Sjögren Syndrome

Excerpted from "Questions and Answers about Sjögren Syndrome,"
National Institute of Arthritis and Musculoskeletal and Skin
Diseases (NIAMS), May 2010.

What Is Sjögren Syndrome?

Sjögren syndrome is an autoimmune disease; that is, a disease in which the immune system turns against the body's own cells. Normally, the immune system works to protect us from disease by destroying harmful invading organisms like viruses and bacteria. In the case of Sjögren syndrome, disease-fighting cells attack various organs, most notably the glands that produce tears and saliva (the lacrimal and salivary glands). Damage to these glands causes a reduction in both the quantity and quality of their secretions. This results in symptoms that include dry eyes and dry mouth. In technical terms, the form of eye dryness associated with Sjögren syndrome is called keratoconjunctivitis sicca, or KCS, and the symptoms of dry mouth are called xerostomia. Your doctor may use these terms when talking to you about Sjögren syndrome.

You might hear Sjögren syndrome called a rheumatic disease. This means it causes inflammation in joints, muscles, skin, and other organs. Like rheumatoid arthritis and systemic lupus erythematosus, it is also considered one of the autoimmune connective tissue diseases.

Primary Versus Secondary Sjögren Syndrome

Sjögren syndrome is classified as either primary or secondary. Both are systemic diseases, meaning they can affect many systems in the body, and they occur with about equal frequency. The primary form causes early and gradually progressive decreased function in the lacrimal and salivary glands, and can include a variety of extraglandular conditions. The secondary form occurs in people who already have another autoimmune connective tissue disease, most commonly rheumatoid arthritis or systemic lupus erythematosus. These people then develop dry eyes or dry mouth.

What Are the Symptoms of Sjögren Syndrome?

Sjögren syndrome can cause many symptoms. The main ones include the following:

- **Dry eyes:** Eyes affected by Sjögren syndrome may burn or itch. Some people say it feels like they have sand in their eyes. Others have trouble with blurry vision, or are bothered by bright light, especially fluorescent lighting.

- **Dry mouth:** Dry mouth may feel chalky or like your mouth is full of cotton. It may be difficult to swallow, speak, or taste. Because you lack the protective effects of saliva, you may develop more dental decay (cavities) and mouth infections.

What Causes Dryness in Sjögren Syndrome?

In the autoimmune attack causing Sjögren syndrome, white blood cells called lymphocytes often will initially target and damage the glands that produce tears and saliva. Although no one knows exactly how this occurs, the damaged glands produce tears and saliva that are diminished in both quantity and quality, leading to the symptoms of dryness of the eyes and mouth.

Who Gets Sjögren Syndrome?

Sjögren syndrome can affect people of either sex and of any age, but most cases occur in women. The average age for onset is late forties, but in rare cases, Sjögren syndrome is diagnosed in children. In 2008, the number of Americans with primary Sjögren syndrome was estimated to be 1.3 million.

What Causes Sjögren Syndrome?

Researchers think Sjögren syndrome is caused by a combination of genetic and environmental factors. Several different genes appear to be involved, but scientists are not certain exactly which ones are linked to the disease, because different genes seem to play a role in different people.

How Is Sjögren Syndrome Diagnosed?

Some common eye and mouth tests are:

- **Schirmer test:** This test measures tears to see how the lacrimal (tear) glands are working. The doctor puts thin paper strips under the lower eyelids and measures the amount of wetness on the paper after five minutes. People with Sjögren syndrome usually produce less than eight millimeters of tears.

- **Slit lamp examination:** This test, in which an ophthalmologist uses equipment to magnify and carefully examine the eye, shows how severe the dryness is and whether the outside of the eye is inflamed.

- **Staining with vital dyes (rose bengal or lissamine green):** These tests show the extent to which dryness has damaged the surface of the eye. To perform one of these tests, the doctor puts a drop of a liquid containing a dye into the lower eyelid. The dye stains the surface of the eye, highlighting any areas of injury, thereby allowing the doctor to see with the slit lamp how much damage has occurred on the surface of the eye.

- **Mouth exam:** The doctor will look outside the mouth for signs of major salivary gland swelling and inside the mouth for signs of dryness. Signs of dry mouth include a dry, sticky lining (called oral mucosa); dental caries (cavities) in characteristic locations; thick saliva, or none at all coming out of the major salivary ducts; redness of the mouth lining, often associated with a smooth, burning tongue; and sores at the corners of the lips. The doctor might also try to get a sample of saliva, to check its quality and see how much of it the glands are producing.

- **Lip biopsy:** This test is the best way to find out whether dry mouth is caused by Sjögren syndrome. To perform this test the doctor removes tiny minor salivary glands from the inside of the lower lip and examines them under the microscope. If the glands contain white blood cells in a particular pattern, the test is positive for the salivary component of Sjögren syndrome.

Because there are many causes of dry eyes and dry mouth (including many common medications, other diseases, or previous treatment such as radiation of the head or neck), the doctor needs a thorough history from the patient, and additional tests to see whether other parts of the body are affected. These tests may include:

- **Routine blood tests:** The doctor will take a blood sample to look for levels of different types of blood cells, check blood sugar level, and see how the liver and kidneys are working.

- **Other blood tests:** Various blood tests may be performed to check for antibodies and other immunological substances often found in the blood of people with Sjögren syndrome.

- **Chest x ray:** Sjögren syndrome can cause inflammation in the lungs, so the doctor may want to take an x ray to check them.

- **Urinalysis:** The doctor will probably test a sample of your urine to see how well the kidneys are working.

How Is Sjögren Syndrome Treated?

Treatment can vary from person to person, depending on what parts of the body are affected. But in all cases, the doctor will help relieve your symptoms, especially dryness.

What Can I Do about Dry Mouth?

There are many remedies for dry mouth. You can try some of them on your own. Your doctor may prescribe others. Here are some many people find useful:

- **Chewing gum and hard candy:** If your salivary glands still produce some saliva, you can stimulate them to make more by chewing gum or sucking on hard candy. However, gum and candy must be sugar-free, because dry mouth makes you extremely prone to progressive dental decay (cavities).

- **Water:** Take sips of water or another sugar-free, noncarbonated drink throughout the day to wet your mouth, especially when you are eating or talking. Note that drinking large amounts of liquid throughout the day will not make your mouth any less dry and will make you urinate more often. You should only take small sips of liquid, but not too often. If you sip liquids every few minutes, it may reduce or remove the mucus coating inside your mouth, increasing the feeling of dryness.

- **Lip balm:** You can soothe dry, cracked lips by using oil- or petroleum-based lip balm or lipstick. If your mouth hurts, your doctor may give you medicine in a mouth rinse, ointment, or gel to apply to the sore areas to control pain and inflammation.

- **Saliva substitutes:** If you produce very little saliva or none at all, your doctor might recommend a saliva substitute. These products mimic some of the properties of saliva, which means they make the mouth feel wet. Gel-based saliva substitutes tend to give the longest relief, but as with all saliva products, their effectiveness is limited by the fact that you eventually swallow them. It is best to use these products rather than water when awakening from sleep: They reduce oral symptoms more effectively, and they do not cause excessive urine formation.

- **Prescription medications:** At least two prescription drugs stimulate the salivary glands to produce saliva. These are pilocarpine and cevimeline. The effects last for a few hours, and you can take them three or four times a day. However, they are not suitable for everyone, so talk to your doctor about whether they might help you. In trials of these drugs, patients have also experienced some reduction in their dry eye symptoms.

The Importance of Oral Hygiene

Natural saliva contains substances that rid the mouth of the bacteria that cause dental decay (cavities) and mouth infections, so good oral hygiene is extremely important when you have dry mouth. Here's what you can do to prevent cavities and infections:

- Visit a dentist regularly, at least twice a year, to have your teeth examined and cleaned.
- Rinse your mouth with water several times a day. Don't use mouthwash that contains alcohol, because alcohol is drying.
- Use toothpaste that contains fluoride to gently brush your teeth, gums, and tongue after each meal and before bedtime. Nonfoaming toothpaste is less drying.
- Floss your teeth every day.
- Avoid sugar between meals. That means choosing sugar-free gum, candy, and soda. If you do eat or drink sugary foods, brush your teeth immediately afterward.
- See a dentist right away if you notice anything unusual or have continuous burning or other oral symptoms.
- Ask your dentist whether you need to take fluoride supplements, use a fluoride gel at night, or have a varnish put on your teeth to protect the enamel.

Other Autoimmune Connective Tissue Diseases

Patients who have an autoimmune connective tissue disease other than Sjögren syndrome may subsequently develop the dry eyes and or dry mouth of Sjögren syndrome. They would then be diagnosed as having secondary Sjögren syndrome, along with their primary connective tissue disease. These other autoimmune connective tissue diseases include polymyositis, rheumatoid arthritis (RA), scleroderma, and systemic lupus erythematosus (SLE).

Does Sjögren Syndrome Cause Lymphoma?

A small percentage of people with Sjögren syndrome develop lymphoma, which involves salivary glands, lymph nodes, the gastrointestinal tract, or the lungs. Persistent enlargement of a major salivary gland should be carefully and regularly observed by your doctor and investigated further if it changes in size in a short period of time. Other symptoms may include the following:

- unexplained fever,
- night sweats,
- constant fatigue,
- unexplained weight loss,
- itchy skin,
- reddened patches on the skin.

Medicines and Dryness

Certain drugs can contribute to eye and mouth dryness. If you take any of the drugs listed below, ask your doctor whether they could be causing symptoms. However, don't stop taking them without asking your doctor—he or she may already have adjusted the dose to help protect you against drying side effects or chosen a drug that's least likely to cause dryness. Drugs that can cause dryness include:

- antihistamines,
- decongestants,
- diuretics,
- some antidiarrhea drugs,
- some antipsychotic drugs,
- tranquilizers,
- some blood pressure medicines,
- antidepressants.

Chapter 41

Jaw Problems

Chapter Contents

385

Section 41.1

Jaw Dislocation or Fracture

A broken jaw is a break in the jaw bone. A dislocated jaw means the lower part of the jaw has moved out of its normal position at one or both joints where the jaw bone connects to the skull (temporomandibular joints).

Considerations

A broken or dislocated jaw usually heals completely after treatment. However, the jaw may become dislocated again in the future.

Complications may include the following:

- Airway blockage
- Bleeding
- Breathing blood or food into the lungs
- Difficulty eating (temporary)
- Difficulty talking (temporary)
- Infection of the jaw or face
- Jaw joint (TMJ) pain and other problems
- Problems aligning the teeth

Causes

The most common cause of a broken or dislocated jaw is injury to the face. This may be due to:

- assault,
- industrial accident,
- motor vehicle accident,
- recreational or sports injury.

Symptoms

Symptoms of a dislocated jaw include these:

- Bite that feels "off" or crooked
- Difficulty speaking
- Drooling because of inability to close the mouth
- Inability to close the mouth
- Jaw that may protrude forward
- Pain in the face or jaw, located in front of the ear on the affected side, and gets worse with movement
- Teeth that do not line up properly

Symptoms of a fractured (broken) jaw include these:

- Bleeding from the mouth
- Difficulty opening the mouth widely
- Facial bruising
- Facial swelling
- Jaw stiffness
- Jaw tenderness or pain, worse with biting or chewing
- Loose or damaged teeth
- Lump or abnormal appearance of the cheek or jaw
- Numbness of the face (particularly the lower lip)
- Very limited movement of the jaw (with severe fracture)

First Aid

A broken or dislocated jaw requires immediate medical attention because of the risk of breathing problems or significant bleeding. Call your local emergency number (such as 911) or local hospital for further advice.

Hold the jaw gently in place with your hands while traveling to the emergency room. A bandage may also be wrapped over the top of the head and under the jaw. However, such a bandage should be easily removable in case you need to vomit.

If breathing problems or heavy bleeding occurs, or if there is severe facial swelling, a tube may be placed into your airways to help you breathe.

Dislocated Jaw

If the jaw is dislocated, the health care provider may be able to place it back into the correct position using the thumbs. Numbing medications (anesthetics) and muscle relaxants may be needed to relax the strong jaw muscles.

The jaw may need to be stabilized. This usually involves bandaging the jaw to keep the mouth from opening widely. In some cases, surgery may be needed to do this, particularly if repeated jaw dislocations occur.

After dislocating your jaw, you should not open your mouth widely for at least six weeks. Support your jaw with one or both hands when yawning and sneezing.

Fractured Jaw

Temporarily bandaging the jaw (around the top of the head) to prevent it from moving may help reduce pain.

The specific treatment for a fractured jaw depends on how badly the bone is broken. If you have a minor fracture, you may only need pain medicines and to follow a soft or liquid diet for a while.

Surgery is often needed for moderate to severe fractures. The jaw may be wired to the teeth of the opposite jaw to improve stability. Jaw wires are usually left in place for 6–8 weeks. Small rubber bands (elastics) are used to hold the teeth together. After a few weeks, some of the elastics are removed to allow motion and reduce joint stiffness.

If the jaw is wired, you can only drink liquids or eat very soft foods. Have blunt scissors readily available to cut the elastics in the event of vomiting or choking. If the wires must be cut, consult a health care provider promptly so they can be replaced.

Do Not

Do not attempt to correct the position of the jaw.

When to Contact a Medical Professional

A broken or dislocated jaw requires immediate medical attention. Emergency symptoms include difficulty breathing or heavy bleeding.

Prevention

Safe practices in work, sports, and recreation, such as wearing a proper helmet when playing football, may prevent some accidental injuries to the face or jaw.

Section 41.2

Temporomandibular Joint and Muscle (TMJ) Disorders

Excerpted from "TMJ Disorders," National Institute of Dental and Craniofacial Research (NIDCR), NIH Publication No. 10–3487, March 2010.

Temporomandibular joint and muscle disorders, commonly called TMJ, are a group of conditions that cause pain and dysfunction in the jaw joint and the muscles that control jaw movement. We don't know for certain how many people have TMJ disorders, but some estimates suggest that over ten million Americans are affected. The condition appears to be more common in women than men.

What is the temporomandibular joint?

The temporomandibular joint connects the lower jaw, called the mandible, to the bone at the side of the head—the temporal bone. If you place your fingers just in front of your ears and open your mouth, you can feel the joints. Because these joints are flexible, the jaw can move smoothly up and down and side to side, enabling us to talk, chew, and yawn. Muscles attached to and surrounding the jaw joint control its position and movement.

The temporomandibular joint is different from the body's other joints. The combination of hinge and sliding motions makes this joint among the most complicated in the body. Also, the tissues that make up the temporomandibular joint differ from other load-bearing joints, like the knee or hip. Because of its complex movement and unique makeup, the jaw joint and its controlling muscles can pose a tremendous challenge to both patients and health care providers when problems arise.

What are TMJ disorders?

Disorders of the jaw joint and chewing muscles—and how people respond to them—vary widely. Researchers generally agree that the conditions fall into three main categories:

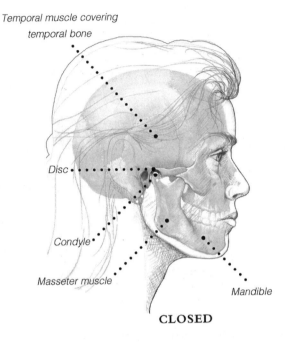

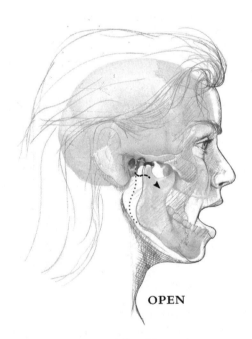

Figure 41.1. *Temporomandibular Joint*

1. Myofascial pain, the most common temporomandibular disorder, involves discomfort or pain in the muscles that control jaw function.

2. Internal derangement of the joint involves a displaced disc, dislocated jaw, or injury to the condyle.

3. Arthritis refers to a group of degenerative/inflammatory joint disorders that can affect the temporomandibular joint.

What are the signs and symptoms?

A variety of symptoms may be linked to TMJ disorders. Pain, particularly in the chewing muscles and/or jaw joint, is the most common symptom. Other likely symptoms include:

- radiating pain in the face, jaw, or neck;
- jaw muscle stiffness;
- limited movement or locking of the jaw;
- painful clicking, popping, or grating in the jaw joint when opening or closing the mouth;
- a change in the way the upper and lower teeth fit together.

How are TMJ disorders diagnosed?

There is no widely accepted, standard test now available to correctly diagnose TMJ disorders. Because the exact causes and symptoms are not clear, identifying these disorders can be difficult and confusing.

How are TMJ disorders treated?

Because more studies are needed on the safety and effectiveness of most treatments for jaw joint and muscle disorders, experts strongly recommend using the most conservative, reversible treatments possible. Conservative treatments do not invade the tissues of the face, jaw, or joint, or involve surgery. Reversible treatments do not cause permanent changes in the structure or position of the jaw or teeth. Even when TMJ disorders have become persistent, most patients still do not need aggressive types of treatment.

What are conservative treatments?

Because the most common jaw joint and muscle problems are temporary and do not get worse, simple treatment is all that is usually needed to relieve discomfort.

391

Self-care practices: There are steps you can take that may be helpful in easing symptoms, such as:

- eating soft foods,

- applying ice packs,

- avoiding extreme jaw movements (such as wide yawning, loud singing, and gum chewing),

- learning techniques for relaxing and reducing stress,

- practicing gentle jaw stretching and relaxing exercises that may help increase jaw movement. Your health care provider or a physical therapist can recommend exercises if appropriate for your particular condition.

Pain medications: For many people with TMJ disorders, short-term use of over-the-counter pain medicines or nonsteroidal anti-inflammatory drugs (NSAIDs), such as ibuprofen, may provide temporary relief from jaw discomfort. When necessary, your dentist or doctor can prescribe stronger pain or anti-inflammatory medications, muscle relaxants, or anti-depressants to help ease symptoms.

Stabilization splints: Your doctor or dentist may recommend an oral appliance, also called a stabilization splint or bite guard, which is a plastic guard that fits over the upper or lower teeth. Stabilization splints are the most widely used treatments for TMJ disorders. Studies of their effectiveness in providing pain relief, however, have been inconclusive. If a stabilization splint is recommended, it should be used only for a short time and should not cause permanent changes in the bite.

Botox (botulinum toxin type A) is a drug made from the same bacterium that causes food poisoning. Used in small doses, Botox injections can actually help alleviate some health problems. Botox has not been approved by the Food and Drug Administration (FDA) for use in TMJ disorders. Research is under way to learn how Botox specifically affects jaw muscles and their nerves. The findings will help determine if this drug may be useful in treating TMJ disorders.

What are irreversible treatments?

Irreversible treatments that have not been proven to be effective—and may make the problem worse—include orthodontics to change the bite; crown and bridge work to balance the bite; grinding down teeth to bring the bite into balance, called occlusal adjustment; and repositioning splints, also called orthotics, which permanently alter the bite.

Surgery: Other types of treatments, such as surgical procedures, invade the tissues. Surgical treatments are controversial, often irreversible, and should be avoided where possible. If surgery is recommended, be sure to have the doctor explain to you, in words you can understand, the reason for the treatment, the risks involved, and other types of treatment that may be available.

Implants: Surgical replacement of jaw joints with artificial implants may cause severe pain and permanent jaw damage. Some of these devices may fail to function properly or may break apart in the jaw over time. If you have already had temporomandibular joint surgery, be very cautious about considering additional operations. Persons undergoing multiple surgeries on the jaw joint generally have a poor outlook for normal, pain-free joint function. Before undergoing any surgery on the jaw joint, it is extremely important to get other independent opinions and to fully understand the risks.

What if you think you have a TMJ disorder?

Remember that for most people, discomfort from TMJ disorders will eventually go away on its own. Simple self-care practices are often effective in easing symptoms. If treatment is needed, it should be based on a reasonable diagnosis, be conservative and reversible, and be customized to your special needs. Avoid treatments that can cause permanent changes in the bite or jaw. If irreversible treatments are recommended, be sure to get a reliable, independent second opinion.

Because there is no certified specialty for TMJ disorders in either dentistry or medicine, finding the right care can be difficult. Look for a health care provider who understands musculoskeletal disorders (affecting muscle, bone, and joints) and who is trained in treating pain conditions. Pain clinics in hospitals and universities are often a good source of advice, particularly when pain continues over time and interferes with daily life.

Section 41.3

Osteonecrosis of the Jaw

Osteonecrosis of the jaw, commonly called ONJ, occurs when the jaw bone is exposed and begins to starve from a lack of blood. As the name indicates (*osteo* meaning bone and *necrosis* meaning death), the bone begins to weaken and die, which usually, but not always, causes pain. ONJ is associated with cancer treatments (including radiation), infection, steroid use, or potent antiresorptive therapies that help prevent the loss of bone mass. Examples of potent antiresorptive therapies include bisphosphonates such as alendronate (Fosamax); risedronate (Actonel and Atelvia); ibandronate (Boniva); and denosumab (Prolia). While ONJ is associated with these conditions, it also can occur without any identifiable risk factors.

Fast Facts

- ONJ may occur in patients taking strong antiresorptive therapies such as bisphosphonates or receptor activator of nuclear factor kappa-B ligand (RANKL) inhibitors. ONJ has not been reported with other antiresorptive therapies such as selective estrogen receptor modulators (SERM) or calcitonin. SERMs include therapies like raloxifene (Evista).

- The risk of ONJ in patients taking bisphosphonates may depend on the dose of medication, the length of time it is taken, and the medical condition for which the bisphosphonate is prescribed. As a result, cancer patients taking higher doses of bisphosphonates, particularly by intravenous (IV), are at higher risk.

- The number of ONJ cases in patients taking bisphosphonates by mouth is estimated to be between one in 1,000 and one in 100,000 for each year of exposure to the medication.

- Most patients with ONJ who are taking antiresorptive therapy for osteoporosis can be healed with conservative treatment and often do not require surgery.

- Most cases of ONJ happen after a dental extraction.

- Good oral hygiene and regular dental care is the best way to lower the risk of ONJ.

What Is ONJ?

ONJ is a condition in which an area of jawbone is not covered by the gums. The condition must last for more than eight weeks to be called ONJ. ONJ has occurred in patients with herpes zoster virus infections, in those who are undergoing radiation therapy of the head and neck (radiation osteonecrosis), osteomyelitis (bone infection) and in persons taking steroid therapy chronically. Patients taking antiresorptive therapy to reduce fracture risk also may experience ONJ. In this latter case, ONJ most often develops after an invasive (surgical) dental procedure such as dental extraction. ONJ also may occur spontaneously over boney growths in the roof or inner parts of the mouth.

What Causes ONJ?

Why some patients taking antiresorptive therapy get ONJ is unknown. It may be due to: 1) a decrease the bone's ability to repair itself; 2) a decrease in blood vessel formation; or 3) possible effects of infection.

Who Gets ONJ?

ONJ associated with bisphosphonate use, also referred to as BON, may develop in patients after taking the medication for as little as 12 months. The risk increases the longer bisphosphonates are taken. Most cases occur after prolonged therapy (more than five years).

For osteoporosis patients who do not have cancer and who are treated with osteoporosis medications, the risk of ONJ is low. Study results vary from less than one in 100,000 getting ONJ from bisphosphonate therapy to one patient in 263,158. One recent study suggested no increased incidence of ONJ with osteoporosis medication. However, the risk of ONJ in patients on bisphosphonates who have invasive dental work such as dental extraction may be higher. The risk of ONJ in patients taking denosumab (Prolia) is less well studied.

Cancer patients are at particular risk for ONJ. The doses of IV bis-phosphonates used to treat cancer can be ten times higher or more than the doses used for osteoporosis. Furthermore, cancer patients receive IV bisphosphonates as often as every 3–4 weeks, while osteoporosis patients receive only a single IV dose yearly. As a result, the risk of ONJ in cancer patients varies, but it is higher. Even with many risk factors, the incidence of ONJ in some European countries for cancer patients receiving IV bisphosphonates and other cancer treatments may be as high as one in ten patients. ONJ has been most commonly observed in cancer patients with multiple myeloma and breast cancer.

Besides cancer, other risk factors include advanced age, steroid use, diabetes, gum disease, and smoking.

How Is ONJ Diagnosed?

There is no diagnostic test to determine if an individual patient is at increased risk for ONJ. The condition itself is diagnosed only by the presence of exposed bone, lasting more than eight weeks. Patients typically complain of pain, which is often related to infection, soft tissue swelling, drainage, and exposed bone.

How Is ONJ Treated?

Most patients with osteoporosis who develop ONJ are treated conservatively with rinses, antibiotics, and oral analgesics. In the IV trial in osteoporosis mentioned, both cases resolved within months on such conservative treatment.

Prevention

A health program of oral hygiene and regular dental care is the optimal approach for lowering ONJ risk. Patients should inform their dentists that they are taking potent antiresorptive therapy. Dentists should consider conservative invasive dental care in patients taking potent antiresorptive therapies.

For instance, endodontic (root canal) treatment is preferred to dental extraction if the tooth can be saved. If dental extraction is needed, full mouth dental extractions or periodontal surgery should be avoided. (It may be better to assess healing by doing individual extractions.)

Patients with periodontal disease should consider non-surgical therapy before agreeing to surgical treatment. Many patients taking bisphosphonates may undergo dental implants without problems. Although some dentists recommend the use of blood tests to decide who is at risk, this practice is controversial due to a very limited evidence base and should not be used at this time.

Those on oral bisphosphonates are at low risk for BON. However, they are not without risk. Any problems developing in the mouth should signal the need for dental review. There is no data to suggest that bisphosphonates should be stopped prior to a dental procedure. However, patients about to start bisphosphonate therapy should consider waiting until any immediate invasive dental surgery is completed.

Points to Remember

- Up to one out of every two women over 50 will break a bone (such as wrist, spine, or hip) due to osteoporosis in their lifetime. Each year, about 250,000 will break a hip due to osteoporosis. Of these, up to 24% will die, and less than 25% regain full function. Vertebral (spine) fractures, which occur twice as often as hip fractures, also cause back pain and increased mortality.

- Up to one out of four men over 50 will break a bone due to osteoporosis in their lifetime. Each year, about 80,000 men will break a hip.

- Oral or IV bisphosphonates have been shown to prevent 50–70% of vertebral fractures in postmenopausal women and 40–50% of hip fractures in clinical trials. Denosumab (Prolia) has been shown to reduce vertebral fractures in 70% of postmenopausal women and 40% of hip fractures.

- Given the risk of osteoporotic fracture, and the low risk of ONJ associated with potent antiresorptive therapy use, the benefit of preventing osteoporotic fracture clearly far exceeds the risk of ONJ.

The Role of the Rheumatologist

Rheumatologists are specialists in musculoskeletal disorders including osteoporosis and, therefore, are best qualified to review the risks and benefits of antiresorptive therapy for osteoporosis. They can also advise patients about the best treatment options available.

Chapter 42

Mouth Sores

Chapter Contents

Section 42.1

Types, Causes, and Prevention of Mouth Sores

Different types of sores can appear anywhere in the mouth, including the inner cheeks, gums, tongue, lips, or palate.

Causes

Mouth sores may be caused by irritation from:

- a sharp or broken tooth or poorly fitting dentures;
- biting your cheek, tongue, or lip;
- burning your mouth from hot food or drinks;
- braces;
- chewing tobacco.

Cold sores are caused by the herpes simplex virus and are very contagious. Usually, you will have tenderness, tingling, or burning before the actual sore appears. Cold sores usually begin as blisters and then crust over. The herpes virus can live in your body for years. It only appears as a mouth sore when something triggers it, such as:

- another illness, especially if there is a fever;
- hormone changes (such as menstruation);
- stress;
- sun exposure.

Canker sores are not contagious. They can appear as a single pale or yellow ulcer with a red outer ring, or as a cluster of these sores. Women seem to get them more than men. The cause of canker sores is not clear, but may be related to:

- a weakness in your immune system (for example, from the cold or flu),

- hormone changes,

- stress,

- lack of certain vitamins and minerals in the diet, including vitamin B_{12} or folate.

Less commonly, mouth sores can be a sign of an illness, tumor, or reaction to a medication. This can include:

- autoimmune disorders (including systemic lupus erythematosus),

- bleeding disorders,

- cancer of the mouth,

- infections such as hand-foot-mouth disease,

- weakened immune system—for example, if you have autoimmune deficiency syndrome (AIDS) or are taking medication after a transplant.

Drugs that may cause mouth sores include aspirin, chemotherapy, penicillin, sulfa drugs, and phenytoin (used for seizures).

Home Care

Mouth sores often go away in 10 to 14 days, even if you don't do anything. They sometimes last up to six weeks. The following steps can make you feel better:

- Avoid hot beverages and foods, spicy and salty foods, and citrus.

- Gargle with salt water or cool water.

- Eat popsicles. This is helpful if you have a mouth burn.

- Take pain relievers like acetaminophen.

For canker sores:

- Apply a thin paste of baking soda and water to the sore.

- Mix one part hydrogen peroxide with one part water and apply this mixture to the sores using a cotton swab.

- For more severe cases, treatments include fluocinonide gel (Lidex), anti-inflammatory amlexanox paste (Aphthasol), or chlorhexidine gluconate (Peridex) mouthwash.

401

Over-the-counter medications, such as Orabase, can protect a sore ⋅ inside the lip and on the gums. Blistex or Campho-Phenique may provide some relief of canker sores and fever blisters, especially if applied when the sore first appears. To help cold sores or fever blisters, you can also apply ice to the sore.

When to Contact a Medical Professional

Call your doctor if:

- the sore begins soon after you start a new medication;
- you have large white patches on the roof of your mouth or your tongue (this may be thrush or another type of infection);
- your mouth sore lasts longer than two weeks;
- you have a weakened immune system (for example, from human immunodeficiency virus (HIV) or cancer);
- you have other symptoms like fever, skin rash, drooling, or difficulty swallowing.

What to Expect at Your Office Visit

Your doctor will perform a physical examination, focusing on your mouth and tongue. You will be asked questions about your medical history and symptoms.

Treatment may include the following:

- A medicine that numbs the area when applied such as lidocaine may be used to relieve pain. This should be avoided in children.
- An antiviral medication to treat herpes sores (although some experts don't believe medication will make the sores go away sooner)
- Steroid gel applied to the sore
- A paste that reduces swelling or inflammation (such as Aphthasol)
- A special type of mouthwash such as chlorhexidine gluconate (such as Peridex)

Prevention

You may reduce your chance of getting common mouth sores by:

- avoiding very hot foods or beverages,

- reducing stress and practicing relaxation techniques like yoga or meditation,

- chewing slowly,

- using a soft-bristle toothbrush,

- visiting your dentist right away if you have a sharp or broken tooth or misfit dentures.

If you seem to get canker sores often, talk to your doctor about taking folate and vitamin B_{12} to prevent outbreaks.

To prevent cancer of the mouth:

- Do not smoke or use tobacco.

- Limit alcohol to two drinks per day.

- Wear a wide-brimmed hat to shade your lips. Wear a lip balm with SPF 15 at all times.

Section 42.2

Canker Sores

About one in five people regularly gets bothersome canker sores, which can make eating, drinking, and even brushing teeth a real pain. But just because they're relatively common doesn't mean these small open sores inside the mouth should be ignored.

About Canker Sores

Also known as aphthous ulcers, canker sores are small sores that can occur inside the mouth, cheeks, lips, throat, or sometimes on the tongue. But don't confuse canker sores with cold sores or fever blisters, which are sores that are caused by the herpes simplex virus and are found outside the mouth around the lips, on the cheeks or chin, or inside the nostrils. Whereas cold sores are contagious, canker sores are not contagious—so kissing cannot spread them.

Although canker sores aren't contagious, the tendency to have outbreaks of canker sores can run in a family. If you're prone to canker sores, your child has a 90% chance of getting them as well.

Although no one knows exactly what causes canker sores, many factors are thought to put a person at risk. Diet may be a factor. People who have nutritional deficiencies of folic acid, vitamin B_{12}, and iron seem to develop canker sores more often, as do people who have food allergies. Canker sores may also indicate that a person has an immune system problem.

Mouth injuries, such as biting the inside of your lip or even brushing too hard and damaging the delicate lining inside the mouth, also seem to bring on canker sores. Even emotional stress seems to be a factor. One study of college students showed that they had more canker sores during stressful periods, such as around exam time, than they did during less stressful times, such as summer break.

Although anyone can get them, young people in their teens and early twenties seem to get them most often, and women are twice as likely to develop them as men. Some girls and women find that they get canker sores at the start of their menstrual periods.

Signs and Symptoms

Canker sores usually appear as painful, red spots that can be up to one inch (2.5 centimeters) across, although most of them are much smaller. Sometimes the area will tingle or burn before a spot actually appears. Once it does, the canker sore may swell and burst in about a day. The open sore may then have a white or yellowish coating over it as well as a red "halo" around it. Most often, canker sores pop up alone, but they can also occur in small clusters.

Although uncommon, canker sores can be accompanied by such symptoms as fever, swollen lymph nodes, and a lethargic or slightly ill feeling.

It takes about two weeks for canker sores to heal. During this time, the sores can be painful, although the first three to four days are usually the worst.

If your child develops canker sores that last longer than two weeks or is unable to eat or drink because of the pain, contact your doctor. Also, call the doctor if the sores appear more than two or three times a year.

Diagnosis

If your child has recurrent canker sores, the doctor may want to perform tests to look for possible nutritional deficiencies (which can be corrected with dietary changes or using prescription vitamin supplements), immune system deficiencies, and food or other allergies.

Treatment

Often, canker sores can be easily treated with over-the-counter or even home remedies. Carbamide peroxide is a combination of peroxide and glycerin that cleans out the sore while coating it to protect the wound.

Many over-the-counter remedies have benzocaine, menthol, and eucalyptol in them. These may sting at first and need to be applied repeatedly, but they can reduce pain and shorten the duration of the sore.

You can also have your child rinse his or her mouth with a homemade solution for about a minute, four times a day, as needed. It's extremely important to remember, though, that these rinses should not be swallowed, so they shouldn't be used in kids too young to understand not to swallow.

You can try these rinse recipes:

- Two ounces (59 milliliters) of hydrogen peroxide and two ounces (59 milliliters) of water

- Four ounces (118 milliliters) of water mixed with one teaspoon (five milliliters) of salt and one teaspoon (five milliliters) of baking soda

Another option to help reduce discomfort and speed healing is dabbing a mixture of equal parts water and hydrogen peroxide directly on the sore, followed by a bit of milk of magnesia.

Some doctors suggest applying wet black tea bags to the sore. Black tea contains tannin, an astringent that can help relieve pain. You can also get tannin in over-the-counter medications. Ask the pharmacist for more information.

If the doctor prescribes a medicine that should be applied directly to the canker sore, first dry the area with a tissue. Use a cotton swab to apply a small amount of the medication. Finally, have your child avoid eating or drinking for at least 30 minutes to make sure that the medicine isn't immediately washed away and has time to work.

In some cases of severe mouth sores, the doctor may prescribe immunosuppressive drugs or mouth rinses or gels that contain steroids.

Caring for Your Child

Help make canker sores less painful and prevent them from recurring by encouraging your child to:

- avoid eating abrasive foods, such as potato chips and nuts, which can irritate gums and other delicate mouth tissues;

- try brushing and rinsing with toothpastes and mouthwashes that do not contain sodium lauryl sulfate (SLS);

- use only soft-bristle toothbrushes and be careful not to brush too hard;

- avoid any foods he or she is allergic to;

- avoid spicy, salty, and acidic foods (such as lemons and tomatoes), which can aggravate tender mouth sores.

Although they can certainly be a pain, in most cases, canker sores aren't a huge problem. Many people have learned to deal with them— and your child can, too.

Section 42.3

Cold Sores

About Cold Sores

Cold sores are small and painful blisters that can appear around the mouth, face, or nose. Sometimes referred to as fever blisters, they're caused by herpes simplex virus type 1 (HSV-1). Kids can get cold sores by kissing or sharing eating utensils with an infected person.

Colds sores in the mouth are very common, and many kids get infected with HSV-1 during the preschool years. The sores usually go away on their own within about a week.

Symptoms

Most kids who get cold sores get infected by eating or drinking from the same utensils as someone who is infected with the herpes virus or by getting kissed by an infected adult.

The cold sores first form blisters on the lips and inside the mouth. The blisters then become sores. In some cases, the gums become red and swollen. In other cases, the virus also leads to a fever, muscle aches, eating difficulties, a generally ill feeling, irritability, and swollen neck glands. These symptoms can last up to two weeks.

After a child is initially infected, the virus can lie dormant without causing any symptoms. But it can reactivate later, typically after some sort of stress like a cold, an infection, hormonal change, menstrual periods, or even before a big test at school. If the virus is reactivated it can cause tingling and numbness around the mouth and a blister.

Treatment

Usually, HSV-1 causes cold sores in the mouth or face, and herpes simplex virus type 2 (HSV-2) causes lesions in the genital area, resulting in genital herpes. But sometimes, HSV-1 can cause genital lesions as well, especially if someone has received oral sex from an infected partner.

Cold sores from HSV-1 usually go away on their own within five to seven days. Although no medications can make the infection go away, some treatments are available that can shorten the length of the outbreak and make the cold sores less painful.

Cool foods and drinks can help relieve discomfort, and acetaminophen may also ease the pain. Aspirin should not be given to kids with viral infections since it has been associated with Reye syndrome.

Call the doctor if your child:

- has another health condition that has weakened the immune system, which could allow the HSV infection to spread and cause problems in other parts of the body;

- has sores that don't heal by themselves within seven to ten days;

- has any sores near the eyes;

- gets cold sores frequently.

Since the virus that causes cold sores is so contagious, it's important to prevent it from spreading to other family members. Precautions to take with kids who have cold sores include:

- keeping their drinking glasses and eating utensils separate from those used by other family members and washing these items thoroughly after use;

- teaching them not to kiss others until the sores heal;

- having them wash their hands frequently and as soon as possible after touching the cold sores;

- trying to keep them from touching their eyes—if HSV infects the eyes, it can be very serious.

If you're caring for a child with a cold sore, you also should be sure to wash your hands frequently so that you don't contract the virus or spread it to others.

Chapter 43

Oral Allergy Syndrome

What Is Food Allergy?

Food allergy is an abnormal response to a food triggered by the body's immune system. There are several types of immune responses to food. This chapter focuses on one type of adverse reaction to food— that in which the body produces a specific type of antibody called immunoglobulin E (IgE).

The binding of IgE to specific molecules present in a food triggers the immune response. The response may be mild or in rare cases it can be associated with the severe and life-threatening reaction called anaphylaxis. Therefore, if you have a food allergy, it is extremely important for you to work with your healthcare professional to learn what foods cause your allergic reaction. Sometimes, a reaction to food is not an allergy at all but another type of reaction called food intolerance.

What Is an Allergic Reaction to Food?

A food allergy occurs when the immune system responds to a harmless food as if it were a threat. The first time a person with food allergy is exposed to the food, no symptoms occur; but the first exposure primes the body to respond the next time. When the person eats the food again, an allergic response can occur.

Excerpted from "Food Allergy: An Overview," National Institute of Allergy and Infectious Diseases (NIAID), November 2010.

The Allergic Reaction Process

An allergic reaction to food is a two-step process.

Step 1: The first time you are exposed to a food allergen, your immune system reacts as if the food were harmful and makes specific IgE antibodies to that allergen. The antibodies circulate through your blood and attach to mast cells and basophils. Mast cells are found in all body tissues, especially in areas of your body that are typical sites of allergic reactions. Those sites include your nose, throat, lungs, skin, and gastrointestinal (GI) tract. Basophils are found in your blood and also in tissues that have become inflamed due to an allergic reaction.

Step 2: The next time you are exposed to the same food allergen, it binds to the IgE antibodies that are attached to the mast cells and basophils. The binding signals the cells to release massive amounts of chemicals such as histamine. Depending on the tissue in which they are released, these chemicals will cause you to have various symptoms of food allergy. The symptoms can range from mild to severe. A severe allergic reaction can include a potentially life-threatening reaction called anaphylaxis.

Generally, you are at greater risk for developing a food allergy if you come from a family in which allergies are common. These allergies are not necessarily food allergies but perhaps other allergic diseases, such as asthma or eczema (atopic dermatitis). If you have two parents who have allergies, you are more likely to develop food allergy than someone with one parent who has allergies.

An allergic reaction to food usually takes place within a few minutes to several hours after exposure to the allergen. The process of eating and digesting food and the location of mast cells both affect the timing and location of the reaction.

Symptoms of Food Allergy

If you are allergic to a particular food, you may experience all or some of the following symptoms:

- Itching in your mouth
- Swelling of lips and tongue
- Gastrointestinal symptoms, such as vomiting, diarrhea, or abdominal cramps and pain
- Hives
- Worsening of eczema

- Tightening of the throat or trouble breathing
- A drop in blood pressure

What Is Oral Allergy Syndrome?

Oral allergy syndrome (OAS) is an allergy to certain raw fruits and vegetables, such as apples, cherries, kiwis, celery, tomatoes, and green peppers. OAS occurs mostly in people with hay fever, especially spring hay fever due to birch pollen and late summer hay fever due to ragweed pollen.

Eating the raw food causes an itchy, tingling sensation in the mouth, lips, and throat. It can also cause swelling of the lips, tongue, and throat; watery, itchy eyes; runny nose; and sneezing. Just handling the raw fruit or vegetable may cause a rash, itching, or swelling where the juice touches the skin.

Cooking or processing easily breaks down the proteins in the fruits and vegetables that cause OAS. Therefore, OAS typically does not occur with cooked or baked fruits and vegetables or processed fruits, such as in applesauce.

What Is Anaphylaxis?

If you have a food allergy, there is a chance that you may experience a severe form of allergic reaction known as anaphylaxis. Anaphylaxis may begin suddenly and may lead to death if not immediately treated.

Anaphylaxis includes a wide range of symptoms that can occur in many combinations. Some symptoms are not life-threatening, but the most severe restrict breathing and blood circulation.

Symptoms may begin within several minutes to several hours after exposure to the food. Sometimes the symptoms go away, only to return 2–4 hours later or even as many as eight hours later. When you begin to experience symptoms, you must seek immediate medical attention because anaphylaxis can be life-threatening.

Anaphylaxis caused by an allergic reaction to a certain food is highly unpredictable. The severity of a given attack does not predict the severity of subsequent attacks. The response will vary depending on several factors, such as these:

- Your sensitivity to the food
- How much of the food you are exposed to
- How the food entered your body

Any anaphylactic reaction may become dangerous and must be evaluated by a healthcare professional. Food allergy is the leading cause of anaphylaxis. However, medications, insect stings, and latex can also cause an allergic reaction that leads to anaphylaxis.

Diagnosing Food Allergy

Detailed history: Your healthcare professional will begin by taking a detailed medical history to find out whether your symptoms are caused by an allergy to specific foods, a food intolerance, or other health problems.

A detailed history is the most valuable tool for diagnosing food allergy. Your healthcare professional will ask you several questions and listen to your history of food reactions to decide whether the facts fit a diagnosis of food allergy.

Your healthcare professional is likely to ask some of the following questions:

- Did your reaction come on quickly, usually within minutes to several hours after eating the food?

- Is your reaction always associated with a certain food?

- How much of this potentially allergenic food did you eat before you had a reaction?

- Have you eaten this food before and had a reaction?

- Did anyone else who ate the same food get sick?

- Did you take allergy medicines, and if so, did they help? Antihistamines should relieve hives, for example.

Other ways to diagnose food allergy include: a diet diary, an elimination diet, skin prick tests, a blood test, and oral food challenges.

Prevention of Food Allergies

There is currently no cure for food allergies. You can only prevent the symptoms of food allergy by avoiding the allergenic food. After you and your healthcare professional have identified the food(s) to which you are sensitive, you must remove them from your diet.

Chapter 44

Oral Cancer

Chapter Contents

Section 44.1

Detecting Oral Cancer

Text in this section includes excerpts from "Detecting Oral Cancer: A
Guide for Health Care Professionals," National Institute of Dental and
Craniofacial Research (NIDCR), March 2011; and "The Oral Cancer
Exam," National Institutes of Health (NIH), NIH Publication No.
08–5032, September 2008.

Detecting Oral Cancer

Incidence and Survival

Oral cancer accounts for roughly 2% of all cancers diagnosed annually
in the United States. Approximately 36,500 people will be diagnosed with
oral cancer each year and about 7,900 will die from the disease. On average, 61% of those with the disease will survive more than five years.

Early Detection Saves Lives

With early detection and timely treatment, deaths from oral cancer
could be dramatically reduced. The 5-year survival rate for those with
localized disease at diagnosis is 83% compared with only 32% for those
whose cancer has spread to other parts of the body. Early detection of
oral cancer is often possible. Tissue changes in the mouth that might
signal the beginnings of cancer often can be seen and felt easily.

Warning Signs

Lesions that might signal oral cancer: Two lesions that could be
precursors to cancer are leukoplakia (white lesions) and erythroplakia
(red lesions). Any white or red lesion that does not resolve itself in
two weeks should be reevaluated and considered for biopsy to obtain
a definitive diagnosis.

Other possible signs and symptoms: Possible signs and symptoms of oral cancer include: a lump or thickening in the oral soft tissues, soreness or a feeling that something is caught in the throat,
difficulty chewing or swallowing, ear pain, difficulty moving the jaw

or tongue, hoarseness, numbness of the tongue or other areas of the mouth, or swelling of the jaw that causes dentures to fit poorly or become uncomfortable.

If these problems persist for more than two weeks, a thorough clinical examination and laboratory tests as necessary should be performed to obtain a definitive diagnosis. If a diagnosis cannot be obtained, referral to the appropriate specialist is indicated.

Risk Factors

Tobacco/alcohol use: Most cases of oral cancer are linked to cigarette smoking, heavy alcohol use, or the use of both tobacco and alcohol together. Using tobacco plus alcohol poses a much greater risk than using either substance alone.

Human papilloma virus (HPV): Infection with the sexually transmitted human papillomavirus (specifically the HPV 16 type) has been linked to a subset of oral cancers.

Age: Risk increases with age. Oral cancer most often occurs in people over the age of 40.

Sun exposure: Cancer of the lip can be caused by sun exposure.

Diet: A diet low in fruits and vegetables may play a role in oral cancer development.

What You Can Do

A thorough head and neck examination should be a routine part of each patient's dental visit and general medical examination. Clinicians should be particularly vigilant in checking those who use tobacco or excessive amounts of alcohol.

The Oral Cancer Exam

An oral cancer exam is painless and quick—it takes only a few minutes. Your regular dental checkup is an excellent opportunity to have the exam.

Here's what to expect:

1. If you have dentures (plates) or partials, you will be asked to remove them.

2. Your health care provider will inspect your face, neck, lips, and mouth to look for any signs of cancer.

3. With both hands, he or she will feel the area under your jaw and the side of your neck, checking for lumps that may suggest cancer.

4. He or she will then look at and feel the insides of your lips and cheeks to check for possible signs of cancer, such as red or white patches.

5. Next, your provider will have you stick out your tongue so it can be checked for swelling or abnormal color or texture.

6. Using gauze, he or she will then gently pull your tongue to one side, then the other, to check the base of your tongue. The underside of your tongue will also be checked.

7. In addition, he or she will look at the roof and floor of your mouth, as well as the back of your throat.

8. Finally, your provider will put one finger on the floor of your mouth and, with the other hand under your chin, gently press down to check for lumps or sensitivity.

Section 44.2

What You Need to Know about Oral Cancer

Excerpted from "What You Need to Know about Oral Cancer," National Cancer Institute (NCI), December 23, 2009.

Oral cancer can develop in any part of the oral cavity (the mouth and lips) or the oropharynx (the part of the throat at the back of the mouth). Each year in the United States, more than 21,000 men and 9,000 women are diagnosed with oral cancer. Most are over 60 years old.

The Mouth and Throat

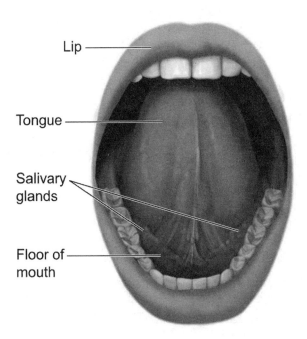

Figure 44.1. *This picture shows the parts of your mouth, including the area under the tongue.*

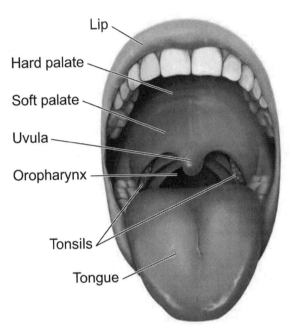

Lip

Hard palate

Soft palate

Uvula

Oropharynx

Tonsils

Tongue

Figure 44.2. This picture shows the parts of your mouth and throat.

Cancer Cells

Almost all oral cancers begin in the flat cells (squamous cells) that cover the surfaces of the mouth, tongue, and lips. These cancers are called squamous cell carcinomas.

Oral cancer cells can spread by breaking away from the original tumor. They enter blood vessels or lymph vessels, which branch into all the tissues of the body. The cancer cells often appear first in nearby lymph nodes in the neck. The cancer cells may attach to other tissues and grow to form new tumors that may damage those tissues. The spread of cancer is called metastasis.

Risk Factors

When you get a diagnosis of cancer, it's natural to wonder what may have caused the disease. Doctors can't always explain why one person gets oral cancer and another doesn't. However, we do know that people with certain risk factors may be more likely than others to develop oral cancer. A risk factor is something that may increase the chance of getting a disease.

Studies have found the following risk factors for oral cancer:

Tobacco use causes most oral cancers.

Heavy alcohol use: People who are heavy drinkers are more likely to develop oral cancer than people who don't drink alcohol.

HPV infection: Some members of the HPV family of viruses can infect the mouth and throat. These viruses are passed from person to person through sexual contact.

Sun: Cancer of the lip can be caused by exposure to the sun.

A personal history of oral cancer: People who have had oral cancer are at increased risk of developing another oral cancer. Smoking increases this risk.

Diet: Some studies suggest that not eating enough fruits and vegetables may increase the chance of getting oral cancer.

Betel nut use: Betel nut use is most common in Asia, where millions chew the product. It's a type of palm seed wrapped with a betel leaf and sometimes mixed with spices, sweeteners, and tobacco. Chewing betel nut causes oral cancer. The risk increases even more if the person also drinks alcohol and uses tobacco.

Number of risk factors: The more risk factors that a person has, the greater the chance that oral cancer will develop. However, most people with known risk factors for oral cancer don't develop the disease.

Symptoms

Symptoms of oral cancer may include:

- Patches inside your mouth or on your lips:
  - White patches (leukoplakia) are the most common. White patches sometimes become malignant.
  - Mixed red and white patches (erythroleukoplakia) are more likely than white patches to become malignant.
  - Red patches (erythroplakia) are brightly colored, smooth areas that often become malignant.
- A sore on your lip or in your mouth that doesn't heal
- Bleeding in your mouth
- Loose teeth

- Difficulty or pain when swallowing
- Difficulty wearing dentures
- A lump in your neck
- An earache that doesn't go away
- Numbness of lower lip and chin

Most often, these symptoms are not from oral cancer. Another health problem can cause them. Anyone with these symptoms should tell their doctor or dentist so that problems can be diagnosed and treated as early as possible.

Staging

If oral cancer is diagnosed, your doctor needs to learn the extent (stage) of the disease to help you choose the best treatment.

Early cancer: Stage I or II oral cancer is usually a small tumor (smaller than a walnut), and no cancer cells are found in the lymph nodes.

Advanced cancer: Stage III or IV oral cancer is usually a large tumor (as big as a lime). The cancer may have invaded nearby tissues or spread to lymph nodes or other parts of the body.

Treatment

People with early oral cancer may be treated with surgery or radiation therapy. People with advanced oral cancer may have a combination of treatments. For example, radiation therapy and chemotherapy are often given at the same time. Another treatment option is targeted therapy.

Surgery

Surgery to remove the tumor in the mouth or throat is a common treatment for oral cancer. Sometimes the surgeon also removes lymph nodes in the neck. Other tissues in the mouth and neck may be removed as well. You may have surgery alone or in combination with radiation therapy.

Radiation Therapy

Radiation therapy uses high-energy rays to kill cancer cells. It's an option for small tumors or for people who can't have surgery. Or, it may be used before surgery to shrink the tumor. Doctors use two types of radiation therapy to treat oral cancer. Some people with oral cancer have both types: external radiation therapy that comes from a machine; and, internal radiation therapy, which is not commonly used for oral cancer, that comes from radioactive material in seeds, wires, or tubes put directly in the mouth or throat tissue.

Chemotherapy

Chemotherapy uses drugs to kill cancer cells. The drugs that treat oral cancer are usually given through a vein (intravenous). The drugs enter the bloodstream and travel throughout your body. Chemotherapy and radiation therapy are often given at the same time.

Targeted Therapy

Some people with oral cancer receive a type of drug known as targeted therapy. It may be given along with radiation therapy or chemotherapy. Cetuximab (Erbitux) was the first targeted therapy approved for oral cancer. Cetuximab binds to oral cancer cells and interferes with cancer cell growth and the spread of cancer. You may receive cetuximab through a vein once a week for several weeks at the doctor's office, hospital, or clinic.

Second Opinion

Before starting treatment, you might want a second opinion about your diagnosis, the stage of cancer, and the treatment plan. You may even want to talk to several different doctors about all of the treatment options, their side effects, and the expected results.

Nutrition

Your diet is an important part of your treatment for oral cancer. You need the right amount of calories, protein, vitamins, and minerals to maintain your strength and to heal. However, when you have oral cancer, it may be difficult to eat. You may be uncomfortable or tired, and you may have a dry mouth, have trouble swallowing, or not feel like eating. You also may have nausea, vomiting, constipation, or diarrhea from cancer treatment or pain medicine. Tell your health care team if you're having any problems eating, drinking, or digesting your food. If you're losing weight, a dietitian can help you choose the foods and nutrition products that will meet your needs.

Reconstruction

Some people with oral cancer may need to have plastic or reconstructive surgery to rebuild the bones or tissues of the mouth. Research has led to many advances in the way bones and tissues can be rebuilt. Some people may need dental implants. Or they may need to have grafts (tissue moved from another part of the body). Skin, muscle, and bone can be moved to the mouth from the chest, arm, or leg. The plastic surgeon uses this tissue for repair.

If you're thinking about reconstruction, you may wish to consult with a plastic or reconstructive surgeon before your treatment for oral cancer begins. You can have reconstructive surgery at the same time as you have the cancer removed, or you can have it later on. Talk with your doctor about which approach is right for you.

Rehabilitation

Your health care team will help you return to normal activities as soon as possible. The goals of rehabilitation depend on the extent of the disease and type of treatment.

If oral cancer or its treatment leads to problems with talking, speech therapy will generally begin as soon as possible. A speech therapist may see you in the hospital to plan therapy and teach speech exercises. Speech therapy may continue after you return home.

Some people will need a prosthesis to help them talk and eat as normally as possible. A prosthesis is an artificial device that replaces the missing teeth or tissues of the mouth. For example, if part of the palate is removed, a dentist with special training (a prosthodontist) may be able to fit you with a plastic device that replaces the missing tissue.

Section 44.3

Smokeless Tobacco's Connection to Cancer

Excerpted from "Smokeless Tobacco and Cancer: Key Points,"
National Cancer Institute (NCI), October 25, 2010.

Smokeless tobacco is tobacco that is not burned. It is also known as chewing tobacco, oral tobacco, spit or spitting tobacco, dip, chew, and snuff. Most people chew or suck (dip) the tobacco in their mouth and spit out the tobacco juices that build up, although spit-less, smokeless tobacco has also been developed. Nicotine in the tobacco is absorbed through the lining of the mouth.

There are two main types of smokeless tobacco:

- **Chewing tobacco** is available as loose leaves, plugs (bricks), or twists of rope. A piece of tobacco is placed between the cheek and lower lip, typically toward the back of the mouth. It is either chewed or held in place. Saliva is spit or swallowed.

- **Snuff** is finely cut or powdered tobacco. It may be sold in different scents and flavors. It is packaged moist or dry; most American snuff is moist. It is available loose, in dissolvable lozenges or strips, or in small pouches similar to tea bags. The user places a pinch or pouch of moist snuff between the cheek and gums or behind the upper or lower lip. Another name for moist snuff is snus (pronounced snoose). Some people inhale dry snuff into the nose.

Are there harmful chemicals in smokeless tobacco?

Yes. There is no safe form of tobacco. At least 28 chemicals in smokeless tobacco have been found to cause cancer. The most harmful chemicals in smokeless tobacco are tobacco-specific nitrosamines that are formed during the growing, curing, fermenting, and aging of tobacco.

Does smokeless tobacco cause cancer?

Yes. Smokeless tobacco causes oral cancer, esophageal cancer, and pancreatic cancer.

Does smokeless tobacco cause other diseases?

Yes. Using smokeless tobacco may also cause heart disease, gum disease, and oral lesions other than cancer, such as leukoplakia (precancerous white patches in the mouth).

Can a user get addicted to smokeless tobacco?

Yes. All tobacco products, including smokeless tobacco, contain nicotine which is addictive. Users of smokeless tobacco and users of cigarettes have comparable levels of nicotine in the blood. In users of smokeless tobacco, nicotine is absorbed through the mouth tissues directly into the blood where it goes to the brain. Even after the tobacco is removed from the mouth, nicotine continues to be absorbed into the bloodstream. Also, the nicotine stays in the blood longer for users of smokeless tobacco than for smokers.

The level of nicotine in the blood depends on the amount of nicotine in the smokeless tobacco product, the tobacco cut size, the product's pH (a measure of its acidity or basicity), and other factors. A Centers for Disease Control and Prevention (CDC) study of the 40 most widely used popular brands of moist snuff showed that the amount of nicotine per gram of tobacco ranged from 4.4 milligrams to 25.0 milligrams. Other studies have shown that moist snuff had between 4.7 and 24.3 milligrams per gram of tobacco, dry snuff had between 10.5 and 24.8 milligrams per gram of tobacco, and chewing tobacco had between 3.4 and 39.7 milligrams per gram of tobacco.

Is using smokeless tobacco less hazardous than smoking cigarettes?

Because all tobacco products are harmful and cause cancer, the use of all of these products should be strongly discouraged. There is no safe level of tobacco use. People who use any type of tobacco product should be urged to quit.

Should smokeless tobacco be used to help a person quit smoking?

No. There is no scientific evidence that using smokeless tobacco can help a person quit smoking. Because all tobacco products are harmful and cause cancer, the use of all tobacco products is strongly discouraged. There is no safe level of tobacco use. People who use any type of tobacco product should be urged to quit. For help with quitting, ask your doctor about individual or group counseling, telephone quit-lines, or other methods.

Chapter 45

Taste Disorders

How common are taste disorders?

Many of us take our sense of taste for granted, but a taste disorder can have a negative effect on a person's health and quality of life. If you are having a problem with your sense of taste, you are not alone. More than 200,000 people visit a doctor each year for problems with their chemical senses, which include taste and smell. The senses of taste and smell are very closely related. Some people who go to the doctor because they think they have lost their sense of taste are surprised to learn that they have a smell disorder instead.

What are the taste disorders?

The most common taste disorder is phantom taste perception; that is, a lingering, often unpleasant taste even though you have nothing in your mouth. We also can experience a reduced ability to taste sweet, sour, bitter, salty, and umami (a savory taste)—a condition called hypogeusia. Some people cannot detect any tastes, which is called ageusia. True taste loss, however, is rare. Most often, people are experiencing a loss of smell instead of a loss of taste.

Text in this chapter is excerpted from "Taste Disorders," National Institute of Deafness and Other Communication Disorders (NIDCD), NIH Publication No. 09-3231A, Updated July 2009; and, an excerpt titled "Most Common Causes of Taste Disorders," from "Problems with Taste," National Institutes of Health (NIH), May 17, 2011.

In other disorders of the chemical senses, an odor, a taste, or a flavor may be distorted. Dysgeusia is a condition in which a foul, salty, rancid, or metallic taste sensation will persist in the mouth. Dysgeusia is sometimes accompanied by burning mouth syndrome, a condition in which a person experiences a painful burning sensation in the mouth. Although it can affect anyone, burning mouth syndrome is most common in middle-aged and older women.

What causes taste disorders?

Some people are born with taste disorders, but most develop them after an injury or illness. Among the causes of taste problems are:

- upper respiratory and middle ear infections;
- radiation therapy for cancers of the head and neck;
- exposure to certain chemicals, such as insecticides and some medications, including some common antibiotics and antihistamines;
- head injury;
- some surgeries to the ear, nose, and throat (for example, third molar, wisdom tooth, extraction and middle ear surgery);
- poor oral hygiene and dental problems.

Most Common Causes of Taste Disorders

The most common causes of taste disorders are medications, infections, head trauma, and dental problems. Most people who have a problem with taste are taking certain medications or they have had a head or neck injury. Gum disease, dry mouth, and dentures can contribute to taste problems, too. Other causes are radiation therapy for head and neck cancers, heavy smoking, vitamin deficiencies, Bell's palsy, and Sjögren syndrome. [Source: "Problems with Taste," National Institutes of Health, May 17, 2011.]

How are taste disorders diagnosed?

Both taste and smell disorders are diagnosed by an otolaryngologist, a doctor of the ear, nose, throat, head, and neck. An otolaryngologist can determine the extent of your taste disorder by measuring the lowest concentration of a taste quality that you can detect or recognize. You may also be asked to compare the tastes of different substances or to note how the intensity of a taste grows when a substance's concentration is increased.

Scientists have developed taste testing in which the patient responds to different chemical concentrations. This may involve a simple sip, spit, and rinse test, or chemicals may be applied directly to specific areas of the tongue.

An accurate assessment of your taste loss will include, among other things, a physical examination of your ears, nose, and throat; a dental examination and assessment of oral hygiene; a review of your health history; and a taste test supervised by a health care professional.

Are taste disorders serious?

Taste disorders can weaken or remove an early warning system that most of us take for granted. Taste helps us detect spoiled food or liquids and, for some people, the presence of ingredients to which they are allergic.

Loss of taste can create serious health issues. A distorted sense of taste can be a risk factor for heart disease, diabetes, stroke, and other illnesses that require sticking to a specific diet. When taste is impaired, a person may change his or her eating habits. Some people may eat too little and lose weight, while others may eat too much and gain weight.

Loss of taste can cause us to eat too much sugar or salt to make our food taste better. This can be a problem for people with certain medical conditions, such as diabetes or high blood pressure. In severe cases, loss of taste can lead to depression.

Loss of taste and smell can also be a sign of certain degenerative diseases of the nervous system, such as Parkinson disease or Alzheimer disease. If you are experiencing a taste disorder, talk with your physician.

Can taste disorders be treated?

Many types of taste disorders are curable. For those that are not, counseling is available to help people adjust to their problem.

Diagnosis by an otolaryngologist is important to identify and treat the underlying cause of your disorder. If a certain medication is the cause, stopping or changing your medicine may help eliminate the problem. (Do not stop taking your medications unless directed by your doctor, however.) Some people, notably those with respiratory infections or allergies, regain their sense of taste when these conditions are resolved. Often, the correction of a general medical problem also can correct the loss of taste. Occasionally, a person may recover his or her sense of taste spontaneously. Proper oral hygiene is important to regaining and maintaining a well-functioning sense of taste.

If you lose some or all of your sense of taste, there are things you can do to make your food taste better:

- Prepare foods with a variety of colors and textures.

- Use aromatic herbs and hot spices to add more flavor; however, avoid adding more sugar or salt to foods.

- If your diet permits, add small amounts of cheese, bacon bits, butter, olive oil, or toasted nuts on vegetables.

- Avoid combination dishes, such as casseroles, that can hide individual flavors and dilute taste.

Chapter 46

Thrush

Candidiasis of the mouth and throat, also known as a thrush or oropharyngeal candidiasis (OPC), is a fungal infection that occurs when there is overgrowth of fungus called candida. Candida is normally found on skin or mucous membranes. However, if the environment inside the mouth or throat becomes imbalanced, Candida can multiply. When this happens, symptoms of thrush appear. Candida overgrowth can also develop in the esophagus, and is called candida esophagitis, or esophageal candidiasis.

How common is OPC and who can get it?

OPC, or thrush, can affect normal newborns, persons with dentures, and people who use inhaled corticosteroids. It occurs more frequently and more severely in people with weakened immune systems, particularly in persons with autoimmune deficiency syndrome (AIDS) and people undergoing treatment for cancer. Candida esophagitis usually occurs in people with weakened immune systems. It is very unusual in otherwise healthy people.

How do I get thrush (OPC)?

Most cases of thrush (OPC) are caused by the person's own Candida organisms which normally live in the mouth or digestive tract. A person has symptoms when overgrowth of Candida organisms occurs.

Excerpted from "Candidiasis," Centers for Disease Control and Prevention (CDC), July 6, 2010.

What are the symptoms of OPC?

People with OPC (thrush) infection usually have painless, white patches in the mouth. Others may have redness and soreness of the inside of the mouth. Cracking at the corners of the mouth, known as angular cheilitis, may occur. Symptoms of candida esophagitis may include pain and difficulty swallowing. Other conditions can cause similar symptoms, so it is important to see your doctor.

How is thrush (OPC) diagnosed?

Thrush, also called OPC, is often diagnosed based on the clinical appearance of the mouth and by taking a scraping of the white patches and looking at it under a microscope. A culture may also be performed. Because Candida organisms are normal inhabitants of the human mouth, a positive culture by itself does not make the diagnosis.

How is OPC treated?

Prescription treatments include clotrimazole troches or lozenges and nystatin suspension. Another commonly prescribed treatment is oral fluconazole. For infection which does not respond to these treatments, there are a number of other antifungal drugs that are available.

What will happen if a person does not seek treatment for a OPC?

Symptoms, which may be uncomfortable, may persist. In rare cases, invasive candidiasis may occur.

Can thrush (OPC) become resistant to treatment?

Yes, thrush (OPC) and candida esophagitis can become resistant to antifungal treatment over time. Therefore, it is important to see your doctor for evaluation if you think you have OPC or Candida esophagitis.

What is invasive candidiasis?

Invasive candidiasis is a fungal infection that occurs when candida species enter the blood, causing bloodstream infection and then spreading throughout the body. The symptoms of invasive candidiasis are not specific. Fever and chills that do not improve after antibiotic therapy are the most common symptoms. If the infection spreads to deep organs such as kidneys, liver, bones, muscles, joints, spleen, or eyes, additional specific symptoms may develop, which vary depending on the site of infection. If the infection does not respond to treatment, the patient's organs may fail and cause death.

How is invasive candidiasis transmitted?

Invasive candidiasis is extremely rare in persons without risk factors. In persons at risk, invasive candidiasis may result when a person's own Candida organisms, normally found in the digestive tract, enter the bloodstream. On rare occasions, it can also occur when medical equipment or devices become contaminated with Candida. In either case, the infection may spread throughout the body.

Chapter 47

Tongue Disorders

Chapter Contents

433

Section 47.1

Tongue Tie (Ankyloglossia)

"Tongue Tie," © 2012 A.D.A.M., Inc. Reprinted with permission.

Tongue tie is a condition in which the bottom of the tongue is attached to the floor of the mouth by a band of tissue called the lingual frenulum. This connection restricts the free movement (range of motion) of the tongue's tip.

Causes

The exact cause of tongue tie is not known. Genes may be involved because tongue tie is reported more often in some families.

Symptoms

In a newborn or infant, the symptoms of tongue tie are similar to the symptoms in any child who is having problems with breast feeding, including these:

- Acting irritable or fussy, even after feeding.
- Difficulty creating or maintaining suction. The infant may become tired in one or two minutes, or fall asleep before eating enough.
- Poor weight gain or weight loss.
- Problems latching onto the nipple. The infant may just chew on the nipple instead.

The breast-feeding mother may have problems with breast pain, plugged milk ducts, or painful breasts, and may feel frustrated.

Exams and Tests

Most experts do not recommend that health care providers examine newborns for tongue tie unless there are breast-feeding problems. Most health care providers only consider tongue tie when:

- the mother and baby have had problems establishing breast-feeding;

- the mother has received at least two to three days of support from a breast-feeding (lactation) specialist.

Treatment

Most breast-feeding problems can be easily managed with a variety of strategies. If you run into any problems, talk to a lactation consultant (a person who specializes in breast feeding).

Surgery is seldom necessary, but if it is needed, it involves cutting the tissue under the tongue. This surgery is called a frenulotomy. Most often, this procedure is done in the doctor's office. Infection or bleeding afterwards are possible, but rare.

Surgery for more severe cases is done in a hospital operating room. A surgical reconstruction procedure called a z-plasty closure may be needed to prevent scar tissue from forming.

Possible Complications

On rare occasions, tongue tie has been associated with tooth, swallowing, or speech problems.

Section 47.2

Tongue Pain and Other Problems

"Tongue Problems," © 2012 A.D.A.M., Inc. Reprinted with permission.

Tongue Problems

Tongue problems include pain, swelling, or a change in how the tongue looks.

Considerations

The tongue is mainly made up of muscles. It is covered with a mucus membrane. Small bumps (papillae) cover the upper surface of the tongue.

- Between the papillae are the taste buds, which allow you to taste.

- The tongue moves food to help you chew and swallow.

- The tongue also helps you form words.

There are many different reasons for changes in the tongue's function and appearance.

Problems Moving the Tongue

Tongue movement problems are most often caused by nerve damage. Rarely, problems moving the tongue may also be caused by a disorder where the band of tissue that attaches the tongue to the floor of the mouth is too short. This is called ankyloglossia.

Tongue movement disorders may result in:

- breastfeeding problems in newborns,

- difficulty moving food during chewing and swallowing,

- speech difficulties.

Taste Problems

Taste problems can be caused by damage to the taste buds, nerve problems, side effects of medications, an infection, or other condition. The tongue normally senses sweet, salty, sour, and bitter tastes. Other tastes are actually a function of the sense of smell.

Increased Size of the Tongue

Tongue swelling occurs with:

- acromegaly,
- amyloidosis,
- Down syndrome,
- myxedema,
- rhabdomyoma.

The tongue may get wider in persons who have no teeth and do not wear dentures. Sudden swelling of the tongue can happen due to an allergic reaction or a side effect of medications.

Color Changes

Color changes may occur when the tongue becomes inflamed (glossitis). Papillae (bumps on the tongue) are lost, causing the tongue to appear smooth. Geographic tongue is a patchy form of glossitis where the location of inflammation and the appearance of the tongue change from day to day.

Hairy Tongue

Hairy tongue is a harmless condition in which the tongue looks hairy or furry. The disorder usually goes away with antibiotics.

Black Tongue

Sometimes the upper surface of the tongue turns black or brown in color. This is an unsightly condition but it is not harmful.

Pain in the Tongue

Pain may occur with glossitis and geographic tongue. Tongue pain may also occur with:

- diabetic neuropathy,

- leukoplakia,

- mouth ulcers,

- oral cancer.

After menopause, some women have a sudden feeling that their tongue has been burned. This is called burning tongue syndrome or idiopathic glossopyrosis. There is no specific treatment for burning tongue syndrome, but capsaicin (the ingredient that makes peppers spicy) can offer relief to some patients.

Causes

Minor infections or irritations are the most common cause of tongue soreness. Injury, such as biting the tongue, can cause painful sores. Heavy smoking can irritate the tongue and make it painful.

A viral ulcer, also called a canker sore, commonly appears on the tongue (or anywhere in the mouth) for no obvious reason. Some doctors believe that these ulcers are linked to emotional stress or fatigue, although this has not been proved.

Possible causes of tongue pain:

- Anemia

- Cancer

- Dentures that irritate the tongue

- Oral herpes (ulcers)

- Neuralgia

- Pain from teeth and gums

- Pain from the heart

Possible causes of tongue tremor:

- Neurological disorder

- Overactive thyroid

Possible causes of white tongue:

- Local irritation

- Smoking and alcohol use

438

Possible causes of smooth tongue:

- Anemia
- Vitamin B_{12} deficiency

Possible causes of red (ranging from pink to magenta) tongue:

- Folic acid and vitamin B_{12} deficiency
- Pellagra
- Pernicious anemia
- Plummer-Vinson syndrome
- Sprue

Possible causes of tongue swelling:

- Acromegaly
- Allergic reaction to food or medicine
- Amyloidosis
- Angioedema
- Beckwith syndrome
- Cancer of the tongue
- Congenital micrognathia
- Down syndrome
- Hypothyroidism
- Infection
- Leukemia
- Lymphangioma
- Neurofibromatosis
- Pellagra
- Pernicious anemia
- Strep infection
- Tumor of the pituitary gland

Possible causes of a hairy tongue:

- Autoimmune immunodeficiency syndrome (AIDS)

- Antibiotic therapy
- Drinking coffee
- Dyes in drugs and food
- Chronic medical conditions
- Overuse of mouthwashes containing oxidizing or astringent ingredients
- Radiation of the head and neck
- Tobacco use

Possible cause of grooves in the tongue:

- Birth defect—normally occurs in 10% of population

Home Care

Practice good oral hygiene for hairy tongue and black tongue. Be sure to eat a well-balanced diet. Canker sores will heal on their own. See your dentist if you have a tongue problem caused by dentures.

Antihistamines can help relieve a swollen tongue caused by allergies. You should avoid the food or drug that causes the tongue swelling. Seek medical attention right away if swelling is starting to make breathing difficult.

When to Contact a Medical Professional

Make an appointment with your doctor if your tongue problem persists.

What to Expect at Your Office Visit

The doctor will perform a physical examination, look closely at the tongue, and ask questions such as:

- When did you first notice the problem?
- Have you had similar symptoms before?
- Do you have pain, swelling, breathing problems, or difficulty swallowing?
- Do you have a tongue tremor?
- What makes the problem worse (eating, drinking, swallowing, talking)?

- Do you wear dentures?

- What have you tried that helps?

- Are there problems with the teeth, gums, lips, or throat?

- Does the tongue bleed?

- Do you have a rash or fever?

- Do you have allergies?

- Are there problems with speaking or moving the tongue?

- Have you noticed changes in taste?

- What medications do you take?

- Do you smoke cigarettes, cigars, or a pipe?

- Do you use alcohol excessively?

Blood tests may be done to check for conditions, including systemic causes of tongue disorders. A tongue biopsy may be needed in some cases.

Treatment depends on the cause of the tongue problem:

- If nerve damage has caused a tongue movement problem, the condition must be treated. Therapy may be needed to improve speech and swallowing.

- Ankyloglossia may not need to be treated, unless you have speech or swallowing problems. Surgery to release the tongue can relieve the problem.

- Medicine may be prescribed for mouth ulcers, leukoplakia, oral cancer, and other mouth sores.

- Anti-inflammatory medicines may be prescribed for glossitis and geographic tongue.

Part Six

Health Conditions That Affect Oral Health

Chapter 48

Cancer Treatment Oral Complications

Chapter Contents

Section 48.1

Three Good Reasons to See a Dentist before Cancer Treatment

Text in this section is excerpted from "Three Good Reasons to See a Dentist BEFORE Cancer Treatment," National Institute of Dental and Craniofacial Research (NIDCR), NIH Publication No. 09–5494, March 25, 2011.

1. **Feel better:** Cancer treatment can cause side effects in your mouth. A dental checkup before treatment starts can help prevent painful mouth problems.

2. **Save teeth and bones:** A dentist will help protect your mouth, teeth, and jaw bones from damage caused by head and neck radiation and chemotherapy. Children also need special protection for their growing teeth and facial bones.

3. **Fight cancer:** Serious side effects in the mouth can delay, or even stop, cancer treatment. To fight cancer best, your cancer care team should include a dentist.

Protect Your Mouth during Cancer Treatment

Brush gently, brush often:

- Brush your teeth—and your tongue—gently with an extra-soft toothbrush.
- Soften the bristles in warm water if your mouth is very sore.
- Brush after every meal and at bedtime.

Floss gently—do it daily:

- Floss once a day to remove plaque.
- Avoid areas of your gums that are bleeding or sore, but keep flossing your other teeth.

Keep your mouth moist:

- Rinse often with water.

- Do not use mouthwashes that contain alcohol.
- Use a saliva substitute to help moisten your mouth.

Eat and drink with care:

- Choose soft, easy-to-chew foods.
- Protect your mouth from spicy, sour, or crunchy foods.
- Choose lukewarm foods and drinks instead of hot or icy-cold.
- Avoid alcoholic drinks.

Stop using tobacco:

- Ask your cancer care team to help you stop smoking or chewing tobacco. People who quit smoking or chewing tobacco have fewer mouth problems.

Tips to Help You Care for Mouth Problems

Sore mouth, sore throat: To help keep your mouth clean, rinse often with 1/4 teaspoon each of baking soda and salt in one quart of warm water. Follow with a plain water rinse. Ask your cancer care team about medicines that can help with the pain.

Dry mouth: Rinse your mouth often with water, use sugar-free gum or candy, and talk to your dentist about saliva substitutes.

Infections: Call your cancer care team right away if you see a sore, swelling, bleeding, or a sticky, white film in your mouth.

Eating problems: Your cancer care team can help by giving you medicines to numb the pain from mouth sores and showing you how to choose foods that are easy to swallow.

Bleeding: If your gums bleed or hurt, avoid flossing the areas that are bleeding or sore, but keep flossing other teeth. Soften the bristles of your toothbrush in warm water.

Stiffness in chewing muscles: Three times a day, open and close your mouth as far as you can without pain. Repeat 20 times.

Vomiting: Rinse your mouth after vomiting with 1/4 teaspoon of baking soda in one cup of warm water.

Cavities: Brush your teeth after meals and before bedtime. Your dentist might have you put fluoride gel on your teeth to help prevent cavities.

When Should You Call Your Cancer Care Team about Mouth Problems?

Take a moment each day to check how your mouth looks and feels. Call your cancer care team when:

- you first notice a mouth problem,

- an old problem gets worse,

- you notice any changes you are not sure about.

Section 48.2

Chemotherapy and Your Mouth

Excerpted from "Chemotherapy and Your Mouth," National Institute of Dental and Craniofacial Research (NIDCR), NIH Publication No. 11-4361, March 25, 2011.

How does chemotherapy affect the mouth?

Chemotherapy is the use of drugs to treat cancer. These drugs kill cancer cells, but they may also harm normal cells, including cells in the mouth. Side effects include problems with your teeth and gums; the soft, moist lining of your mouth; and the glands that make saliva (spit). It is important to know that side effects in the mouth can be serious.

- Side effects can hurt and make it hard to eat, talk, and swallow.

- You are more likely to get an infection, which can be dangerous when you are receiving cancer treatment.

- If the side effects are bad, you may not be able to keep up with your cancer treatment. Your doctor may need to cut back on your cancer treatment or may even stop it.

What mouth problems does chemotherapy cause?

You may have certain side effects in your mouth from chemotherapy. Another person may have different problems. The problems depend on the chemotherapy drugs and how your body reacts to them. You may have these problems only during treatment or for a short time after treatment ends.

- Painful mouth and gums
- Dry mouth
- Burning, peeling, or swelling tongue
- Infection
- Change in taste

Why should I see a dentist?

You may be surprised that your dentist is important in your cancer treatment. If you go to the dentist before chemotherapy begins, you can help prevent serious mouth problems. Side effects often happen because a person's mouth is not healthy before chemotherapy starts. Not all mouth problems can be avoided but the fewer side-effects you have, the more likely you will stay on your cancer treatment schedule.

It is important for your dentist and cancer doctor to talk to each other about your cancer treatment. Be sure to give your dentist your cancer doctor's phone number.

When should I see a dentist?

You need to see the dentist one month, if possible, before chemotherapy begins. If you have already started chemotherapy and did not go to a dentist, see one as soon as possible.

Do children get mouth problems too?

Chemotherapy causes other side effects in children, depending on the child's age. Problems with teeth are the most common. Permanent teeth may be slow to come in and may look different from normal teeth. Teeth may fall out. The dentist will check your child's jaws for any growth problems.

Before chemotherapy begins, take your child to a dentist. The dentist will check your child's mouth carefully and pull loose teeth or those that may become loose during treatment. Ask the dentist or hygienist what you can do to help your child with mouth care.

Section 48.3

Head and Neck Radiation Treatment and Your Mouth

Excerpted from "Head and Neck Radiation Treatment and Your Mouth," National Institute of Dental and Craniofacial Research (NIDCR), NIH Publication No. 11-4362, May 12, 2011.

Doctors use head and neck radiation to treat cancer because it kills cancer cells. But radiation to the head and neck can harm normal cells, including cells in the mouth. Side effects include problems with your teeth and gums; the soft, moist lining of your mouth; glands that make saliva (spit); and jaw bones. It is important to know that side effects in the mouth can be serious.

- Side effects can hurt and make it hard to eat, talk, and swallow.

- You are more likely to get an infection, which can be dangerous when you are receiving cancer treatment.

- If the side effects are bad, you may not be able to keep up with your cancer treatment. Your doctor may need to cut back on your cancer treatment or may even stop it.

You may have certain side effects in your mouth from head and neck radiation. Another person may have different problems. Some problems go away after treatment. Others last a long time, while some may never go away. Possible side effects include the following:

- Dry mouth
- A lot of cavities
- Loss of taste
- Sore mouth and gum
- Infections
- Jaw stiffness
- Jaw bone changes

Important Notes

- Visit your dentist before your head and neck radiation treatment starts.

- Take good care of your mouth during treatment.

- Talk to your dentist about using fluoride gel to help prevent all the cavities that head and neck radiation causes.

- Talk regularly with your cancer doctor and dentist about any mouth problems you have during and after head and neck radiation treatment.

Section 48.4

What the Oncology Team Can Do

Excerpted from "Oral Complications of Cancer Treatment: What the Oncology Team Can Do," National Institute of Dental and Craniofacial Research (NIDCR), NIH Publication No. 09-4372, March 25, 2011.

Radiation to the head and neck and chemotherapy for any malignancy can cause a range of oral side effects. For some patients, these complications may become dose-limiting and slow—or even halt—cancer treatment. Preventing and managing oral complications help support optimal cancer therapy, enhancing both patient survival and quality of life.

Who Has Oral Complications?

Oral side effects occur in virtually all patients receiving radiation for head and neck malignancies, in approximately 80% of transplant recipients, and in about 40% of patients receiving primary chemotherapy. Risk for oral complications varies with the treatment regimen. Patients administered minimally myelosuppressive or non-myelosuppressive therapy are at low risk. As chemotherapy becomes more aggressive, the likelihood of oral complications increases. Also at high risk are patients undergoing head and neck radiation for oral and pharyngeal cancer.

Most oral complications resolve when cancer treatment ends and the patient's overall condition improves. Others, such as xerostomia, may persist for years. Unfortunately, patients do not always receive medically necessary dental care that could help avert or minimize oral complications. Ensuring that your patients receive timely oral care helps them maintain the prescribed cancer regimen and complete treatment.

By adding oral care to the pretreatment regimen, you can:

- prevent, eliminate, or control oral pain;
- prevent oral infections that could lead to serious systemic infections;
- optimize nutritional support;
- preserve or improve oral health;
- prevent or reduce the incidence of bone necrosis in patients receiving radiation therapy to the head and neck;
- improve the quality of life;
- decrease the cost of care;
- improve the likelihood that the patient will successfully complete planned cancer treatment.

Oral Care during Treatment

Regular oral assessment and care are necessary during cancer therapy. Planning and communication between the oncology and dental teams can minimize the risk of oral complications and maximize the efficacy of dental and supportive care.

Follow-Up Oral Care

Once all complications of chemotherapy have resolved and blood counts have recovered, most patients may resume their normal dental care schedule. It is essential that the dentist know the patient's hematologic status before initiating any dental treatment or surgery. Advise the dentist if a patient has received intravenous bisphosphonate therapy due to its association with osteonecrosis of the jaw.

Once radiation therapy has been completed and acute oral complications have abated, the patient should be evaluated by a dentist every 4–8 weeks for the first six months. Thereafter, the dentist can determine a schedule based on the needs of the individual patient.

Long-Term Problems Following Head and Neck Radiation Therapy

Radiation therapy to the head and neck can cause oral complications that continue or emerge long after treatment has ended. Although patients may no longer be under an oncologist's care at that time, what they learn about oral health during their treatment will affect how they deal with subsequent complications. Patients receiving radiation therapy need to know about its risks:

- Radiation treatment carries a lifelong risk of osteonecrosis, xerostomia, and dental cavities.

- Because of the risk of osteonecrosis, people who have received radiation should avoid invasive surgical procedures (including extractions) that involve irradiated bone.

- Radiation to the head and neck may permanently reduce the quantity and quality of normal saliva, so ongoing oral care is crucial to optimize oral health. Daily fluoride tray application, good nutrition, and oral hygiene are especially important.

- Radiation may alter oral tissues, so dentures may need to be reconstructed after treatment is completed and the tissues have stabilized. Some people may not be able to wear dentures again.

- Craniofacial and dental structures may develop abnormally in younger children who receive high-dose radiation to those areas.

Hematopoietic Stem Cell Transplantation

Because of the pronounced immunosuppression that accompanies hematopoietic stem cell transplant procedures, patients have a high risk of developing acute oral complications, particularly mucositis, ulcerations, hemorrhage, infection, and xerostomia. Although these problems begin to resolve when hematologic status improves, immunosuppression may last for up to a year after the transplant, so the risk of complications continues. The oral cavity and salivary glands are also commonly involved in graft-versus-host disease in allograft recipients. Careful attention to oral care in the post-transplant period is important to the overall health of these patients.

Section 48.5

What the Dental Team Can Do

Excerpted from "Oral Complications of Cancer Treatment: What the Dental Team Can Do," National Institute of Dental and Craniofacial Research (NIDCR), NIH Publication No. 09-4372, 2009.

Oral complications from radiation to the head and neck or chemotherapy for any malignancy can compromise patients' health and quality of life, and affect their ability to complete planned cancer treatment. For some patients, the complications can be so debilitating that they may tolerate only lower doses of therapy, postpone scheduled treatments, or discontinue treatment entirely. Oral complications can also lead to serious systemic infections. Medically necessary oral care before, during, and after cancer treatment can prevent or reduce the incidence and severity of oral complications, enhancing both patient survival and quality of life.

Oral Complications Related to Cancer Treatment

Oral complications of cancer treatment arise in various forms and degrees of severity, depending on the individual and the cancer treatment. Chemotherapy often impairs the function of bone marrow, suppressing the formation of white blood cells, red blood cells, and platelets (myelosuppression). Following are lists of side effects common to both chemotherapy and radiation therapy, and complications specific to each type of treatment.

Oral Complications Common to Chemotherapy and Radiation

- **Oral mucositis:** Inflammation and ulceration of the mucous membranes; can increase the risk for pain, oral and systemic infection, and nutritional compromise.

- **Infection:** Viral, bacterial, and fungal; results from myelosuppression, xerostomia, and/or damage to the mucosa from chemotherapy or radiotherapy.

- **Xerostomia/salivary gland dysfunction:** Dryness of the mouth due to thickened, reduced, or absent salivary flow; increases the risk of infection and compromises speaking, chewing, and swallowing. Medications other than chemotherapy can also cause salivary gland dysfunction. Persistent dry mouth increases the risk for dental caries.

- **Functional disabilities:** Impaired ability to eat, taste, swallow, and speak because of mucositis, dry mouth, trismus, and infection.

- **Taste alterations:** Changes in taste perception of foods, ranging from unpleasant to tasteless.

- **Nutritional compromise:** Poor nutrition from eating difficulties caused by mucositis, dry mouth, dysphagia, and loss of taste.

- **Abnormal dental development:** Altered tooth development, craniofacial growth, or skeletal development in children secondary to radiotherapy and/or high doses of chemotherapy before age nine.

Other Complications of Chemotherapy

- **Neurotoxicity:** Persistent, deep aching and burning pain that mimics a toothache, but for which no dental or mucosal source can be found. This complication is a side effect of certain classes of drugs.

- **Bleeding:** Oral bleeding from the decreased platelets and clotting factors associated with the effects of therapy on bone marrow.

Other Complications of Radiation Therapy

- **Radiation caries:** Lifelong risk of rampant dental decay that may begin within three months of completing radiation treatment if changes in either the quality or quantity of saliva persist.

- **Trismus/tissue fibrosis:** Loss of elasticity of masticatory muscles that restricts normal ability to open the mouth.

- **Osteonecrosis:** Blood vessel compromise and necrosis of bone exposed to high-dose radiation therapy; results in decreased ability to heal if traumatized.

The Role of Pretreatment Oral Care

With a pretreatment oral evaluation, the dental team can identify and treat problems such as infection, fractured teeth or restorations, or periodontal disease that could contribute to oral complications when cancer therapy begins. The evaluation also establishes baseline data for comparing the patient's status in subsequent examinations.

Follow-Up Oral Care

Chemotherapy: Once all complications of chemotherapy have resolved, patients may be able to resume their normal dental care schedule. However, if immune function continues to be compromised, determine the patient's hematologic status before initiating any dental treatment or surgery. This is particularly important to remember for patients who have undergone stem cell transplantation. Ask if the patient has received intravenous bisphosphonate therapy.

Radiation therapy: Once the patient has completed head and neck radiation therapy and acute oral complications have abated, evaluate the patient regularly (every 4–8 weeks, for example) for the first six months. Keep in mind that oral complications can continue or emerge long after radiation therapy has ended.

Special Considerations for Hematopoietic Stem Cell Transplant Patients

The intensive conditioning regimens of transplantation can result in pronounced immunosuppression, greatly increasing a patient's risk of mucositis, ulceration, hemorrhage, infection, and xerostomia. The complications begin to resolve when hematologic status improves. Although the complete blood count and differential may be normal, immunosuppression may last for up to a year after the transplant, along with the risk of infections. Also, the oral cavity and salivary glands are commonly involved in graft-versus-host disease in allograft recipients. This can result in mucosal inflammation, ulceration, and xerostomia, so continued monitoring is necessary. Careful attention to oral care in the immediate and long-term post-transplant period is important to patients' overall health.

Chapter 49

Celiac Disease and Dental Enamel Defects

Celiac disease manifestations can extend beyond the classic gastrointestinal problems, affecting any organ or body system. One manifestation—dental enamel defects—can help dentists and other health care providers identify people who may have celiac disease and refer them to a gastroenterologist. Ironically, for some people with celiac disease, a dental visit, rather than a trip to the gastroenterologist, was the first step toward discovering their illness.

Not all dental enamel defects are caused by celiac disease, although the problem is fairly common among people with the condition, particularly children, according to Alessio Fasano, MD, medical director at the University of Maryland Center for Celiac Research. And dental enamel defects might be the only presenting manifestations of celiac disease.

Dental enamel problems stemming from celiac disease involve permanent dentition and include tooth discoloration—white, yellow, or brown spots on the teeth—poor enamel formation, pitting or banding of teeth, and mottled or translucent-looking teeth. The imperfections are symmetrical and often appear on the incisors and molars.

Tooth defects resulting from celiac disease are permanent and do not improve after adopting a gluten-free diet—the primary treatment for celiac disease. But dentists may use bonding, veneers, and other cosmetic solutions to cover dental enamel defects in older children and adults.

"Dental Enamel Defects and Celiac Disease," National Institute of Diabetes and Digestive and Kidney Diseases (NIDDK), NIH Publication No. 11–7379, April 2011.

Similar Symptoms, Different Problem

Tooth defects that result from celiac disease may resemble those caused by too much fluoride or a maternal or early childhood illness.

"Dentists mostly say it is from fluoride, that the mother took tetracycline, or that there was an illness early on," said Peter H.R. Green, MD, director of the Celiac Disease Center at Columbia University. "Celiac disease isn't on the radar screen of dentists in this country. Dentists should be made aware of these manifestations to help them identify people and get them to see their doctors so they can exclude celiac disease."

Green just completed a United States (U.S.) study with his dental colleague, Ted Malahias, DDS, that demonstrates celiac disease is highly associated with dental enamel defects in childhood—most likely due to the onset of celiac disease during enamel formation. The study, which did not identify a similar association in adults, concluded that all physician education about celiac disease should include information about the significance of dental enamel defects.

Other Oral Symptoms

Checking a patient's mouth is something primary care physicians also can do to help identify people who might have celiac disease. While dental enamel defects are the most prominent, a number of other oral problems are related to celiac disease, according to Green.

These include the following:

- Recurrent aphthous stomatitis, or canker sores or ulcers that recur inside the mouth

- Atrophic glossitis, a condition characterized by a red, smooth, shiny tongue

- Dry mouth syndrome

- Squamous cell carcinoma—a type of cancer—of the pharynx and mouth

For More Information

Celiac Disease Awareness Campaign (CDAC)
National Digestive Diseases Information Clearinghouse
2 Information Way
Bethesda, MD 20892-3570

Toll-Free: 800-891-5389
Toll-Free TTY: 866-569-1162
Fax: 703-738-4929
Website: http://www.celiac.nih.gov
E-mail: celiac@info.niddk.nih.gov

Chapter 50

Diabetes and Oral Health

Diabetes: Dental Tips

Diabetes can cause serious problems in your mouth, but you can do something about it. If you have diabetes, make sure you take care of your mouth. People with diabetes are at risk for mouth infections, especially periodontal (gum) disease. Periodontal disease can damage the gum and bone that hold your teeth in place and may lead to painful chewing problems. Some people with serious gum disease lose their teeth. Periodontal disease may also make it hard to control your blood glucose (blood sugar).

Other problems diabetes can cause are dry mouth and a fungal infection called thrush. Dry mouth happens when you do not have enough saliva—the fluid that keeps your mouth wet. Diabetes may also cause the glucose level in your saliva to increase. Together, these problems may lead to thrush, which causes painful white patches in your mouth.

You can keep your teeth and gums healthy. By controlling your blood glucose, brushing and flossing every day, and visiting a dentist regularly, you can help prevent periodontal disease. If your diabetes is not under control, you are more likely to develop problems in your mouth.

This chapter includes an excerpt from "Diabetes: Dental Tips," National Institute of Dental and Craniofacial Research (NIDCR), NIH Publication No. 12–2946, March 25, 2011; and excerpts from "Prevent Diabetes Problems: Keep Your Teeth and Gums Healthy," National Institute of Diabetes and Digestive and Kidney Diseases (NIDDK), NIH Publication No. 08–4280, April 2008.

Keep Your Teeth and Gums Healthy

How can diabetes hurt my teeth and gums?

Tooth and gum problems can happen to anyone. A sticky film full of germs, called plaque, builds up on your teeth. High blood glucose helps germs, also called bacteria, grow. Then you can get red, sore, and swollen gums that bleed when you brush your teeth.

People with diabetes can have tooth and gum problems more often if their blood glucose stays high. High blood glucose can make tooth and gum problems worse. You can even lose your teeth.

Smoking makes it more likely for you to get a bad case of gum disease, especially if you have diabetes and are age 45 or older.

Red, sore, and bleeding gums are the first sign of gum disease. These problems can lead to periodontitis. Periodontitis is an infection in the gums and the bone that holds the teeth in place.

If the infection gets worse, your gums may pull away from your teeth, making your teeth look long.

Call your dentist if you think you have problems with your teeth or gums.

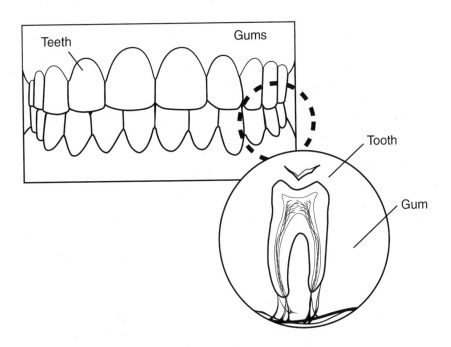

Figure 50.1. *High blood glucose can cause tooth and gum problems.*

How do I know if I have damage to my teeth and gums?

If you have one or more of these problems, you may have tooth and gum damage from diabetes:

- Red, sore, swollen gums
- Bleeding gums
- Gums pulling away from your teeth so your teeth look long
- Loose or sensitive teeth
- Bad breath
- A bite that feels different
- Dentures—false teeth—that do not fit well

How can I keep my teeth and gums healthy?

- Keep your blood glucose as close to normal as possible.
- Use dental floss at least once a day. Flossing helps prevent the buildup of plaque on your teeth. Plaque can harden and grow under your gums and cause problems. Using a sawing motion, gently bring the floss between the teeth, scraping from bottom to top several times.
- Brush your teeth after each meal and snack. Use a soft toothbrush. Turn the bristles against the gum line and brush gently. Use small, circular motions. Brush the front, back, and top of each tooth.
- If you wear false teeth, keep them clean.
- Call your dentist right away if you have problems with your teeth and gums.
- Call your dentist if you have red, sore, or bleeding gums; gums that are pulling away from your teeth; a sore tooth that could be infected; or soreness from your dentures.
- Get your teeth cleaned and your gums checked by your dentist twice a year.
- If your dentist tells you about a problem, take care of it right away.
- Be sure your dentist knows that you have diabetes.
- If you smoke, talk with your doctor about ways to quit smoking.

How can my dentist take care of my teeth and gums?

Your dentist can help you take care of your teeth and gums by

- cleaning and checking your teeth twice a year;
- helping you learn the best way to brush and floss your teeth;
- telling you if you have problems with your teeth or gums and what to do about them;
- making sure your false teeth fit well.

Plan ahead: You may be taking a diabetes medicine that can cause low blood glucose, also called hypoglycemia. Talk with your doctor and dentist before the visit about the best way to take care of your blood glucose during the dental work. You may need to bring some diabetes medicine and food with you to the dentist's office.

If your mouth is sore after the dental work, you might not be able to eat or chew for several hours or days. For guidance on how to adjust your normal routine while your mouth is healing, ask your doctor:

- what foods and drinks you should have,
- how you should change your diabetes medicines, and
- how often you should check your blood glucose.

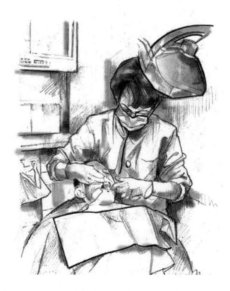

Figure 50.2. Get your teeth cleaned and checked twice a year.

Chapter 51

Disabilities and Oral Care

Chapter Contents

Section 51.1

Practical Oral Care for People with Autism

Excerpted from "Practical Oral Care for People with Autism," National
Institute of Dental and Craniofacial Research (NIDCR), NIH Publication
No. 09–5190, March 25, 2011.

Autism is a complex developmental disability that impairs communication and social, behavioral, and intellectual functioning. Some
people with the disorder appear distant, aloof, or detached from other
people or from their surroundings. Others do not react appropriately
to common verbal and social cues, such as a parent's tone of voice or
smile. Obsessive routines, repetitive behaviors, unpredictable body
movements, and self-injurious behavior may all be symptoms that
complicate dental care.

Health Challenges in Autism and Strategies for Oral Health Care

Communication problems and mental capabilities are central
concerns when treating people with autism. Determine the patient's
intellectual and functional abilities, and then communicate with the
patient at a level he or she can understand. Also, use a "tell-show-do"
approach to providing care. Demonstrations can encourage some patients to be more cooperative.

Behavior problems—which may include hyperactivity and quick
frustration—can complicate oral health care for patients with autism.
The invasive nature of oral care may trigger violent and self-injurious
behavior such as temper tantrums or head banging. Plan a desensitization appointment to help the patient become familiar with the office,
staff, and equipment through a step-by-step process. These steps may
take several visits to accomplish.

Specifically, the familiarity of a toothbrush will help your patient feel
comfortable and provide you with an opportunity to further examine the
mouth. Praise and reinforce good behavior after each step of a procedure.

466

Ignore inappropriate behavior as much as you can. Try to gain cooperation in the least restrictive manner. Use immobilization techniques only when absolutely necessary to protect the patient and staff during dental treatment—not as a convenience. If all other strategies fail, pharmacological options are useful in managing some patients.

People with autism often engage in perseveration, a continuous, meaningless repetition of words, phrases, or movements. Your patient may mimic the sound of the suction, for example, or repeat an instruction over and again.

Unusual responses to stimuli can create distractions and interrupt treatment. People with autism need consistency and can be especially sensitive to changes in their environment. They may exhibit unusual sensitivity to sensory stimuli such as sound, bright colors, and touch. Reactions vary. Some people with autism may overreact to noise and touch, while exposure to pain and heat may not provoke much reaction at all. Use the same staff, dental operatory, and appointment time to sustain familiarity. Also, minimize the number of distractions. Try to reduce unnecessary sights, sounds, odors, or other stimuli that might be disruptive. Allow time for the patient to adjust and become desensitized to the noise of a dental setting. Talk to the caregiver to get a sense of the patient's level of tolerance. People with autism differ in how they accept physical contact. Some are defensive and refuse any contact in or around the mouth, or cradling of the head or face. Others find such cradling comforting.

Section 51.2

Practical Oral Care for People with Cerebral Palsy

Excerpted from "Practical Oral Care for People with Cerebral Palsy," National Institute of Dental and Craniofacial Research (NIDCR), NIH Publication No. 09–5192, March 25, 2011.

Cerebral palsy itself does not cause any unique oral abnormalities. However, several conditions are more common or more severe in people with cerebral palsy than in the general population.

Periodontal disease is common in people with cerebral palsy due to poor oral hygiene and complications of oral habits, physical abilities, and malocclusion. Another factor is the gingival hyperplasia caused by medications.

- Encourage independence in daily oral hygiene. Involve patients in hands-on demonstrations of brushing and flossing.

- Some patients cannot brush and floss independently because of impaired physical coordination or cognitive skills. Talk to caregivers about daily oral hygiene.

- Some patients benefit from the daily use of an antimicrobial agent such as chlorhexidine based on the patient's abilities. Rinsing, for example, may not work for a patient with swallowing difficulties or one who cannot expectorate. Chlorhexidine applied using a spray bottle or toothbrush is equally efficacious.

- If use of particular medications has led to gingival hyperplasia, monitor for possible delayed tooth eruption and emphasize the importance of daily oral hygiene and frequent professional cleanings.

Dental caries are prevalent among people with cerebral palsy, primarily because of inadequate oral hygiene. Other risk factors include mouth breathing, the effects of medication, enamel hypoplasia, and food pouching.

Malocclusion in people with cerebral palsy usually involves more than just misaligned teeth—it is also a musculoskeletal problem. An open bite with protruding anterior teeth is common and is typically associated with tongue thrusting. The inability to close the lips because of an open bite also contributes to excessive drooling.

Unfortunately, correcting malocclusion is almost impossible in people with moderate or severe cerebral palsy. Orthodontic treatment may not be an option because of the risk of caries and enamel hypoplasia. However, a developmental disability in and of itself should not be perceived as a barrier to orthodontic treatment.

Dysphagia, difficulty with swallowing, is often a problem in people with cerebral palsy. Food may stay in the mouth longer than usual, increasing the risk for caries. Additionally, the semi-soft foods caregivers may prepare for people with this problem tend to adhere to the teeth. Coughing, gagging, choking, and aspiration are other related concerns. Caregivers need to inspect the patient's mouth after eating and remove any residual food.

Drooling affects daily oral care as well as social interaction. Hypotonia contributes to drooling, as does an open bite and the inability to close the lips.

Bruxism is common in people with cerebral palsy, especially those with severe forms of the disorder. Bruxism can be intense and persistent and cause the teeth to wear prematurely. Before recommending mouth guards or bite splints, consider that gagging or swallowing problems may make them uncomfortable or unusable.

Hyperactive bite and gag reflexes call for introducing instruments gently into the mouth. A patient with a gagging problem benefits from an early morning appointment, before eating or drinking.

Trauma and injury to the mouth from falls or accidents occur in people with cerebral palsy. Traumas require immediate professional attention.

Section 51.3

Practical Oral Care for People with Developmental Disabilities

Excerpted from "Practical Oral Care for People with Developmental Disabilities," National Institute of Dental and Craniofacial Research (NIDCR), NIH Publication No. 09–5196, February 7, 2012.

People with developmental disabilities typically have more oral health problems than the general population. Focusing on each person's specific needs is the first step toward achieving better oral health.

Dental caries are common in people with developmental disabilities.

- Recommend preventive measures such as fluorides and sealants.

- Caution patients or their caregivers about medicines that reduce saliva or contain sugar. Suggest that patients drink water frequently, take sugar-free medicines when available, and rinse with water after taking any medicine.

- Advise caregivers to offer alternatives to cariogenic foods and beverages as incentives or rewards.

- Educate caregivers about preventing early childhood caries.

- Encourage independence in daily oral hygiene. Ask patients to show you how they brush, and follow up with specific recommendations. Perform hands-on demonstrations to show patients the best way to clean their teeth.

- If necessary, adapt a toothbrush to make it easier to hold. For example, place a tennis ball or bicycle grip on the handle, wrap the handle in tape, or bend the handle by softening it under hot water. Explain that floss holders and power toothbrushes are also helpful.

- Some patients cannot brush and floss independently. Talk to caregivers about daily oral hygiene and do not assume that they know the basics. Use your experiences with each patient to demonstrate oral care techniques and sitting or standing positions for the caregiver. Emphasize that a consistent approach to oral hygiene is important—caregivers should try to use the same location, timing, and positioning.

Periodontal disease occurs more often and at a younger age in people with developmental disabilities. Contributing factors include poor oral hygiene, damaging oral habits, and physical or mental disabilities. Gingival hyperplasia caused by medications such as some anticonvulsants, antihypertensives, and immunosuppressants also increases the risk for periodontal disease. Some patients benefit from the daily use of an antimicrobial agent such as chlorhexidine.

Malocclusion occurs in many people with developmental disabilities and may be associated with intraoral and perioral muscular abnormalities, delayed tooth eruption, underdevelopment of the maxilla, and oral habits such as bruxism and tongue thrusting. Malocclusion can make chewing and speaking difficult and increase the risk of periodontal disease, dental caries, and oral trauma.

Damaging oral habits can be a problem for people with developmental disabilities. Some of the most common of these habits are bruxism, food pouching, mouth breathing, and tongue thrusting. Other oral habits include self-injurious behavior such as picking at the gingiva or biting the lips; rumination, where food is chewed, regurgitated, and swallowed again; and pica, eating objects and substances such as gravel, sand, cigarette butts, or pens.

Oral malformations affect many people with developmental disabilities. Patients may present with enamel defects, high lip lines with dry gingiva, and variations in the number, size, and shape of teeth. Craniofacial anomalies such as facial asymmetry and hypoplasia of the midfacial region are also seen in this population. Identify any malformations and explain to the caregiver the implications for daily oral hygiene and future treatment planning.

Tooth eruption may be delayed in children with developmental disabilities. Eruption times are different for each child, and some children may not get their first primary tooth until they are two years old. In other cases, eruption problems are attributable to the gingival hyperplasia that can result from medications such as phenytoin and cyclosporin. Dental examination by a child's first birthday and regularly thereafter can help identify atypical patterns of eruption.

Physical abuse often presents as oral trauma. Abuse is reported more frequently in people with developmental disabilities than in the general population.

Section 51.4

Practical Oral Care for People with Down Syndrome

Excerpted from "Practical Oral Care for People with Down Syndrome,"
National Institute of Dental and Craniofacial Research (NIDCR), NIH
Publication No. 09–5193, February 7, 2012.

People with Down syndrome have no unique oral health problems. However, some of the problems they have tend to be frequent and severe. Early professional treatment and daily care at home can mitigate their severity and allow people with Down syndrome to enjoy the benefits of a healthy mouth.

Periodontal disease is the most significant oral health problem in people with Down syndrome. Children experience rapid, destructive, periodontal disease. Consequently, large numbers of them lose their permanent anterior teeth in their early teens. Contributing factors include poor oral hygiene, malocclusion, bruxism, conical-shaped tooth roots, and abnormal host response because of a compromised immune system.

- Some patients benefit from the daily use of an antimicrobial agent such as chlorhexidine.

- If use of particular medications has led to gingival hyperplasia, emphasize the importance of daily oral hygiene and frequent professional cleanings.

- Encourage independence in daily oral hygiene. Involve patients in hands-on demonstrations of brushing and flossing.

- Some people with Down syndrome can brush and floss independently, but many need help. Talk to their caregivers about daily oral hygiene. A power toothbrush or a floss holder can simplify oral care.

Dental caries: Children and young adults who have Down syndrome have fewer caries than people without this developmental disability. Additionally, the diets of many children with Down syndrome are closely supervised to prevent obesity; this helps reduce consumption of cariogenic foods and beverages.

472

By contrast, some adults with Down syndrome are at an increased risk of caries due to xerostomia and cariogenic food choices. Also, hypotonia contributes to chewing problems and inefficient natural cleansing action, which allow food to remain on the teeth after eating.

Orofacial features: Several orofacial features are characteristic of people with Down syndrome. The midfacial region may be underdeveloped, affecting the appearance of the lips, tongue, and palate.

Malocclusion is found in most people with Down syndrome because of the delayed eruption of permanent teeth and the underdevelopment of the maxilla. A smaller maxilla contributes to an open bite, leading to poor positioning of teeth and increasing the likelihood of periodontal disease and dental caries. In and of itself, Down syndrome is not a barrier to orthodontic care. The ability of the patient or caregiver to maintain good daily oral hygiene is critical to the feasibility and success of treatment.

Tooth anomalies are common in Down syndrome:

- Congenitally missing teeth occur more often in people with Down syndrome than in the general population.

- Delayed eruption of teeth, often following an abnormal sequence, affects some children with Down syndrome.

- Irregularities in tooth formation, such as microdontia and malformed teeth, are also seen in people with Down syndrome. Severe illness or prolonged fevers can lead to hypoplasia and hypocalcification. A child should be examined by his or her first birthday and regularly thereafter to help identify unusual tooth formation and patterns of eruption.

Section 51.5

Practical Oral Care for People with Intellectual Disability

Excerpted from "Practical Oral Care for People with Intellectual Disability," National Institute of Dental and Craniofacial Research (NIDCR), NIH Publication No. 09–5194, February 7, 2012.

In general, people with intellectual disability have poorer oral health and oral hygiene than those without this condition. Data indicate that people who have intellectual disability have more untreated caries and a higher prevalence of gingivitis and other periodontal diseases than the general population.

Periodontal disease: Medications, malocclusion, multiple disabilities, and poor oral hygiene combine to increase the risk of periodontal disease in people with intellectual disability.

- Encourage independence in daily oral hygiene. Ask patients to show you how they brush, and follow up with specific recommendations on brushing methods or toothbrush adaptations.

- Some patients cannot brush and floss independently due to impaired physical coordination or cognitive skills. Talk to their caregivers about daily oral hygiene.

- Some patients benefit from the daily use of an antimicrobial agent such as chlorhexidine.

- If use of particular medications has led to gingival hyperplasia, emphasize the importance of daily oral hygiene and frequent professional cleanings.

Dental caries: People with intellectual disability develop caries at the same rate as the general population. The prevalence of untreated dental caries, however, is higher among people with intellectual disability, particularly those not living in institutional settings.

Missing permanent teeth, delayed eruption, and enamel hypoplasia are more common in people with intellectual disability and coexisting conditions than in people with intellectual disability alone.

Damaging oral habits are a problem for some people with intellectual disability. Common habits include bruxism; mouth breathing; tongue thrusting; self-injurious behavior such as picking at the gingiva or biting the lips; and pica, eating objects and substances such as gravel, cigarette butts, or pens. If a mouth guard can be tolerated, one may be prescribed for patients who have problems with self-injurious behavior or bruxism.

Section 51.6

Caregiver's Guide for Every Day Dental Care

Excerpted from "Dental Care Every Day: A Caregiver's Guide," National Institute of Dental and Craniofacial Research (NIDCR), NIH Publication No. 12–5191, February, 2012.

Taking care of someone with a developmental disability requires patience and skill. As a caregiver, you know this as well as anyone does. You also know how challenging it is to help that person with dental care. It takes planning, time, and the ability to manage physical, mental, and behavioral problems. Dental care isn't always easy, but you can make it work for you and the person you help. This chapter will show you how to help someone brush, floss, and have a healthy mouth.

Everyone needs dental care every day. Brushing and flossing are crucial activities that affect our health. In fact, dental care is just as important to your client's health and daily routine as taking medications and getting physical exercise. A healthy mouth helps people eat well, avoid pain and tooth loss, and feel good about themselves.

Getting Started

Location: The bathroom isn't the only place to brush someone's teeth. For example, the kitchen or dining room may be more comfortable.

475

Instead of standing next to a bathroom sink, allow the person to sit at a table. Place the toothbrush, toothpaste, floss, and a bowl and glass of water on the table within easy reach. No matter what location you choose, make sure you have good light. You can't help someone brush unless you can see inside that person's mouth.

Behavior: Problem behavior can make dental care difficult. Try these ideas and see what works for you.

- At first, dental care can be frightening to some people. Try the "tell-show-do" approach to deal with this natural reaction. Tell your client about each step before you do it. For example, explain how you'll help him or her brush and what it feels like. Show how you're going to do each step before you do it. Also, it might help to let your client hold and feel the toothbrush and floss. Do the steps in the same way that you've explained them.

- Give your client time to adjust to dental care. Be patient as that person learns to trust you working in and around his or her mouth.

- Use your voice and body to communicate that you care. Give positive feedback often to reinforce good behavior.

- Have a routine for dental care. Use the same technique at the same time and place every day. Many people with developmental disabilities accept dental care when it's familiar. A routine might soothe fears or help eliminate problem behavior.

- Be creative. Some caregivers allow their client to hold a favorite toy or special item for comfort. Others make dental care a game or play a person's favorite music. If none of these ideas helps, ask your client's dentist or dental hygienist for advice.

Three Steps to a Healthy Mouth

Like everyone else, people with developmental disabilities can have a healthy mouth if these three steps are followed:

1. **Brush gently every day:** If the person you care for is unable to brush, these suggestions might be helpful.

   - First, wash your hands and put on disposable gloves. Sit or stand where you can see all of the surfaces of the teeth.

   - Be sure to use a regular or power toothbrush with soft bristles.

- Use a pea-size amount of toothpaste with fluoride, or none at all. Toothpaste bothers people who have swallowing problems. If this is the case for the person you care for, brush with water instead.

- Brush the front, back, and top of each tooth. Gently brush back and forth in short strokes.

- Gently brush the tongue after you brush the teeth.

- Help the person rinse with plain water. Give people who can't rinse a drink of water or consider sweeping the mouth with a finger wrapped in gauze.

2. **Floss every day:** Flossing cleans between the teeth where a toothbrush can't reach. Many people with disabilities need a caregiver to help them floss. If you have trouble flossing, try using a floss holder instead of holding the floss with your fingers. Also, the dentist may prescribe a special rinse for your client. Fluoride rinses can help prevent cavities. Chlorhexidine rinses fight germs that cause gum disease.

3. **Visit a dentist regularly:** Your client should have regular dental appointments. Professional cleanings are just as important as brushing and flossing every day. Regular examinations can identify problems before they cause unnecessary pain.

Prepare for Every Dental Visit

Be prepared for every appointment. You're an important source of information for the dentist. If you have questions about what the dentist will need to know, call the office before the appointment. Know the person's dental history and remember to bring a complete medical history; and bring all insurance, billing, and legal information.

Remember

Brushing and flossing every day and seeing the dentist regularly can make a big difference in the quality of life of the person you care for. If you have questions or need more information, talk to a dentist.

Chapter 52

Eating Disorders and Oral Health

Eating Disorders

What are eating disorders?

An eating disorder is an illness that causes serious disturbances to your everyday diet, such as eating extremely small amounts of food or severely overeating. A person with an eating disorder may have started out just eating smaller or larger amounts of food, but at some point, the urge to eat less or more spiraled out of control. Severe distress or concern about body weight or shape may also characterize an eating disorder.

Eating disorders frequently appear during the teen years or young adulthood but may also develop during childhood or later in life. Common eating disorders include anorexia nervosa, bulimia nervosa, and binge-eating disorder.

It is unknown how many adults and children suffer with other serious, significant eating disorders, including one category of eating disorders called eating disorders not otherwise specified (EDNOS). EDNOS includes eating disorders that do not meet the criteria for anorexia or bulimia nervosa. Binge-eating disorder is a type of eating

This chapter begins with an excerpt from "Eating Disorders," National Institute of Mental Health (NIMH), NIH Publication No. 11-4901, Revised 2011; and concludes with "Eating Concerns and Oral Health," reprinted with permission from the National Eating Disorders Association, © 2005. For more information, visit www.nationaleatingdisorders.org. Reviewed in April 2012 by David A. Cooke, MD, FACP.

disorder called EDNOS. EDNOS is the most common diagnosis among people who seek treatment.

Eating disorders are real, treatable, medical illnesses. They frequently coexist with other illnesses such as depression, substance abuse, or anxiety disorders. Other symptoms can become life-threatening if a person does not receive treatment. People with anorexia nervosa are 18 times more likely to die early compared with people of similar age in the general population.

What are the types of eating disorders?

Anorexia nervosa: Many people with anorexia nervosa see themselves as overweight, even when they are clearly underweight. Eating, food, and weight control become obsessions. People with anorexia nervosa typically weigh themselves repeatedly, portion food carefully, and eat very small quantities of only certain foods. Some people with anorexia nervosa may also engage in binge-eating followed by extreme dieting, excessive exercise, self-induced vomiting, and/or misuse of laxatives, diuretics, or enemas.

Bulimia nervosa is characterized by recurrent and frequent episodes of eating unusually large amounts of food and feeling a lack of control over these episodes. This binge-eating is followed by behavior that compensates for the overeating such as forced vomiting, excessive use of laxatives or diuretics, fasting, excessive exercise, or a combination of these behaviors.

Unlike anorexia nervosa, people with bulimia nervosa usually maintain what is considered a healthy or normal weight, while some are slightly overweight. But like people with anorexia nervosa, they often fear gaining weight, want desperately to lose weight, and are intensely unhappy with their body size and shape. Usually, bulimic behavior is done secretly because it is often accompanied by feelings of disgust or shame. The binge-eating and purging cycle happens anywhere from several times a week to many times a day.

Binge-eating disorder: With binge-eating disorder, a person loses control over his or her eating. Unlike bulimia nervosa, periods of binge eating are not followed by purging, excessive exercise, or fasting. As a result, people with binge-eating disorder often are overweight or obese. People with binge-eating disorder who are obese are at higher risk for developing cardiovascular disease and high blood pressure. They also experience guilt, shame, and distress about their binge-eating which can lead to more binge eating.

Eating Concerns and Oral Health

Dietary habits can and do play a role in oral health. Everyone has heard from their dentist that eating too much sugar can lead to cavities, but did you know that high intake of acidic diet foods can have an equally devastating effect on your teeth?

In fact, while up to 89% of bulimic patients show signs of the tooth erosion usually associated with regurgitation, some studies have found similar prevalence rates in patients with highly restrictive dietary habits. The harmful habits and nutritional deficiencies that often accompany disordered eating can have severe consequences on one's dental health. It is often the pain and discomfort associated with dental complications that causes individuals with eating disorders to seek treatment.

Signs and Symptoms

- Loss of tissue and erosive lesions on the surface of teeth due to the effects of acid. These lesions can appear as early as six months from the start of the problem.

- Changes in the color, shape, and length of teeth. Teeth can become brittle, translucent, and weak.

- Increased sensitivity to temperature. In extreme cases the pulp can be exposed and cause infection, discoloration, or even pulp death.

- Enlargement of the salivary glands, dry mouth, and reddened, dry, cracked lips.

- Tooth decay, which can actually be aggravated by extensive tooth brushing or rinsing following vomiting.

- Unprovoked, spontaneous pain within a particular tooth.

Changes in the mouth are often times the first physical signs of an eating disorder. If you are experiencing any of these symptoms, talk with your dentist about ways to care for your teeth and mouth. There are methods for improving your oral health while you are seeking help to change harmful eating habits.

Chapter 53

Growth Hormone Deficiency Causes Dental Problems

Dental problems are not the typical issue parents think about when their child has a growth disorder, particularly growth hormone deficiency. Yet, dental development and dental problems often occur for these children. The following information was prepared by one of the country's only specialists on the topic of "Dental Problems Associated with Growth Hormone Deficiency."

Dental Aspects of Growth Hormone Deficiency

Deficiency of growth hormone is a widespread problem, which affects more than just your child's height. Normal levels of growth hormone are necessary for the normal growth and development of your child's teeth and jaws. Routine dental care and timely dental screenings and assessments are important to your child's future dental health.

The lack of growth hormone causes a lag in the growth of bones, which is clearly evident in a child's height. Less evident to most people are the effects of growth hormone deficiency on your child's face and teeth. Growth hormone deficiency commonly causes a lag in the growth of your child's teeth and facial bones. For instance, in the absence of growth hormone, it is common to keep the baby (primary) teeth longer (2–5 years usually) than average, so a child might be 10–12 years old before losing any baby teeth. This can cause problems with the eruption (coming into the mouth) of the adult (permanent) teeth. These children are also more likely to be missing adult teeth, which may require braces (orthodontics) and/or bridges/implants/crowns (replacement teeth) to correct. If you should suspect these conditions it is best to take your child to your dentist, who may take x-rays (radiographs) of your child's jaws to check on these conditions.

Growth hormone has a strong effect on bone growth, including the bones of the upper and lower jaws. In growth hormone deficiency it is common to see a growth disorder of the jaws. This growth disorder is commonly seen as a small lower jaw or chin since the lower jaw seems to be more dependent than the upper jaw on normal growth hormone levels. There are treatments that can, in most cases, correct these problems if the jaws are still growing. These treatments may involve plastic retainer-like devices (functional appliances), glued in metal spreaders (expanders) or other devices, and/or braces, and are usually performed by dentists who specialize in braces (orthodontists) or in children's dentistry (pedodontists). Since the jaws usually begin to grow in response to the growth hormone prescribed by your doctors, this is often the best time for this type of treatment. The dental specialist (orthodontist or pedodontist) treating your child may determine that the jaws are in good relationship to each other and only braces are needed. In this case, they may wait to begin braces until most or all of your child's adult teeth are present in the mouth, and/or the jaws have reached most of their adult size. If the differences in size between the jaws are too large for braces alone, then surgery may be needed later. Because of the effects of the growth hormone administered by your doctor on jaw growth, it is important for your treating doctor (endocrinologist) and dentist (orthodontist and/or pedodontist) to have good communication with each other. Too much growth hormone can cause an overgrowth of the lower jaw, commonly seen in adults with tumors of the gland that makes growth hormone, so your dentist/orthodontist and endocrinologist should be aware of this possibility and monitoring your child as they near the end of their childhood growth. Although all the effects of growth hormone on the jaws and teeth are not presently known, research is being directed at this problem.

Because the teeth of children with growth hormone deficiency may be softer than normal or not formed normally, they can be very susceptible to cavities. For this reason, it is very important to see your dentist or children's dental specialist (pedodontist) at least every six months for checkups and teeth cleaning. Fluoride (in toothpaste, varnish ["paint" applied by the dentist], mouth rinses, and/or tablets) is often very good for these children (beware of too much fluoride swallowed though—

follow your doctor's and dentist's recommendations) and plastic placed on the tops of the teeth (sealants) is frequently indicated. A smile children can be proud of can be a very positive influence in their life as they deal with the other problems of growth hormone deficiency.

—Contributing author: Kirt E. Simmons, DDS, PhD,
Director of Craniofacial Orthodontics, Arkansas Children's
Hospital, Department of Surgery, University of Arkansas
Medical Sciences, Little Rock, Arkansas.

Chapter 54

Heart Disease Patients, Anticoagulants, and Dental Care

Antiplatelet and Anticoagulant Agents and Dental Procedures

An increasing number of dental patients are taking blood thinner medications for various medical conditions. These drugs interfere with the body's normal clotting (stopping blood flow) mechanism. There are two main processes by which the body normally forms a blood clot at the site of tissue injury. The first involves small blood cells called platelets which clump together at the wound to form a mechanical plug. This plug slows the flow of blood through the vessel and forms a matrix for the next phase of coagulation. During coagulation chemicals in the blood interact with each other to fill in the spaces between the platelets, stabilize the clot, and make it more solid until the process stops the bleeding.

Antiplatelet agents such as aspirin, Ticlid (ticlopidine), and Plavix (clopidogrel), target the first phase of clot formation by preventing platelets from sticking together and adhering to blood vessels. These agents do this by creating permanent changes in the platelets which last throughout the lifetime of the platelet (7–10 days). These effects can only be countered as the body produces new platelets that have not been exposed to the drug.

Anticoagulant agents such as warfarin (Coumadin) inhibit the second phase of clotting by blocking production of proteins that stabilize the clot. Warfarin can only affect these blood proteins when they are being made. This means that it takes several days for the drug to reach full effect and that anticoagulation also goes away slowly when the medication is stopped. Consequently, when changing the levels of anticoagulation, this process must occur gradually. Another important fact is that the effect of warfarin is influenced by many foods and other drugs, resulting in the need for frequent monitoring by the physician.

Many procedures in dentistry can produce bleeding. Most of the time this bleeding is not difficult to control even in patients who are taking anticoagulation and antiplatelet medications. However, both the effect of these medicines on clotting and the potential for bleeding associated with particular dental procedures is variable. Consequently, it is essential that for each procedure that the risk of bleeding be weighed against the risk of altering the dose or discontinuing the medication.

Some Dental Procedures Associated with Bleeding

- Dental prophylaxis (teeth cleaning)
- Scaling and root planing (deep teeth cleaning)
- Periodontal (gum) surgery
- Tooth extractions
- Dental implant placement
- Biopsies

Your dentist will want you to provide a thorough and complete medical history. Factors that he or she may ask you to provide include: all current medications, name of your physician, purpose of antiplatelet and/or anticoagulation therapy, anticipated time that you will be on these medications, the results of any laboratory monitoring of the effects of these agents, and any problems that you have had with your medicines. Your dentist may want to consult with your physician and it may be necessary to run some tests before your treatment. Furthermore, precautions may be made before, during, and after the dental procedure to reduce the risk of significant oral bleeding. Do not discontinue or alter your medications without the advice of your physician and dentist.

International Normalized Ratio (INR)

The INR is the primary method that health care providers use to measure the degree of anticoagulation that patients have as a result of taking warfarin (Coumadin). This test has generally replaced the pro-thrombin time (PT). For most medical indications, the expected range for anticoagulation as measured by the INR is 2.0–3.5. This number gives an approximation of how long someone taking these medications needs to clot in comparison to a normal individual. For example, an INR of 2.0 roughly equates to a coagulation time of twice normal.

Questions and Answers about Antiplatelet and Anticoagulant Medications

Is it necessary to check my clotting times before a dental appointment?

Depending upon the type of medication you are taking and the type of dental procedure that is to be performed, you may need to obtain specific blood tests that your dentist orders shortly before your dental procedure. This will give your doctor an idea of how your medication is affecting your ability to clot. On the rare occasion when it is recommended that a medication be discontinued, this decision is typically made by discussion between your dentist and your physician. They will determine when and for how long any medication should be discontinued, and when it should be resumed. These orders should be followed explicitly.

Why not stop my blood thinners before dental care just to be safe?

In the past, these medications were discontinued prior to dental procedures because of fear of potential bleeding. However, many studies have since proven that the risks of discontinuing these medications can be very dangerous, and serious bleeding from most dental procedures is very uncommon. Additionally, bleeding can be controlled in the dental office in many ways (pressure, stitches, medications, socket packing, and so forth). Therefore, even with surgical procedures these important medications are seldom stopped in modern dentistry.

What measures can I take to minimize bleeding after a dental procedure?

Most invasive dental procedures result in bleeding that is well controlled if simple procedures are followed. For example, after surgical treatment applying firm pressure on the bleeding sites for 30 minutes with moist gauze or tea bags will usually stop the bleeding. Patients should refrain from spitting, rinsing, using a straw, drinking hot beverages, and smoking for at least the first 24 hours. Also, patients should avoid eating hard or sharp foods (such as pretzels, chips, nuts) for the first two to three days. Your dentist may also prescribe certain medications that can help minimize bleeding. Follow the instructions given to you by your dentist.

At what point do I seek help for oral bleeding and whom should I contact?

If at any time you have a concern regarding bleeding after surgery, you should feel free to contact your dentist or oral surgeon. If all the local precautions described are taken and there is significant blood loss; meaning continuous bleeding that occurs for more than several hours, or the formation of a very large blood clot (a liver clot), then you clearly should seek help. Your dentist or oral surgeon should provide you with a means of contact after hours (for example, an office number or on-call pager), and failing that, you should visit your local emergency room.

What other precautions should I take if I am on antiplatelet or anticoagulant medications?

If you are prescribed a new medication while taking anticoagulants, make sure your prescribing doctor understands you are on these medications. Your pharmacy will also check for drug interactions, and if you have any doubts, consult your physician or dentist to ensure there is no conflict. Be aware also that over-the-counter medications such as Motrin, Advil, and Aleve, can result in antiplatelet effects. Additionally herbal or non-traditional medications can interfere with, or increase, the effects of your anticoagulant medications. Before you take any new medication whether prescribed or over-the-counter, you should check with the provider that prescribed your anticoagulant medications.

Chapter 55

Immune System Disorders and Oral Health

Chapter Contents

Section 55.1

Latex Allergy and Dental Treatment

Excerpted from "Contact Dermatitis and Latex Allergy," Centers for
Disease Control and Prevention (CDC), September 9, 2011.

What is contact dermatitis?

Occupationally related contact dermatitis can develop from frequent
and repeated use of hand hygiene products, exposure to chemicals, and
glove use. Contact dermatitis is classified as either irritant or allergic. Irritant contact dermatitis is common, nonallergic, and develops
as dry, itchy, irritated areas on the skin around the area of contact.
By comparison, allergic contact dermatitis (type IV hypersensitivity)
can result from exposure to accelerators and other chemicals used in
the manufacture of rubber gloves as well as from exposure to other
chemicals found in the dental practice setting. Allergic contact dermatitis often manifests as a rash beginning hours after contact and, like
irritant dermatitis, is usually confined to the areas of contact.

What is latex allergy?

Latex allergy (type I hypersensitivity to latex proteins) can be a
more serious systemic allergic reaction. It usually begins within minutes of exposure but can sometimes occur hours later. It produces
varied symptoms, which commonly include runny nose, sneezing, itchy
eyes, scratchy throat, hives, and itchy burning sensations. However,
it can involve more severe symptoms including asthma marked by
difficult breathing, coughing spells, and wheezing; cardiovascular and
gastrointestinal ailments; and, in rare cases, anaphylaxis and death.

Dental health care personnel experiencing contact dermatitis or
latex allergy symptoms should seek a definitive diagnosis by an experienced health care professional (dermatologist, allergist) to determine
the specific etiology and appropriate treatment for their condition, as
well as to determine what work restrictions or accommodations may
be necessary.

What are some considerations if dental health care personnel are allergic to latex?

Dental health care personnel who are allergic to latex will need to take precautions at work and outside the workplace since latex is used in a variety of other common products in addition to gloves. The following recommendations are based on those issued by the National Institute for Occupational Health and Safety (NIOSH). If definitively diagnosed with allergy to natural rubber latex (NRL) protein:

- Avoid, as far as feasible, subsequent exposure to the protein and only use nonlatex (nitrile or vinyl) gloves.

- Make sure that other staff members in the dental practice wear either nonlatex or reduced protein, powder-free, latex gloves.

- Use only synthetic or powder-free rubber dams.

Dental personnel can further reduce occupational exposure to NRL protein by taking the following steps:

- Using reduced protein, powder-free, latex gloves.

- Frequently changing ventilation filters and vacuum bags used in latex contaminated areas.

- Checking ventilation systems to ensure they provide adequate fresh or recirculating air.

- Frequently cleaning all work areas contaminated with latex dust.

- Educating dental staff on the signs and symptoms of latex allergies.

Why are powder-free gloves recommended?

Proteins responsible for latex allergies are attached to glove powder. When powdered gloves are worn, more latex protein reaches the skin. Also, when gloves are put on or removed, particles of latex protein powder become aerosolized and can be inhaled, contacting mucous membranes. As a result, allergic dental health care personnel and patients can experience symptoms related to cutaneous, respiratory, and conjunctival exposure. Dental health care personnel can become sensitized to latex proteins after repeated exposure. Work areas where only powder-free, low-allergen (reduced-protein) gloves are used show low or undetectable amounts of allergy-causing proteins.

What are some considerations for providing dental treatment to patients with latex allergy?

Patients with a latex allergy should not have direct contact with latex-containing materials and should be treated in a latex-safe environment. Such patients also may be allergic to the chemicals used in manufacturing natural rubber latex gloves, as well as to metals, plastics, or other materials used to provide dental care. By obtaining thorough patient health histories and preventing patients from having contact with potential allergens, dental health care professionals can minimize the possibility of patients having adverse reactions. Considerations in providing safe treatment for patients with possible or documented latex allergy include (but are not limited to) the following:

- Screen all patients for latex allergy (for example: obtain their health history, provide medical consultation when latex allergy is suspected).

- Be aware of some common predisposing conditions (such as spina bifida; urogenital anomalies; or, allergies to avocados, kiwis, nuts, or bananas).

- Be familiar with the different types of hypersensitivity— immediate and delayed—and the risks that these pose for patients and staff.

- Consider sources of latex other than gloves. Dental patients with a history of latex allergy may be at risk from a variety of dental products including, but not limited to, prophylaxis cups, rubber dams, and orthodontic elastics.

- Provide an alternative treatment area free of materials containing latex. Ensure a latex-safe environment or one in which no personnel use latex gloves and no patient contact occurs with other latex devices, materials, and products.

- Remove all latex-containing products from the patient's vicinity. Adequately cover or isolate any latex-containing devices that cannot be removed from the treatment environment.

- Be aware that latent allergens in the ambient air can cause respiratory and or anaphylactic symptoms in people with latex hypersensitivity. Therefore, to minimize inadvertent exposure to airborne latex particles among patients with latex allergy, try to give them the first appointments of the day.

- Frequently clean all working areas contaminated with latex powder or dust.

- Frequently change ventilation filters and vacuum bags used in latex-contaminated areas.

- Have latex-free kits (dental treatment and emergency kits) available at all times.

- Be aware that allergic reactions can be provoked from indirect contact as well as direct contact (such as being touched by someone who has worn latex gloves). Hand hygiene, therefore, is essential.

- Communicate latex allergy procedures (for example: verbal instructions, written protocols, posted signs) to other personnel to prevent them from bringing latex-containing materials into the treatment area.

- If latex-related complications occur during or after the procedure, manage the reaction and seek emergency assistance as indicated. Follow current medical emergency response recommendations for management of anaphylaxis.

Section 55.2

Mouth Problems with HIV

Excerpted from "Mouth Problems and HIV,"
National Institute of Dental and Craniofacial Research
(NIDCR), March 25, 2011.

Oral problems are very common in people with human immuno-deficiency virus (HIV). More than a third of people living with HIV have oral conditions that arise because of their weakened immune system. And even though combination antiretroviral therapy has made some oral problems less common, others are occurring more often with this type of treatment. They can be painful, annoying, and lead to other problems.

You may be told that oral problems are minor compared to other things you have to deal with. But, you know that they can cause discomfort and embarrassment and really affect how you feel about yourself. Oral problems can also lead to trouble with eating. If mouth pain or tenderness makes it difficult to chew and swallow, or if you can't taste food as well as you used to, you may not eat enough. And, your doctor may tell you to eat more than normal so your body has enough energy to deal with HIV.

They can be treated: The most common oral problems linked with HIV can be treated. So, talk with your doctor or dentist about what treatment might work for you. Remember, with the right treatment, your mouth can feel better. And that's an important step toward living well, not just longer, with HIV.

If You Have Dry Mouth

Dry mouth happens when you do not have enough saliva, or spit, to keep your mouth wet. Saliva helps you chew and digest food, protects teeth from decay, and prevents infections by controlling bacteria and fungi in the mouth. Without enough saliva, you could develop tooth decay or other infections and might have trouble chewing and swallowing. Your mouth might also feel sticky, dry, and have a burning feeling. And, you may have cracked, chapped lips.

To help with a dry mouth, try the following:

- Sip water or sugarless drinks often

- Chew sugarless gum or suck on sugarless hard candy

- Avoid tobacco

- Avoid alcohol

- Avoid salty foods

- Use a humidifier at night

Talk to your doctor or dentist about prescribing artificial saliva, which may help keep your mouth moist.

Section 55.3

Oral Hypersensitivity Reactions

"Oral Hypersensitivity Reactions," © 2011 American Academy of Oral Medicine (www.aaom.com). All rights reserved. Reprinted with permission.

Hypersensitivity reactions are abnormal reactions of the immune system that occur in response to exposure to otherwise harmless substances. These reactions encompass true allergic and other non-allergic reactions, and their severity can range from mild to life-threatening. The most severe hypersensitivity reaction is called anaphylaxis, and this allergic reaction usually begins immediately after exposure to the allergen. Hypersensitivity reactions in and around the mouth may produce a wide range of clinical appearances including redness or whiteness of the mucosa; swelling of the lips, tongue, and cheeks; and/or ulcers and blisters.

Types of Oral Hypersensitivity Reactions

Stomatitis: Typical signs of stomatitis are redness and swelling that may involve any part of the mouth including the tongue, roof of the mouth, cheeks, and lips (cheilitis). There is occasional formation of blisters and ulcers. Affected individuals may complain of a burning sensation and mouth sensitivity to cold, hot, and spicy foods.

Lichenoid reactions: These lesions resemble lichen and consist of slightly raised, thin, whitish lines that blend together to form a lacelike pattern. Sometimes ulcers are located within the lesion and surrounded by the whitish lines. Lichenoid lesions are found most commonly on the mucosa of the cheeks but may occur throughout the mouth.

Angioedema: Angioedema is a soft, painless, non-itchy swelling that usually involves the lips, tongue, or cheeks. It typically develops rapidly and can become a serious event requiring emergency treatment, if the swelling spreads to the larynx and results in severe breathing difficulty.

Erythema multiforme: In erythema multiforme, both the skin and the mouth may be affected. Mouth lesions begin as swelling and redness of the oral mucosa, followed by the formation of blisters which break and leave areas of ulceration. The lips may become swollen and develop bloody crusts. The typical skin lesion is the target or iris lesion that consists of concentric rings of red skin surrounded by areas of normal colored skin. The extent of involvement can be so severe as to require hospitalization.

Plasma cell gingivitis: Plasma cell gingivitis appears as a bright redness and swelling of the gums without ulceration (loss of skin cells). This characteristic appearance is due to the gathering of specific white blood cells, called plasma cells, in the gums. Other areas that may be involved include the tongue or lips. This reversible condition is different than gum disease, and symptoms resolve once the cause is removed.

Questions and Answers about Oral Hypersensitivity Reactions

What should I do if I think that I am experiencing a hypersensitivity reaction?

You should seek out a professional evaluation by a dentist or other health care provider to determine the diagnosis and obtain appropriate treatment. Mild allergic reactions are often treated with antihistamine drugs or topical steroids. If you experience difficulty in breathing, you should go immediately to an emergency treatment facility.

What can cause a hypersensitivity reaction in the mouth?

A large number of substances. The most common causes are food, food additives, drugs, oral hygiene products, and dental materials.

Are there any specific foods that are more commonly implicated in intraoral hypersensitivity reactions?

Yes. Nuts (walnuts, cashew nuts, almonds, hazelnuts), fruits and vegetables (banana, avocado, kiwi, mango, tomato, potato), milk, eggs, soybeans, fish (cod, tuna, salmon) and shellfish (snails, mussels, oysters, lobster, crabs, shrimps) are the most commonly implicated food allergens worldwide. Gums and candies are often flavored with agents like cinnamon, peppermint, or menthol, which can trigger hypersensitivity reactions in susceptible individuals.

What is the Latex-Fruit Syndrome?

A large number of individuals who are allergic to latex products show hypersensitivity to some foods especially fresh fruits. This association of latex allergy with fruit allergy is called "Latex-Fruit Syndrome." Fruits such as avocado, banana, passion fruit, kiwi, papaya, mango, peach, fig, melon, and pineapple, are all associated with this syndrome. You should inform your dentist if you are allergic to any of these fruits, because of your increased risk of being allergic to latex.

Which drugs are responsible for intraoral hypersensitivity manifestations?

The truth is that almost any drug can cause such a hypersensitivity reaction in the mouth, though some are more common than others. If you suspect you suffer from a hypersensitivity reaction, you should discuss it with your prescribing doctor.

What oral hygiene products are considered as causes of hypersensitivity reactions?

Virtually any. Many toothpastes and mouthwashes are flavored with potential allergens such as cinnamon, peppermint, eugenol, and menthol. Even dental floss and denture cleansers may contain ingredients known to cause a hypersensitivity reaction.

How can dental treatment trigger a hypersensitivity reaction?

Some dental materials used by the dentist can cause a hypersensitivity reaction in certain individuals. Potential allergens include the metals in amalgam (silver) fillings, crowns and bridges, and orthodontic wires; the plastic or acrylic in dentures; composite restorations; bonding agents; impression materials; varnishes; and rubber products such as gloves and rubber dams.

The roof of my mouth under my denture is red and burns. Is this an allergy?

A true allergic reaction to the substances in a denture is uncommon. Your symptoms are much more likely the result of inflammation caused by the denture being too loose or a yeast infection.

Can local anesthetics cause allergic reactions?

Yes, they can, although it is rare. Only 1% of the adverse reactions due to local anesthetics are considered truly allergic, and most of these are due to an allergic response to the preservatives used to prolong the shelf life of the anesthetic and not the anesthetic itself. The vast majority of adverse reactions attributed to local anesthetics are in reality caused by either patient anxiety or as a response to the vasoconstrictor present in the anesthetic solution.

How can I determine if I have an allergy?

It can be a challenge, particularly when you are experiencing mild allergic reactions. Your healthcare provider will often ask if you can identify a relationship between your exposure to a particular food, drug, or other product and the onset of your symptoms. If necessary, your provider may refer you to an allergist for a more comprehensive evaluation.

Can I prevent a hypersensitivity reaction from occurring?

Maybe. The best way to prevent a hypersensitivity reaction is to avoid any agent that provokes it. While this is easy when the causative agent is known; in many cases, it is difficult to conclusively identify the causative agent. For example, the foods you eat may contain small amounts of ingredients capable of causing a hypersensitivity reaction.

Chapter 56

Marfan Syndrome and Dental Problems

Many people with Marfan syndrome have narrow jaws and high, arched palates which can create dental and orthodontic problems. There is limited research regarding specific management of the orthodontic problems commonly seen in people with Marfan syndrome, but seeking orthodontic care is an important part of Marfan syndrome management, particularly in children.

In addition, people with mitral valve prolapse and artificial heart valves are at risk for endocarditis (infection of the heart and heart valves) when they have dental work, and should follow the recommendations regarding endocarditis prophylaxis.

Following are answers to frequently asked questions regarding orthodontics and other dental concerns.

When should children with Marfan syndrome visit an orthodontist?

According to the American Association of Orthodontists, children should see an orthodontist by the age of seven years. This is particularly true for children with Marfan syndrome. Many treatment options are possible for a growing child. However, as a patient becomes a teenager and an adult, the number of treatment options becomes more limited.

What is the most common orthodontic problem affecting children with Marfan syndrome)?

When a child is seven or eight years, it is possible to recognize a narrow upper jaw which is a common characteristic in children with Marfan syndrome. A narrow upper jaw causes the upper teeth on the side of the mouth to be set inside the lower teeth creating a posterior crossbite. Normally, the upper teeth overlap the lower teeth.

How is a posterior crossbite treated?

A posterior crossbite can be treated by widening the upper arch with an orthodontic expander. In a young child, the suture (where the bones of the palate come together) is not fused. As a child gets older, these areas become less flexible and fuse. Typically, when a child becomes a teenager, simple orthodontic expansion is not possible without surgical assistance to make the bones flexible again. However, due to the nature of Marfan syndrome and the continued growth that people with the disorder experience, the time frame for correcting the posterior crossbite with an orthodontic expander varies, and can extend beyond the preteen years. If expansion is done early to take advantage of the flexible palate, it is often beneficial to follow this treatment with full braces. If braces are not started right away, there are other options such as a transpalatal arch to hold the space until braces are appropriate.

It is important to consult with your orthodontist to determine the timing that is best for your situation and, if there is any question, get a second opinion from another orthodontist who has treated people with Marfan syndrome.

If a posterior crossbite cannot be corrected with an expander, are there other options?

For people who are past the growth period, and not likely to benefit from the use of a skeletal orthodontic expansion appliance, a surgical procedure can assist in the widening of the upper arch. Any surgical procedure introduces certain risks to people with Marfan syndrome who already have cardiovascular complications. The patient's cardiologist should be consulted to evaluate the risk-benefit for this elective surgical procedure. If the cardiologist and the patient do not deem it to be worth the potential risks, the posterior crossbite cannot be treated. Then, the orthodontist will separately—and nonsurgically—address other orthodontic issues, such as a crowding, overbite, or underbite.

Is the extraction of teeth an option to correct orthodontic problems for people with Marfan syndrome?

Extractions of teeth for orthodontic treatment can be done safely in people with Marfan syndrome as long as antibiotic medication is given one hour before the procedure. A prescription for the antibiotic can be obtained from a cardiologist or pediatrician. The usual one-time, high dose of antibiotics should be double-checked with the patient's cardiologist.

What are some of the other orthodontic concerns facing people with Marfan syndrome?

If orthodontic bands (rings) are fitted over the molar teeth, then meticulous oral hygiene is needed to prevent dental plaque accumulation around the gum line. Plaque around the gums is a source of bacteria that could enter the blood stream and potentially infect the heart. Regular tooth brushing in a circular motion around the gums can prevent gum inflammation and bleeding. Flossing with floss threaders and brushing after every meal is the minimum care needed to maintain good oral hygiene. Oral irrigators can also help to keep braces and orthodontic expanders clean.

Patients who are at risk of developing infections from dental procedures need antibiotic coverage during band placement and band removal procedures. If it is possible, bands should be avoided and replaced with brackets that are placed above the gums. If a child has a posterior crossbite, then usually two to four teeth will need orthodontic bands to make an orthodontic expander.

What is endocarditis?

Endocarditis is the inflammation of the lining of the heart cavity and valves. People with mitral valve prolapse or an artificial heart valve can develop endocarditis during dental procedures and other medical situations where there is an increased likelihood that bacteria can enter the blood stream. Endocarditis is a terrible complication for anyone, but particularly so in a patient who has had surgical reconstruction of the aorta with placement of an artificial valve. This is a condition that is almost incurable by medicine alone, and nearly always requires surgery to remove the artificial valve and Dacron graft. Not only is the operation itself of much higher risk than the original operation, but there remains a substantial chance that not all of the infected tissue will be removed, and that recurrent endocarditis will occur. Endocarditis prophylaxis is the prevention of endocarditis before it occurs.

How can I prevent infections of the heart and valves (endocarditis)?

Precautions must be taken prior to any procedure that may introduce bacteria into the bloodstream. This includes routine dental work. Many dental procedures go below the gum line and provide an opportunity for bacteria to enter the blood stream. People with Marfan syndrome should advise their dentist of their heart problems so that the dentist can consult with the cardiologist about the need for antibiotics prior to beginning the dental work.

Is TMJ (Temporomandibular Joint Syndrome) associated with Marfan syndrome?

TMJ disease is common in Marfan syndrome because TMJ is a joint. People with Marfan syndrome have deficiency of elastic fiber in many joints in the body, and the temporomandibular joint, which connects the jaw to the skull, is no exception. The TMJ is also more pronounced in Marfan syndrome. A prosthodontist should be consulted for TMJ and jaw problems.

Are people with Marfan syndrome more likely to get cavities?

There is no evidence that people with Marfan syndrome are more likely to get cavities than the general population.

Chapter 57

Meth (Methamphetamine) Mouth

Methamphetamine Abuse Undermines Dental Health

Clinicians have long observed that methamphetamine users often have extreme dental decay. Now researchers have, for the first time, provided scientific evidence of this condition and shed light on how the method of drug administration influences dental disease patterns. The National Institute on Drug Abuse (NIDA)-funded research—conducted by Dr. Vivek Shetty and colleagues at the University of California, Los Angeles—was in response to the growing body of anecdotal observations and media reports about the oral health effects of methamphetamine abuse. The team of dental, addiction, and public health researchers evaluated comprehensive medical and oral health information collected from 301 adults who had received treatment for methamphetamine abuse and 301 comparable nonusers participating in the National Health and Nutrition Examination Survey III.

Increased dental disease was one of the most common health conditions among methamphetamine abusers, found in 41%. Methamphetamine abusers also had more teeth missing than nonusers (average five versus two). People who injected methamphetamine were twice as likely to have missing teeth as smokers of the drug. Their higher rates likely reflect more severe addiction and accompanying neglect of self-care.

This chapter begins with "Methamphetamine Abuse Undermines Dental Health," *NIDA Notes*, National Institute on Drug Abuse (NIDA), July 2011. Text beginning at "Methamphetamine" consists of excerpts from *NIDA InfoFacts: Methamphetamine*, NIDA, updated March 2010.

505

Dr. Shetty and colleagues concluded that dental disease is a distinctive side effect of methamphetamine abuse and that rates and patterns of dental disease may be useful in the early identification of such abuse. The study also found that 29% of methamphetamine abusers expressed concern about their dental appearance. Dentists may be able to use this concern to motivate stimulant abusers to participate in targeted behavioral interventions in the dental office or seek help at addiction treatment programs, the researchers say.

Facts about Methamphetamine

Methamphetamine is a central nervous system stimulant drug that is similar in structure to amphetamine. Due to its high potential for abuse, methamphetamine is classified as a Schedule II drug and is available only through a prescription that cannot be refilled. Although methamphetamine can be prescribed by a doctor, its medical uses are limited, and the doses that are prescribed are much lower than those typically abused. Most of the methamphetamine abused in this country comes from foreign or domestic super labs, although it can also be made in small, illegal laboratories, where its production endangers the people in the labs, neighbors, and the environment.

How is methamphetamine abused?

Methamphetamine is a white, odorless, bitter-tasting crystalline powder that easily dissolves in water or alcohol and is taken orally, intranasally (snorting the powder), by needle injection, or by smoking.

How does methamphetamine affect the brain?

Methamphetamine increases the release and blocks the reuptake of the brain chemical (or neurotransmitter) dopamine, leading to high levels of the chemical in the brain—a common mechanism of action for most drugs of abuse. Dopamine is involved in reward, motivation, the experience of pleasure, and motor function. Methamphetamine's ability to release dopamine rapidly in reward regions of the brain produces the intense euphoria, or rush, that many users feel after snorting, smoking, or injecting the drug.

Chronic methamphetamine abuse significantly changes how the brain functions. Noninvasive human brain imaging studies have shown alterations in the activity of the dopamine system that are associated with reduced motor skills and impaired verbal learning. Recent studies in chronic methamphetamine abusers have also revealed severe structural and functional changes in areas of the brain associated with emotion and memory, which may account for many of the emotional and cognitive problems observed in chronic methamphetamine abusers.

Repeated methamphetamine abuse can also lead to addiction—a chronic, relapsing disease characterized by compulsive drug seeking and use, which is accompanied by chemical and molecular changes in the brain. Some of these changes persist long after methamphetamine abuse is stopped. Reversal of some of the changes, however, may be observed after sustained periods of abstinence (for example, more than one year).

What other adverse effects does methamphetamine have on health?

Taking even small amounts of methamphetamine can result in many of the same physical effects as those of other stimulants, such as cocaine or amphetamines, including increased wakefulness, increased physical activity, decreased appetite, increased respiration, rapid heart rate, irregular heartbeat, increased blood pressure, and hyperthermia.

Long-term methamphetamine abuse has many negative health consequences, including extreme weight loss, severe dental problems (meth mouth), anxiety, confusion, insomnia, mood disturbances, and violent behavior. Chronic methamphetamine abusers can also display a number of psychotic features, including paranoia, visual and auditory hallucinations, and delusions (for example, the sensation of insects crawling under the skin).

Transmission of human immunodeficiency virus (HIV) and hepatitis B and C can be consequences of methamphetamine abuse. The intoxicating effects of methamphetamine, regardless of how it is taken, can also alter judgment and inhibition and can lead people to engage in unsafe behaviors, including risky sexual behavior. Among abusers who inject the drug, HIV/acquired immunodeficiency syndrome (AIDS) and other infectious diseases can be spread through contaminated needles, syringes, and other injection equipment that is used by more than one person. Methamphetamine abuse may also worsen the progression of HIV/AIDS and its consequences. Studies of methamphetamine abusers who are HIV-positive indicate that HIV causes greater neuronal injury and cognitive impairment for individuals in this group compared with HIV-positive people who do not use the drug.

Monitoring the Future Survey

Methamphetamine use among teens appears to have dropped significantly in recent years, according to data revealed by the *2009*

Monitoring the Future survey. The number of high-school seniors reporting past-year use is now only at 1.2%, which is the lowest since questions about methamphetamine were added to the survey in 1999; at that time, it was reported at 4.7%. Lifetime use among eighth-graders was reported at 1.6% in 2009, down significantly from 2.3% in 2008. In addition, the proportion of tenth-graders reporting that crystal methamphetamine was easy to obtain has dropped to 14%, down from 19.5% five years ago.

Table 57.1. Methamphetamine Prevalence of Abuse, Monitoring the Future Survey, 2009

Grade	8th grade	10th grade	12th grade
Lifetime**	1.6%	2.8%	2.4%
Past Year	1.0%	1.6%	1.2%
Past Month	0.5%	0.6%	0.5%

**Lifetime refers to use at least once during a respondent's lifetime. Past year refers to use at least once during the year preceding an individual's response to the survey. "Past month" refers to use at least once during the 30 days preceding an individual's response to the survey.

Chapter 58

Organ Transplantation May Affect Your Mouth

Organ Transplantation and Your Mouth

If you are an organ transplant patient, you are at risk for serious mouth problems. Your medical condition and side effects from your transplant medications can affect your oral health and complicate dental care. This chapter identifies problems you may encounter and explains how you can help keep your mouth healthy.

Pre-Transplant Dental Check-Up

A dental check-up is an important part of your pre-transplant evaluation. Because some medications you take after transplant can cause problems in your mouth, you want your mouth to be as healthy as possible before your transplant procedure. Taking care of cavities, periodontal (gum) disease, and any other mouth problems ahead of time can help prevent or reduce the side effects of transplant medicines. Keeping your mouth clean and free of dental disease is important for your general health as well.

Post-Transplant Dental Care

Anti-rejection medications suppress your immune system and make it easier for you to develop infections and other problems in your mouth, including these:

This chapter includes: "Organ Transplantation and Your Mouth," National Institute of Dental and Craniofacial Research (NIDCR), NIH Publication No. 11–6269, reviewed April 2011; and, "Dental Management of the Organ Transplant Patient," NIDCR, NIH Publication No. 11–6270, reviewed April 2011.

- **Dry mouth:** The cotton mouth feeling you get when you don't have enough saliva to keep your mouth moist. Dry mouth increases your risk for tooth decay.

- **Mouth ulcers:** Sores in the soft lining of the mouth that can make chewing, speaking, or swallowing painful.

- **Infections:** Gum disease that can harm the tissues holding the teeth in place; or thrush, a fungus infection that appears as creamy white patches in the mouth.

- **Gingival overgrowth:** Enlarged gums that cover part of the teeth, making brushing and flossing difficult and increasing the risk for bleeding and infection.

- **Tumors:** Mouth cancers that occur in some transplant patients, especially those who have smoked.

Once your transplant has stabilized, your dentist can treat new dental disease and help you manage any side effects of transplant medication that may occur. All mouth problems should be treated.

It's important for your dentist and your transplant doctor to speak with each other before dental treatment. Together, they will work out a dental care plan that safely meets your needs.

For example, they may decide that you need to take antibiotics before dental treatment, or your doctor may adjust your medication.

- Make sure your dentist knows that you are a transplant patient. Give your dentist the contact information for your transplant doctor.

- Bring a list of all your medications, including over-the-counter drugs, to every dental appointment. Remember to tell your dentist if your medications have changed.

- Talk to your dentist about your general health. If you have diabetes or other health conditions, make sure your dentist knows. In the same way, talk to your transplant doctor about your oral health. Tell your doctor if you have mouth problems.

Keeping Your Mouth Healthy

You can do a lot to keep your mouth healthy after your transplant procedure. Look inside your mouth daily and check how it feels with your tongue. Side effects from medications may show as white or red patches, sores, ulcers, or tumors. You may notice dryness in your mouth, a lump, or bleeding gums when you brush. Call your dentist if you notice any changes or problems.

Brush and floss every day. Good daily oral hygiene is vital to keeping your mouth healthy. If you have any questions about brushing and flossing, particularly if your mouth is sore, ask your dentist or dental hygienist.

Remember

- Have a dental check-up before your transplant procedure.

- See your dentist regularly after your transplant has stabilized.

- Call your dentist when you notice any problem or change in your mouth.

- Take care of your mouth every day.

Dental Management of the Organ Transplant Patient

Organ transplant patients need specialized dental care. The compromised health and immune system of patients place them at increased risk for systemic as well as oral infections. This fact must be considered when planning dental treatment before and after transplantation and requires consultation with your patient's physician.

Managing Oral Health before Organ Transplantation

Before treating a prospective transplant recipient, obtain and review the patient's medical and dental histories and perform a non-invasive initial oral examination (without periodontal probing). After the examination, discuss the current status of your patient's health and immune system, and the degree of organ dysfunction with his or her physician. Decisions about the timing of treatment, the need for antibiotic prophylaxis, precautions to prevent excessive bleeding, and appropriate medication and dosage should be considered during your discussion.

Whether a patient can tolerate dental treatment is another crucial concern. In some cases, it will be safer for patients to undergo extensive treatment after transplant as the new organ improves their health.

Preparing for Dental Treatment

Several factors should be considered before starting treatment:

- **Antibiotic prophylaxis:** Decide with the patient's physician whether antibiotic prophylaxis is required to prevent systemic infection from invasive dental procedures. Unless advised otherwise by the physician, the American Heart Association's standard regimen to prevent endocarditis (http://www.heart.org) is an accepted option.

- **Infection:** If the patient presents with an active infection, such as a purulent periodontal infection or an abscessed tooth, antibiotics should be given to the patient before and after dental treatment to prevent systemic infection. Confirm the choice of antibiotic with the patient's physician.

- **Excessive bleeding:** Several factors can cause bleeding problems in organ transplant candidates, such as organ dysfunction or their medications. Many may be anticoagulated, and some may have a decreased platelet count. Patients with end-stage liver disease may have excessive bleeding because the liver is no longer producing sufficient amounts of clotting factors. Before treatment, assess the patient's bleeding potential with the appropriate laboratory tests and take precautions to limit bleeding.

  - Consult with your patient's physician about whether antifibrinolytic drugs, vitamin K, fresh frozen plasma, or other interventions are appropriate. The physician also may decide to temporarily decrease the patient's level of anticoagulation before extensive dental surgeries. Some patients are only suitable for surgery in a hospital setting or dental offices designed to handle emergency medical situations.

  - Use aggressive suctioning techniques when performing extractions or other invasive procedures to prevent your patient from swallowing blood. In a small number of patients with advanced liver disease, swallowed blood may increase risk for hepatic coma.

  - Manage bleeding sites with careful packing and suturing techniques.

- **Medication considerations:** Patients preparing to undergo organ transplantation usually take multiple medications. These include anticoagulants, beta blockers, calcium channel blockers, diuretics, and others. Be aware of the side effects of these medications, which range from xerostomia and gingival hyperplasia to orthostatic hypotension and hyperglycemia, and their interactions with drugs you might prescribe. Likewise, use caution when prescribing medication to patients with end-stage kidney or liver disease. Many medications commonly used in dental practice, including nonsteroidal anti-inflammatory drugs (NSAIDs), opiates, and some antimicrobials, are metabolized by these organs and are not removed from circulation as quickly in patients with markedly reduced kidney or liver function. Prior to dental treatment, consult the patient's physician on appropriate drug selection, dosage, and administration intervals.

- **Other medical problems:** Patients with end-stage organ failure may have other major medical conditions. A person with end-stage kidney disease, for example, may have diabetes and/or significant pulmonary or heart disease. Carefully review the patient's medical history to determine what additional treatment considerations the patient may have.

Dental Treatment

Whenever possible, all active dental disease should be aggressively treated before transplantation, since postoperative immunosuppression decreases a patient's ability to resist systemic infection.

Managing Oral Health after Organ Transplantation

Except for emergency dental care, patients should avoid dental treatment for at least three months following organ transplantation. Dosage of immunosuppressive medications is highest in the early post-transplant period, and patients are at greatest risk for rejection of the transplanted organ and other serious complications during that time. Once the graft has stabilized, typically 3–6 months post-surgery, patients can be treated in the dental office with proper precautions.

Preparing for Dental Treatment

Treatment after transplantation requires consultation with your patient's physician. The medical consult can help to understand the patient's general health and ability to tolerate treatment. Post-transplant patients vary widely in their ability to endure dental treatment and heal following invasive procedures. Discussion needs to address whether the patient requires antibiotic prophylaxis and if the physician will need to adjust other medications before treatment.

Oral Complications

Side effects from immunosuppressive drugs to prevent organ rejection are among the most frequent oral health problems affecting transplant recipients. Common immunosuppressive agents and their side effects include the following:

- **Cyclosporine:** Changes in liver/kidney function, hypertension, bleeding problems, and poor wound healing are among the adverse effects of this potent agent, which also interacts with a number of other drugs. Gingival hyperplasia occurs in some patients; incidence varies and is dependent on each patient and his or her drug regimen. Calcium channel blockers, for example, may exacerbate the problem. Children tend to be more susceptible to gingival overgrowth than adults. Conscientious daily oral hygiene is important for all patients.

- **Tacrolimus:** An immunosuppressive agent used increasingly in place of cyclosporine, tacrolimus causes less gingival overgrowth but is associated with oral ulcerations and numbness or tingling, especially around the mouth.

- **Azathioprine:** Bone marrow suppression and related complications such as stomatitis and opportunistic infections are significant side effects of this drug. A decrease in white blood cell counts and excessive bleeding may occur.

- **Mycophenolate mofetil:** This immunosuppressant is commonly used as an alternative to azathioprine. Adverse effects include decreased white cell counts, opportunistic infections, and gastrointestinal problems.

- **Corticosteroids:** Hypertension and high blood glucose (steroid-induced diabetes) are among the numerous side effects of these drugs, along with increased risk for infection, poor wound healing, and depression. Adrenal suppression may occur, making invasive dental and medical procedures more difficult for your patient. Corticosteroids may also mask the early signs of oral infection. The trend toward using lower doses of corticosteroids in combination with other immunosuppressants for post-transplant maintenance therapy has helped mitigate these side effects.

- **Sirolimus:** Side effects of this anti-rejection drug can include hypertension, joint pain, low white cell count, hypercholesterolemia, and oral ulceration.

Marked Immunosuppression

Several complications associated with marked immunosuppression manifest in the mouth, including oral candidiasis, herpes simplex/

herpes zoster, hairy leukoplakia, aphthous ulcers, and uncommon viral and fungal infections. Progressive periodontal disease, delayed wound healing, and excessive bleeding may also become problems for these patients.

Notify your physician if signs of marked immunosuppression are noticed. In some cases, the dosage of anti-rejection agents prescribed for patients may need to be reduced. This may help control the opportunistic infections and other oral complications. However, there will be patients who must be maintained on high-dose immunosuppression to prevent organ rejection. Treatment of oral opportunistic infection is necessary in any transplanted patient.

Oral Malignancies

All patients should be screened for oral malignancies at every appointment. Kaposi's sarcoma, lymphoma, and squamous cell carcinoma of the lip are among the oral malignancies that sometimes occur in organ transplant patients. Malignancies can occur decades earlier in transplant recipients than in people who are not immunosuppressed.

Organ Rejection

If a patient's body begins to reject a transplanted organ, only emergency dental care may be provided. Talk with the physician about antibiotic prophylaxis or other special needs before dental treatment.

Chapter 59

Osteoporosis Affects Bones and Teeth

Chapter Contents

Section 59.1

Oral Health and Bone Disease

Excerpted from "Oral Health and Bone Disease," National Institute of
Arthritis and Musculoskeletal and Skin Diseases (NIAMS), October 2010.

Osteoporosis and tooth loss are health concerns that affect many older
men and women. Osteoporosis is a condition in which the bones become
less dense and more likely to fracture. This disease can affect any bone in
the body, although the bones in the hip, spine, and wrist are affected most
often. In the United States more than 40 million people either already
have osteoporosis or are at high risk due to low bone mass.

Research suggests a link between osteoporosis and bone loss in the
jaw. The bone in the jaw supports and anchors the teeth. When the
jawbone becomes less dense, tooth loss can occur, a common occurrence
in older adults. Tooth loss affects approximately one-third of adults
age 65 and older.

Skeletal Bone Density and Dental Concerns

The portion of the jawbone that supports our teeth is known as the
alveolar process. Several studies have found a link between the loss of
alveolar bone and an increase in loose teeth (tooth mobility) and tooth
loss. Women with osteoporosis are three times more likely to experience
tooth loss than those who do not have the disease.

Low bone density in the jaw can result in other dental problems as
well. For example, older women with osteoporosis may be more likely
to have difficulty with loose or ill-fitting dentures and may have less
optimal outcomes from oral surgical procedures.

Periodontal Disease and Bone Health

Periodontitis is a chronic infection that affects the gums and the
bones that support the teeth. Bacteria and the body's own immune
system break down the bone and connective tissue that hold teeth in
place. Teeth may eventually become loose, fall out, or have to be removed.
Although tooth loss is a well-documented consequence of periodontitis,

the relationship between periodontitis and skeletal bone density is less clear. Some studies have found a strong and direct relationship among bone loss, periodontitis, and tooth loss. It is possible that the loss of alveolar bone mineral density leaves bone more susceptible to periodontal bacteria, increasing the risk for periodontitis and tooth loss.

Effects of Osteoporosis Treatments on Oral Health

It is not known whether osteoporosis treatments have the same beneficial effect on oral health as they do on other bones in the skeleton. Bisphosphonates, a group of medications available for the treatment of osteoporosis, have been linked to the development of osteonecrosis of the jaw (ONJ), which is cause for concern. The risk of ONJ has been greatest in patients receiving large doses of intravenous bisphosphonates, a therapy used to treat cancer. The occurrence of ONJ is rare in individuals taking oral forms of the medication for osteoporosis treatment.

Section 59.2

Bisphosphonate Therapy Effects

"Bisphosphonate Therapy and the Oral Cavity,"
© 2011 American Academy of Oral Medicine (www.aaom.com).
All rights reserved. Reprinted with permission.

Questions and Answers about Bisphosphonate Therapy

What are bisphosphonates?

Bisphosphonates are a class of drugs that are used to prevent bone loss demineralization (weakening or destruction). These have been used since the 1970s, but technological developments in recent years have continued to reduce the frequency of dosage and made other stronger forms of the drugs available. Some of these drugs can be taken by mouth, while others must be given intravenously at a hospital or clinic. Examples include drugs such as Actonel, Zometa, Fosamax, and Boniva.

What conditions are bisphosphonates prescribed to treat?

Bisphosphonates are approved for the treatment of the following:

- **Osteoporosis:** The loss of bone density often seen in postmenopausal females.

- **Hypercalcemia of malignancy:** Increased calcium in the blood from bone breakdown.

- **Metastatic disease to bone:** Cancer spreading to bone tissue.

Are there side effects to my mouth from taking these drugs?

Yes, there is an important but rare side effect you should know about. Less than five years ago, doctors began reporting cases of individuals having difficulty healing after undergoing tooth extraction or other invasive dental procedures, a phenomenon called osteonecrosis of the jaw. The only common factor in these patients was that they were taking bisphosphonate drugs. As a consequence, most doctors agree that there is an association between osteonecrosis of the jaw and bisphosphonates, although the drugs are not the only factor involved.

How common is this problem?

Since 2003, about 4,000 cases of bisphosphonate-associated osteonecrosis of the jaw have been reported to the U.S. Food and Drug Administration (FDA). Considering the fact that there have been tens of millions of prescriptions written for bisphosphonate drugs, this is a rare side effect. Over 90% of these cases were in patients receiving an intravenous (IV) form of the drug, with a much smaller number in those taking the medication by mouth. Overall, the risk is thought to be less than 1% for patients taking IV bisphosphonates, and at least ten times less likely than that for patients taking the drugs by mouth.

If I take bisphosphonates, am I automatically at risk?

The short answer is yes. Anyone who takes these medications has a chance of developing the condition. However, most reported cases occur after oral trauma (tooth extraction or oral surgical procedure). Tobacco use, treatment with corticosteroids, long-term use of bisphosphonates, treatment with more than one kind of bisphosphonate, and diabetes also may increase the risk of this condition occurring.

What are the signs of bisphosphonate-associated osteonecrosis?

The hallmarks of this condition are gum wounds that heal very slowly or do not heal at all for six weeks or more after a procedure and exposed bone. Some patients report that this begins with a feeling of roughness on the gum tissue. If these open wounds become infected, you may see pus or swelling in the adjacent gum tissue. Many times, this condition is painless in the beginning, and patients only experience pain after the exposed bone becomes infected. If this infection lasts long enough, there may even be numbness, especially in the lower jaw.

What kind of treatment is available for osteonecrosis?

Unfortunately, at this time most reported treatments are slow to resolve osteonecrosis of the jaw, so the best treatment is prevention. Current treatment methods that are used include antiseptic rinses, systemic antibiotics, and cleaning/removal of dead bone from the affected area. Sometimes if treatment is too aggressive it can make the condition worse. If your dentist diagnoses the condition, he or she may send you to a specialist in oral medicine or oral surgery to evaluate the best possible therapy. Generally, therapy focuses on controlling pain and preventing infection so that the body can heal properly.

What can I do to avoid this condition if I am taking bisphosphonates?

You should discuss with your dentist ways to minimize the risk of needing invasive procedures (extractions and oral surgery). Frequent professional cleanings, attention to home care, and careful observation of any changes in your mouth are a good start. It is best to attempt to preserve teeth, when possible, through root canal therapy or other conservative treatments, rather than extractions. You and your dentist should come up with an overall treatment plan for comprehensive and preventive treatment. The best scenario is one where dental work is planned and executed before therapy with bisphosphonates is started.

Is osteonecrosis always associated with a dental procedure?

No, some patients have reported the condition being caused by an irritating denture, or some other injury (sharp food, for example). Some cases appear to have no immediate cause at all.

Should I stop taking my bisphosphonates before dental procedures?

Not without the advice or instruction by your physician. These drugs have been shown to be stored within the bones and slowly released over time. It is believed that, even when not taking the medications, the drugs can persist for decades in bone. There is no evidence that stopping the medication will reduce the risk of developing osteonecrosis of the jaw. The only reason to stop taking your medication is because your physician specifically instructs you to do so.

Section 59.3

Osteogenesis Imperfecta

Dental Care for Persons with Osteogenesis Imperfecta (OI)

Osteogenesis imperfecta (OI) is always associated with bone fragility. In addition, OI may affect the growth of the jaws and may or may not affect the teeth. About half of the people who have OI have teeth that appear normal, and their major concerns are routine care. However, the other half has a defect in the teeth called dentinogenesis imperfecta (DI), sometimes referred to as opalescent teeth or brittle teeth. These teeth may be misshapen, may chip or break easily, and will require special care.

Oral cavity problems related to osteogenesis imperfecta may include the following:

- **A skeletal Class III malocclusion:** The teeth do not correctly match up making biting difficult. This is caused by the size and/or position of the upper jaw or the lower jaw.

- **An open bite:** There is a vertical gap between some of the upper and lower teeth.

- **Impacted teeth:** The first or second permanent molars do not erupt, or they erupt out of the usual location (ectopic).

- **Dental development:** Tooth development may be delayed or advanced in some individuals affected by OI. OI does not affect the presence or absence of gum disease (periodontitis).

Major Parts of the Teeth

The teeth are made up of four distinct parts.

- **Enamel** is the outside part of the crown. It is the hardest substance in the body and the point of contact for chewing.

- **Dentin** is the substance under the enamel that forms the rest of the crown and surrounding the pulp chamber and almost all of the root structure. It is similar to bone.

- **The pulp chamber** is the inner hollow part of the tooth containing blood vessels and nerves.

- The **dentinoenamel junction** (DEJ) is the term for where the enamel and dentin are attached to each other.

Dentinogenesis Imperfecta (DI)

Dentinogenesis imperfecta can be part of osteogenesis imperfecta (DI type I) or it can be a separate inherited dominant trait without OI (DI type II). DI occurring with OI seems to run in families but can vary in severity from one member to another. DI has a variable effect on the color, shape, and wear of both primary and permanent teeth. If someone has OI and DI, all of their teeth may not be affected to the same degree.

Teeth affected by DI have essentially normal enamel, but the DEJ and the dentin are not normal. The enamel tends to crack away from the dentin, which will wear away more quickly than enamel. The dentin makes the teeth look darker or opalescent. The dentin also grows to fill in the pulp chamber, causing a loss of feeling in the tooth. Affected teeth will have an increased incidence of fracture, wear, and decay.

Dentinogenesis imperfecta may be diagnosed with the first baby tooth. If the tooth looks gray, bluish, or brown, DI should be suspected. Children should be taken to a dentist (if possible a specialist in pediatric dentistry) when the first teeth are erupting. This may happen as early as six months to one year of age. Radiographs, or x-rays, can be useful but may be difficult to obtain until the child is older. Sometimes there are changes visible on the x-rays that are not obvious just by looking at the teeth. Crowns appear bulbous and roots may be shorter and more slender than standard. Primary teeth are usually more affected than the permanent teeth.

When, for any reason, crowns are not feasible, a tooth color dental material may be used, such as composites or glass ionomer in conjunction with composites. The sand abrasion method may also be useful because it removes carious dentine only and thus spares dental tissue. In any case, amalgam restorations should not be used because they impose an additional stress on the teeth.

General Care for People with OI and without DI

A dentist should see a child with OI by six months after the eruption of the first baby tooth at the latest. Baby teeth require care. They are important for chewing, speaking, holding space for the permanent teeth to grow in, and growth of the jaws. There appears to be minimal risk of jaw fracture from routine dental care and dental extractions. No particular precautions are needed other than those that would be taken anyway, such as support of a very thin lower jaw when an extraction procedure is being done.

Good care involves brushing and flossing the teeth of young children, then teaching them how to do it themselves and checking them as they grow older. Soft toothbrushes are good for everybody and easier on gums, since gums also need brushing. Mechanical toothbrushes tend to be more effective than brushing by hand. Use of fluoride toothpaste is recommended. Children should use a small dab of toothpaste, or a children's toothpaste, and be taught to spit it out well after brushing so they do not swallow excessive amounts. Before going to bed, children should spit out the toothpaste after brushing, but not rinse their mouths. This will leave more fluoride in the mouth to work overnight. Parents should talk to their child's dentist about the fluoride content of their drinking water and ask if supplemental fluoride is needed from a pill, a non-alcohol fluoride rinse, or a fluoride gel. Sealants placed on the biting surface of the permanent molars in children may reduce the chance of developing cavities in the grooves of the teeth.

Starting when the child is seven years old, an orthodontist should check the child's bite for evidence of an open bite or Class III malocclusion.

General Care for People with OI Plus DI

Children with OI and dentinogenesis imperfecta need the same basic care as discussed above, but they also need to be monitored for cracking, chipping and abrasion of the teeth. Special care will be needed even with the baby teeth. All of the teeth may not be affected by DI, and primary teeth usually are affected to a greater extent than the permanent teeth. Restorative treatment may be needed at some point.

Regular care is needed so the teeth will last as long as possible and to prevent abscesses and pain. Brushing and cleaning have not been shown to cause damage, but will not make teeth affected by DI white. Sealants should be effective on teeth affected with DI as long as the enamel is intact.

Older children and especially adolescents with DI are often embarrassed by their discolored teeth. Different types of veneers can sometimes hide the problem. Bleaching is not recommended because the discoloration is not in the enamel.

If the teeth are wearing excessively, caps (also called crowns), will probably need to be placed on at least some of the teeth. Caps serve to keep the teeth in place and encourage proper development of the jaw. More specialized treatment may be more appropriate for permanent teeth.

Treating Malocclusions with Orthodontia or Orthognathic Surgery

A malocclusion is an abnormal relationship between the upper and lower teeth, which creates problems with how the teeth come together. This may be due to the relationship of the upper and lower jaws to each other, the alignment of the teeth, or both. This type of problem includes crooked teeth, underbite, overbite, and open bite. Treatment is usually provided by an orthodontist. The particular treatment plan depends on the specific problem(s) with the bite and the teeth. If the malocclusion is caused by skeletal discrepancies, then orthognathic (jaw) surgery may be required along with orthodontia.

An orthodontist should examine each child with OI around the age of seven years. At that time early orthodontic interventions in children who are developing a relatively small upper jaw compared to the lower jaw may help decrease the need for later orthognathic surgery.

Although there are only a few case reports and no published studies regarding orthodontia for people with OI, it seems to be safe to treat them if DI is not present. If DI is present, the orthodontist will have to decide if the enamel is strong enough for braces. Unfortunately, it is difficult to determine how strong the enamel is until it is tried. Conventional practice involves gluing brackets to the teeth for the braces and removing the brackets later. Plastic brackets can be used instead of metal brackets because they can be removed with a hand piece without disturbing the fragile enamel. If there is concern about the enamel cracking off and treatment is still desired, placing bands on all the teeth to hold the brackets may work. Although bands are considered an old fashioned method, the technique still works. It may be necessary to seek out an older orthodontist who learned to install braces before the current practice of gluing bands directly to teeth was discovered. The orthodontist will need to minimize forces on the teeth as well as movement of teeth over long distances. The wires which are attached to the bands should initiate slow and light movements. Whenever possible, removable orthodontic appliances are preferred. Caps, or crowns, may also be effective in correcting rotations or mildly malpositioned teeth.

In some children with OI the upper jaw, or maxilla, does not grow as much as the lower jaw, or mandible. Sometimes the way that both jaws grow makes it difficult, if not impossible, to bring the teeth together properly, even after orthodontic braces. If the malocclusion is due to a problem with the growth of one or both jaws, then a combination of orthodontic braces and orthognathic surgery may be used to align the teeth. Some period of orthodontic braces is also usually needed after the jaw surgery. There are a few published reports about these surgeries indicating good postoperative healing of the jaws. The same concerns that one would have with any surgery in people with OI, such as potential bleeding problems and reaction to general anesthesia, still apply. Furthermore, the recent use of bisphosphonates to treat different bone disorders triggers many additional questions regarding maxillofacial surgeries.

Treating Impacted Teeth

The dentist needs to consider if the impacted teeth should be left alone or extracted, or if an attempt should be made to move them into a functional position in the mouth. To move a tooth, a coordinated effort is needed between the oral surgeon and the orthodontist to surgically uncover the impacted tooth and glue an attachment onto the tooth so that light force from the braces can be used to bring the tooth into the proper position. The orthodontist may also use braces prior to surgery to be sure there is space to bring the impacted tooth into the proper position.

Other Treatments

Dental implants are used to replace missing teeth. Theoretically it is possible to do this successfully for a person with OI and there is anecdotal evidence that this has been accomplished. However, there are no controlled studies on the use of dental implants in people with OI and only a few case reports in the literature. The high failure, reported to be 50% within three years of surgery is a concern.

Dental implants are somewhat like screws. In order to function, there must be enough bone in the jaw for the implant to be securely placed. After healing, a post is placed in the implant and an artificial tooth is attached. Good, strong healing around the implant is critical.

Veneers are cosmetic coverings typically placed on the outer surface of the upper anterior teeth. Anterior teeth are seen when a person smiles. Sometimes adults, often older children and especially adolescents with DI resent the color of their teeth. Adults can have veneers or crowns placed to change the appearance of the anterior "smiling teeth," but older children and adolescents are too young to receive permanent restorations. They can be good candidates for composite veneers. Veneers can last for years and have the merit of being relatively inexpensive, versatile, and are effective for hiding unsightly tooth color. However, veneers are not typically made to withstand biting forces. Recommendations for this type of treatment are made on a case by case basis.

Caps and bridges have a variety of uses. Caps, also called crowns, are made of metal or ceramic and cover the entire tooth after the enamel is removed. If teeth are wearing excessively, crowns usually provide the best treatment. Preformed stainless steel crowns are typically used for baby teeth, while cast metal or ceramic crowns are used for adult teeth. If there is not enough tooth left above the gum to place a crown, the individual may need gum surgery to make the part of the tooth showing above the gum larger. The surgeon may place a post down into the root of the tooth to act as a reinforcing rod, and then rebuild part of the tooth above the gum for the crown to sit on. In teeth not affected with DI, root canal treatment may be needed if the nerves and blood vessels inside the tooth are infected from a cavity or if the post needs to go down the center of the root(s).

In teeth with DI, the inside where the nerves and blood vessels are normally located may already be filled with dentine. This makes placing a post in the center of the root and/or root canal treatment difficult, if not impossible. Small reinforcing pins may be placed in the dentine away from the center of the root to help make the new crown of the tooth stronger.

A bridge is at least one artificial tooth attached to one or more crowns. A bridge is sometimes called a fixed partial denture.

Complete dentures are used when there are no teeth remaining in one or both jaws. How well the denture fits depends on how much bone remains after the teeth are lost. There are no studies that compare bone loss under dentures in people with OI to people without OI. The bone loss that occurs when teeth are lost is a resorption of the bone, not a fracture process, so it is not known if bone loss would be more rapid in people with OI. Complete dentures in children and adolescents who are still growing will need to be adjusted and or remade on a routine basis to compensate for growth in the jaw.

Removable partial dentures are used when some teeth remain in one or both jaws. A denture, typically made with a metal framework for strength and retention, is constructed to replace missing teeth.

Bisphosphonates

The class of drugs known as bisphosphonates is being used as a treatment for many bone disorders. An increasing number of children and adults with OI receive bisphosphonates as part of a clinical trial or on an off-label basis. These include: pamidronate (Aredia) and zoledronic acid (Zometa) given by intravenous infusion, and alendronate (Fosamax), risedronate (Actonel), and ibandronate sodium (Boniva) given in tablet (oral) form. There have been reports in medical journals suggesting a link between bisphosphonates and areas of dead bone (osteonecrosis), particularly in the jaw. Osteonecrosis could be caused by the type of bisphosphonate, the dose or the frequency of treatment. All of these factors are currently being studied.

Even though at this time there appears to be no risk of bisphosphonate induced osteonecrosis of the bone (BON) associated with bisphosphonate therapy for OI, it may be prudent to take precautions. People with OI taking a bisphosphonate should be closely monitored by a doctor and a dentist. Good oral hygiene along with regular dental care to prevent infections or periodontal (gum) disease lowers risk. When possible, required dental surgery should be scheduled prior to starting bisphosphonate treatment. Bisphosphonate treatment should not be resumed until after the surgical area is healed. Elective jaw surgery, including dental implants, should be avoided during intravenous bisphosphonate therapy. Extraction of third molars (wisdom teeth) should be deferred until more information is available.

Bisphosphonates work by reducing the remodeling rate in the skeleton. In the short term, reduction of the remodeling rate produces bone with a greater density, although it is not clear if this results in greater strength. It is also not clear what impact this reduction in remodeling will have long term. Because the remodeling rates for bone surrounding teeth are typically higher than for other bones in the body, additional questions arise about the effect of bisphosphonates on the oral cavity. It is also not clear what effect bisphosphonates have on young children whose new teeth are erupting as they grow. Similarly, the effect of bisphosphonates on the necessary remodeling surrounding dental implants is not understood. Separate from the concern about BON is the likelihood that tooth movement from orthodontia will decrease if the patient is taking, or has within some period of time, been taking bisphosphonates.

Locating a Dentist

There is no national list of dentists who treat people with OI. Schools of dentistry or the dental department at major medical centers may be helpful in locating dentists who are familiar with OI and DI. The American Academy of Pediatric Dentistry is a good source of pediatric dentists, although any particular member of this group may or may not see OI patients. Contact the Academy at:

American Academy of Pediatric Dentistry

211 East Chicago Avenue, #700

Chicago, IL 60611-2663

Phone: 312-337-2169

Fax: 312-337-6329

Website: http://www.aapd.org

Dental/orthodontic insurance, or medical insurance that covers dental diagnosis and treatment as a part of having OI, may cover some of the costs of dental care for people with OI. Some states also have financial assistance programs that may provide assistance.

The references included with this summary are an introduction to the professional literature about dental care for people who have OI. Readers are encouraged to share this information with their dentists, orthodontists, and other dental care providers.

References:

Bell RB, White RP Jr. Osteogenesis imperfecta and orthognathic surgery: case report with long-term follow-up, *International Journal of Adult Orthodontics and Orthognathic Surgery; 15:* 171–178. (2000).

Byers P.H. "Osteogenesis Imperfecta," in: *Connective Tissue and its Heritable Disorders. Wiley-Liss, Inc.,* 317–350. (1993).

Feigal R.J., King K.J. "Dental Care for Patients with Osteogenesis Imperfecta," in: *Managing Osteogenesis Imperfecta, A Medical Manual*, P. Wacaster (ed.). Osteogenesis Imperfecta Foundation, Inc. 109–117. (1996).

Gibbard PD. The management of children and adolescents suffering from amelogenesis imperfecta and dentinogenesis imperfecta, *International Journal of Orthodontics: 12:* 15–25. (1974).

Hartsfield JK Jr, WF Hohlt, WE Roberts. Orthodontic treatment and orthognathic surgery in patients with osteogenesis imperfecta, *Seminars in Orthodontics; 12:* 254–271. (2006).

Lee CYS, Ertel SK. Bone graft augmentation and dental implant treatment in a patient with osteogenesis imperfecta: review of the literature with a case report, *Implant Dentistry; 12:* 291–295. (2003).

Lewis MK, Stoker NG. Surgical management of the patient with osteogenesis imperfecta, *Journal of Oral and Maxillofacial Surgery; 45:* 430–437. (1987)

Lund AM, Jensen BL, Nielsen LA, Skovby F. Dental manifestations of osteogenesis imperfecta and abnormalities of collagen I metabolism, *Journal of Craniofacial Genetics and Developmental Biology; 18:* 30–37. (1988).

O'Connell AC, Marini JC. Evaluation of oral problems in an osteogenesis imperfecta population, *Oral Surgery Oral Med Oral Pathol Oral Radiol Endod; 87*: 189–196. (1999).

Ormiston IW, Tideman H. Orthognathic surgery in osteogenesis imperfecta: a case report with management considerations, *J Craniomaxillofacial Surgery; 23*: 261–265. (1995).

Rodrigo C. Anesthesia for maxillary and mandibular osteotomies in osteogenesis imperfecta, *Anesth Prog; 42*:17–20. (1995).

Schwartz, S. "Dental Care for Children with Osteogenesis Imperfecta," in *Interdisciplinary Treatment Approach for Children with Osteogenesis Imperfecta*, R Chiasson, C Munns, L, Zeitlin, (eds). Shriners Hospital for Children (Canada). 137–150. (2004).

Schwartz S, Tsipouras, P. Oral Findings in Patients with Osteogenesis Imperfecta, Oral Surgery. *Oral Med. & Oral Path; 57*:161–7. (1984).

Chapter 60

Periodontal Disease Associated with Chronic Diseases

Increasing evidence suggests that periodontal disease is associated with various chronic conditions. Particular attention has been paid to the possible role of periodontal disease in coronary heart disease (CHD). The notion that improving periodontal health may reduce the risk of cardiovascular disease has public health implications because of the high prevalence of both of these diseases. A recent review provides evidence for the promise of this approach.

Several processes have been proposed through which periodontal disease may contribute to CHD or other chronic diseases. Systemic inflammation, arising in response to periodontal infection, may contribute to the initiation or progression of CHD and other chronic diseases. A review of studies of periodontal disease and CHD notes that both the association of periodontal disease with C-reactive protein and other measures of systemic inflammation and the improvements in these measures following periodontal treatment support the notion that periodontal disease represents a chronic infection resulting in a chronic inflammatory state. In a related process, periodontal pathogens may infect other body systems, as evidenced by the well-established link between oral bacteria and infective endocarditis and by studies that have identified deoxyribonucleic acid (DNA) from periodontal pathogens in atherosclerotic plaques. Only an estimated 40% to 50%

This chapter is excerpted from "Associations of Self-Reported Periodontal Disease with Metabolic Syndrome and Number of Self-Reported Chronic Conditions," *Preventing Chronic Disease, Volume 8: No. 3*, May 2011, Centers for Disease Control and Prevention (CDC).

of the bacteria in the human oral cavity have been cultured, making our understanding of potential pathogens incomplete.

Discussion

Participants who reported having severe periodontal disease reported approximately 40% more chronic conditions than participants who reported having no periodontal disease. To our knowledge, this study is the first to estimate the increased risk of overall chronic illness associated with periodontal disease. The fact that periodontal disease, as a risk factor, is not specific to a single disease but appears to be associated with varied chronic conditions is consistent with the concept that it may contribute to inflammation and damage to various systems.

Our results found associations between need for periodontal treatment and self-reported arthritis, diabetes, a liver condition, and having had a stroke. However, our ability to identify associations of periodontal disease with specific conditions was limited by small numbers. We did not find the expected association between periodontal disease and CHD. Small numbers may also have reduced our ability to identify a link between severe periodontal disease and diabetes, a comparison which achieved significance in our study before, but not after, covariates were added to the model. Major factors potentially limiting the validity of this research are the low response rate and the use of self-reported measures of periodontal disease and chronic disease.

The range of chronic conditions associated with periodontal disease suggests that interventions to increase periodontal health may have far-reaching effects on public health. A review by Maurizio S. Tonetti found that intensive periodontal therapy resulted in a decrease in systemic inflammation and an improvement of endothelial dysfunction in otherwise healthy subjects. Also, a recent study examining the medical costs of diabetes patients found a cost savings in the range of 3% to 8% for patients who were receiving regular dental care compared with those not receiving any preventive or periodontal services.

In conclusion, these results provide evidence that people with severe periodontal disease are more likely to have metabolic syndrome and other chronic conditions compared with people without periodontal disease. These associations did not appear to result from confounding from age, sex, income, smoking, or psychosocial stress. Intervention research about the effectiveness of periodontal treatment to prevent or control various chronic diseases, which have in common an inflammatory process, is needed.

Chapter 61

Pregnancy and Oral Health

Baby Steps to Healthy Pregnancy and On-Time Delivery

The test came back and it's positive—you're pregnant. Your mind is rattled with excitement, and you have created a "to-do" list. While your to-do list and questions continue to grow, it's important to take the necessary steps to ensure an on-time and safe arrival of your most precious cargo yet.

You've probably heard a few old wives' tales about pregnancy including, "A tooth lost for every child." While it seems far-fetched, it actually is based loosely on fact. Your teeth and gums are affected by pregnancy, just as other tissues in your body. You may not be aware that the health of your gums may also affect the health of your baby-to-be.

How does pregnancy affect your teeth and gums?

About half of women experience pregnancy gingivitis. This condition can be uncomfortable and cause swelling, bleeding, redness, or tenderness in the gum tissue. Conversely, a more advanced oral health condition called periodontal disease (a serious gum infection that destroys attachment fibers and supporting bone that hold teeth in the mouth) may affect the health of your baby.

This chapter includes: "Baby Steps to Healthy Pregnancy and On-Time Delivery," © 2011 American Academy of Periodontology (www.perio.org). All rights reserved. Reprinted with permission. Also, "The Kids Are All Right," National Institute of Dental and Craniofacial Research (NIDCR), April 19, 2011.

Is periodontal disease linked to preterm, low birthweight babies?

Studies have shown a possible relationship between periodontal disease and preterm, low birthweight babies. However, the research in this area has been inconclusive. Because pregnant women with periodontal disease may be more likely to have a baby born too early and too small, maintaining periodontal health during pregnancy is a wise precaution.

What if I'm diagnosed with periodontal disease during pregnancy?

If you're diagnosed with periodontal disease, your periodontist will work with you to determine the most appropriate course of treatment. For example, he or she may recommend a common non-surgical procedure called scaling and root planing. During this procedure, your tooth-root surfaces are cleaned to remove plaque and tartar from deep periodontal pockets and smooth the root to remove bacterial toxins. This procedure may also alleviate many of the uncomfortable symptoms associated with pregnancy gingivitis, such as swelling and tenderness of the gums.

As you make your way through the to-do list, remember to check off a visit to the dentist or periodontist. This baby step benefits you and your unborn baby.

Premature Births: The Answers Can't Come Soon Enough

According to the March of Dimes, premature births have soared to become the number one obstetric problem in the United States. Many premature babies come into the world with serious health problems. Those who survive may suffer lifelong consequences, from cerebral palsy and mental retardation to blindness.

The March of Dimes has launched a $75 million, five-year campaign to raise public awareness and reduce rates of preterm birth and increase research to find the cause. Until all of the answers are in, the March of Dimes recommends the following to reduce the risk and/or effects of a premature birth:

- Consume a multivitamin containing 400 micrograms of the B vitamin folic acid before and in the early months of pregnancy.

- Stop smoking.

- Stop drinking and/or using illicit drugs, or prescription or over-the-counter drugs (including herbal preparations) not prescribed by a doctor aware of the pregnancy.

- Once pregnant, get early regular prenatal care, eat a balanced diet with enough calories (usually about 300 more than a woman normally eats), and gain enough weight (25 to 35 pounds is usually recommended).

- Talk to your doctor about signs of premature labor, and what to do if you show any of the warning signs.

The Kids Are All Right

Every day, dentists across the country decide whether or not to provide dental care to a patient who is pregnant. On the one hand, they realize the patient needs to maintain her good oral health, especially if she has periodontal disease, a relatively common and destructive problem during pregnancy. On the other hand, dentists traditionally have lacked the scientific evidence to make informed decisions about the possible effects of dental care, if any, to the developing child. The lack of data has caused many dentists to err strongly on the side of caution, especially during the second trimester when the child's development accelerates and, in theory, exposure to infectious oral bacteria or dental products could have adverse effects. But the fundamental questions remain: Should dentists provide dental care to pregnant women through the second trimester? If so, which types of treatment are safe to provide?

Over the last five years, newer scientific evidence has provided answers to these important questions. The data so far indicate that mothers who receive dental care through the second trimester—both general and periodontal treatment—do not appear to increase their risk of adverse events during pregnancy.

Some of the most scientifically rigorous data come from the National Institute of Dental and Craniofacial Research (NIDCR)-supported Obstetrics and Periodontal Therapy Trial (OPT). In 2006, the OPT reported in the *New England Journal of Medicine* that pregnant women, most with early-to-moderate periodontitis, benefitted from general and periodontal care without an increase in preterm births or other negative pregnancy outcomes. All mothers had been randomly assigned to receive either: (1) scaling and root planing of the teeth prior to the 21st week of pregnancy, then monthly tooth polishings; or, (2) scaling and root planing after delivery, meaning women in this control group did not have their periodontal disease treated during their pregnancies. All women were 16 years or older and between 13 and 17 weeks pregnant upon entry into the study.

Now, as published online in the journal *Pediatrics* on April 11, 2011, the investigators report findings from a follow-up study of the OPT

patients and their children born during the original trial. The researchers evaluated the neurodevelopment of 411 children, including 32
preterm infants, two years after the study. They tested the children
using the *Bayley Scales of Infant and Toddler Development (Third Edition)* and the *Preschool Language Scale (Fourth Edition)*. The former
is a well-recognized assessment instrument for cognitive and motor
functions in young children; the latter is frequently used to assess
language skills in this age group.

The scientists found no difference in the neurodevelopment of children from mothers previously assigned to the treatment or control
group. They also report slight associations between improvements in
a mother's periodontal attachment loss during the original study and
higher cognitive and motor skills in their children. But both the associations are so weak, the scientists considered them "to be of little
or no clinical significance."

Chapter 62

Tobacco Use Associated Oral Changes

The oral changes from tobacco use range from harmless soft tissue changes to a life-threatening oral cancer. Your dentist is trained to perform an oral examination to detect tobacco use related abnormalities. Some of the more common of these are discussed in this chapter.

Smoker's Melanosis

Smoker melanosis is increased tissue pigmentation, or darkening, due to irritation from tobacco smoke. Typically this pigmentation occurs on the gingiva (gums) of the upper and lower front teeth. The amount of pigmentation increases with greater tobacco use, and is more common in females; it occurs in 5%–22% of cigarette and pipe smokers. There is no treatment for smoker's melanosis; however, tissues typically return to normal color in six to 36 months after quitting smoking.

Periodontal Disease

The evidence is overwhelming that smoking contributes to periodontal disease and that continued smoking results in a reduced response to periodontal treatment. There is a greater amount of bone loss around teeth in smokers and individuals who smoke are more likely to lose teeth than nonsmokers. It is reported that more than half of advanced gum disease can be linked to tobacco use.

Nicotinic Stomatitis

In nicotinic stomatitis, the hard palate (roof of the mouth) appears white instead of pink, and numerous, small, raised areas with red centers are found throughout the palate. These red areas are irritated minor salivary glands whose duct openings are inflamed in response to the heat from tobacco products. This type of lesion is most commonly seen in older male tobacco users who smoke pipes, but it also can be found in cigar and cigarette smokers.

There is an increased risk for cancer of the tonsils, posterior mouth, and lungs in individuals who develop nicotinic stomatitis from their tobacco use. However, if the individual stops their tobacco use, the appearance of hard palate typically returns to normal within a few weeks.

Smokeless Tobacco Induced Changes

Use of smokeless tobacco produces a specific change in the area of the mouth where it is held. The area appears more whitish and wrinkled than normal, healthy tissue. This degree of tissue change is directly dependent upon the type of smokeless tobacco (leaf versus fine cut), the specific brand of tobacco, the size of the pinch of tobacco, and the length of time the pinch is in contact with the mouth tissues. Although the use of any tobacco product increases one's risk of developing cancer, the oral cancer risk for smokeless tobacco use is largely unknown. However, use of leaf-type smokeless tobacco for greater than 50 years is associated with the development of a specific oral cancer known as verrucous carcinoma. If the individual stops using the smokeless tobacco, the appearance of the oral tissue typically returns to normal in two to six weeks.

Gingival Recession and Tooth Abrasion

In addition to the development of changes to the oral tissues, the use of smokeless tobacco can damage both the gum tissue and the teeth in the area where it is held in the mouth. Smokeless tobacco can result in localized gum recession and the exposed teeth often develop dental decay due the sweetener in smokeless tobacco. Unfortunately, stopping the tobacco use does not reverse the gum problem or tooth decay.

Black Hairy Tongue

Hairy tongue results from either an overgrowth of the normal tongue papillae or a decrease in the rate that the papillae are removed. With tobacco use, the overgrown papillae can trap pigment from the tobacco and take on a black appearance. This condition has no symptoms; however, it may be a concern due to the appearance and the frequent unpleasant mouth odor from the trapping of particles in the tongue.

Oral Cancer

Use of tobacco products is clearly linked to development of oral cancer. Oral cancers are found primarily in the floor of the mouth (under the tongue), the sides and underside of the tongue, and the soft palate (the back part of the roof of the mouth). The most important key to surviving oral cancer is early detection. The importance of your dentist performing a thorough soft tissue examination cannot be overemphasized. The tissue changes in early cancer can be subtle and it is essential for your dentist to perform a through soft tissue examination to detect cancer at an early stage. He or she may want to take a sample of these tissues (biopsy) for diagnosis, or refer you for this procedure. This is the only way to make a diagnosis of oral cancer, and biopsy can also help in determining your long-term outlook.

As soon as an individual quits smoking, the risk for oral cancer begins to decrease. It is generally acknowledged that it takes around fifteen years after quitting smoking for the risk of a prior smoker to approach that of someone who has never smoked.

Part Seven

Finding and Financing Oral Health in the United States

Chapter 63

Access to Oral Health Care

Chapter Contents

Section 63.1

Oral Health Status and Access

Overview of Oral Health Status and Access to Oral Health Care in the United States

Although there is a wide range of diseases and conditions that manifest themselves in or near the oral cavity itself, this chapter will focus primarily on access to services for the prevention, diagnosis, and treatment of two diseases and their sequelae: dental caries and periodontal diseases. Dental caries, or tooth decay, is caused by a bacterial infection (most commonly *Streptococcus mutans*) that is often passed from person to person (for example, from mother to child). *Oral Health in America* called dental caries the most common chronic disease of childhood (Health and Human Services [HHS], 2000), and it is among the most common diseases in the world. Despite decades of knowledge of how to prevent dental caries, they remain a significant problem for all age groups. Periodontal disease is generally broken into two categories: gingivitis and periodontitis. Gingivitis is an inflammation of the tissue surrounding the teeth that results from a buildup of dental plaque between the tissue and the teeth. It is generally due to poor oral hygiene. Untreated gingivitis can result in periodontitis, the breakdown of the ligament that connects the teeth to the jaw bone, and the destruction of the bone that supports the teeth in the jaw. At least 8.5% of adults (ages 20–64) and 17.2% of older adults (age 65 and older) in the United States have periodontal disease.

Overall Oral Health Status

In April 2007, the National Center for Health Statistics of the Centers for Disease Control and Prevention (CDC) released a comprehensive assessment of the oral health status of the U.S. population.

Using data provided by two iterations of National Health and Nutrition Examination Survey (NHANES III, 1988–1994, and NHANES, 1999–2004), which is the most comprehensive survey on oral health status in the United States, the assessment concluded that "Americans of all ages continue to experience improvements in their oral health." Specifically, the report noted that among older adults, edentulism (complete tooth loss) and periodontitis (gum disease) had declined. Among adults, CDC observed improvements in the prevalence of dental caries, tooth retention, and periodontal health. For adolescents and youth, dental caries decreased, while dental sealants (used to prevent tooth decay) became more prevalent. Encouragingly, the increase in dental sealants was consistent among all racial and ethnic groups, although non-Hispanic Black and Mexican American children and adolescents continue to have a lower prevalence of sealants than white children and adolescents, and low-income children receive fewer dental sealants than those who live above 200% of the federal poverty level (FPL).

While the data from the NHANES surveys showed improvements in certain indicators of oral health status across two intervals of time, Americans' overall health status in the 1999–2004 period remained discouraging. For example, over 25% of adults 20 to 64 years of age and nearly 20% of respondents over age 65 were experiencing untreated dental caries at the time of their examination. Even young children experienced high rates of caries: nearly 28% of children ages 2–5 years had caries experience, and 20% have untreated caries. Moreover, caries prevalence among preschool children increased between 1988–1994 and 1999–2004. In addition, disturbing disparities remain in oral health status for many underserved and vulnerable populations.

Access to Oral Health Care

Limited and uneven access to oral health care contributes to both poor oral health and disparities in oral health. More than half of the population (56%) did not visit a dentist in 2004, and in 2007, 5.5% of the population reported being unable to get or delaying needed dental care, significantly higher than the numbers that reported being unable to get or delaying needed medical care or prescription drugs. Nearly all measures indicate that vulnerable and underserved populations access oral health care in particularly low numbers. For example, poor children are more likely to report unmet dental need than those with higher incomes, non-Hispanic Black and Hispanic children and adults are less likely to have seen a dentist in the past six months than non-Hispanic White populations, and less than 20% of eligible Medicaid beneficiaries received preventive dental services in 2009.

Section 63.2

Vulnerable and Underserved Populations

Oral Health Status and Access to Oral Health Care for Vulnerable and Underserved Populations

While there has been some improvement in the oral health of the U.S. population overall, underserved populations continue to suffer disparities in both their disease burden and access to needed services. For example, dental caries remain a significant problem in certain specific populations such as low-income children and racial and ethnic minorities. According to the National Health and Nutrition Examination Survey (NHANES), twice as many poor children ages 2–11 have at least one untreated decayed tooth, compared to non-poor children. In addition, low-income children also receive fewer dental sealants. Minority children are more likely to have dental decay than white children, and their decay is more severe. When migrant and seasonal farmworkers in Michigan were asked which health care service would benefit them the most, the most common response was dental services, ahead of pediatric care, transportation, and interpretation, among other services. This section will explore the disparities in status and access to care for a variety of vulnerable and underserved populations.

Children and Adolescents

Children: While not all children are underserved, many children are vulnerable to developing oral diseases, particularly dental caries. The U.S. Government Accountability Office (GAO) recently reported that according to NHANES, dental disease in children has not decreased, noting that about one in three children aged 2–18 enrolled in Medicaid had untreated tooth decay, and one in nine had untreated decay in three or more teeth. The lack of adequate dental treatment may affect children's speech, nutrition, growth and function, social development, and quality of life. In spite of these significant problems, according to Medical Expenditure Panel Survey (MEPS), only about 25% of children under the age of six years, 59% of children ages 6–12, and 48% of adolescents ages 13–20 had a dental visit in 2004.

A number of factors are related to the likelihood that a child has visited the dentist in the past year, including insurance status, race, ethnicity, being born outside the United States, language spoken at home, and whether the child's mother has a regular source of dental care. Dentally uninsured children receive fewer dental services than insured children. The data on dental visits for publicly insured children, however, are mixed. Some data indicate that publicly insured children are less likely to receive dental services and receive fewer dental services on average than privately insured children; however, studies that control for race and income (among other factors) indicate that publicly and privately insured children are equally likely to have a preventive dental visit. African American and Latino children are less likely to have had a preventive dental visit or any dental contact in the past year than White children. This may contribute to the low levels of dental visits among publicly insured children in uncontrolled estimates, since African American and Latino children are more likely to be enrolled in Medicaid. Children born outside the United States and children whose primary language at home is not English are both less likely than reference groups to have a preventive dental visit in the past 12 months. In addition, low income children whose parents regularly visit the dentist are more likely to visit the dentist, according to surveys done in Washington state and Detroit.

Adolescents: As previously noted, adolescents, generally those aged 10–19 years, have a high prevalence of oral disease. Risk factors for dental caries are similar to those for other age groups, but adolescents' risk for oral and perioral injury is exacerbated by behaviors such as the use of alcohol and illicit drugs, driving without a seatbelt, cycling without a helmet, engaging in contact sports without a mouth guard, and using firearms. Other concerns among adolescent populations, which are not unique to this age group, include damage caused by the use of all forms of tobacco, erosion of teeth and damage to soft tissues caused by eating disorders, oral manifestations of sexually transmitted infections (soft tissue lesions) as a result of oral sex, and increased risk of periodontal disease during pregnancy. In an online Harris Interactive poll of nearly 1,200 adolescents, respondents frequently mentioned having access to affordable, convenient, and high-quality dental care as what they would most like to change to make health services more helpful.

Homeless Populations

Homeless people have poorer oral health than the general population. However, no national data are available on the oral health status of homeless populations, and the few available studies may skew the results due to sample size, the population surveyed (people who present at a clinic), and inability to reach the chronically homeless, among other factors. In a national survey, homeless veterans reported higher rates of oral pain, more decayed teeth, and fewer filled teeth than the general population. Many homeless veterans reported having oral pain either currently or within the past year. Similarly, in a small survey of homeless adolescents in Seattle, over 50% reported having sensitive teeth, 39% reported a toothache, and 27% reported sore or bleeding gums. In addition, homeless people in these surveys were more likely than the general population to perceive their oral health as poor. Homeless people also struggle to access oral health care. A national survey of homeless people found that dental care was the most commonly reported unmet health need. In fact, homeless people surveyed at a free dental screening had not seen a dentist in, on average, 5.7 years.

Homeless populations face a multitude of barriers to both maintaining good oral health and accessing oral health care. They are more likely to engage in behaviors detrimental to oral health such as smoking and using other types of tobacco products, heavy alcohol use, and substance abuse. They also may lack toothbrushes, toothpaste, clean water, or a place to brush their teeth. Homeless people often lack dental coverage, and homeless children struggle to maintain Medicaid coverage because they do not have a permanent address. Over one-third of homeless people at a free dental screening answered that they did not know where to seek dental care if needed.

Low-Income Populations

Note: For the purposes of this report, poor refers to individuals and families with income below the federal poverty level (FPL); near-poor refers income between 100% and 199% of FPL; and non-poor refers to income above 200% of the FPL.

Socioeconomic status, as measured by poverty status, is a strong determinant of oral health. In every age group, persons in the lower-income group are more likely to have had dental caries experience and more than twice as likely to have untreated dental caries in comparison to their higher-income counterparts. Poor children ages 2–8 have more than twice the rate of dental caries experience as non-poor children.

Despite the fact that most children living below the FPL are eligible to receive dental care through Medicaid, many children in this income group have untreated decay. Among adults, tooth extraction is a common treatment for advanced dental decay when financial resources are limited. Consistently, total tooth loss, or edentulism, among persons 65 years of age and over is more frequent among those living below the FPL than among those living at twice the FPL.

Poor children and adults receive significantly fewer dental services than the population as a whole. The likelihood of visiting a dentist decreases with decreasing income, and people who live below the FPL are less than half as likely to have visited a dentist in the past year as those who make over 400% of the FPL. Children whose families make below 200% of the FPL are less than half as likely to have had a preventive dental visit than children living in higher-income families.

Low-income children also receive fewer dental sealants, although improvements have been made in this area. Between 1988–1994 and 1999–2004, the largest increase in sealant use was among poor children (an increase of 3%–21%). Low-income populations are also more likely to receive episodic or emergency oral health care, rather than receiving preventive care and having a usual source of care.

It is important to note that most children living below the FPL are eligible to receive dental care through Medicaid, and therefore have financing available for oral health care. Indeed, according to the Medical Expenditure Panel Survey (MEPS), 83% of poor children had dental coverage, which is more than any other income group, although they are less likely to have private dental coverage. In contrast, over 60% of poor adults lacked dental coverage. Poor populations face a number of barriers to accessing oral health care. They include inability to pay due to lack of dental coverage or the size of the expense; difficulty finding a dentist who will accept Medicaid; long waits to get appointments; lack of transportation; higher levels of medical care use; and parents who do not receive regular oral health care. Access for low-income populations is also complicated by other factors including age, race, ethnicity, and proximity to oral health providers.

Older Adults

The prevalence of caries and periodontal disease increases steadily with age. Encouragingly, however, the prevalence of both diseases in older adults has decreased over time. In addition, the percentage of older adults who are totally edentulous has decreased over time. Oral health status is related to functional and other health deficiencies. Poor oral health and oral health-related quality of life in older adults are significantly associated with disability and reduction in mobility. In addition, older adults are more likely than other segments of the population to have other diseases that may exacerbate their oral health, and vice versa, such as cardiovascular disease, diabetes, and pneumonia. The Institute of Medicine (IOM) has long recognized issues related to the oral health of older adults. For example, in a 1992 study on various needs of older adults, an entire chapter was devoted to oral health, noting that oral health had improved for older adults, but that adults who retain their teeth continue to be at risk for oral diseases. At that time, the IOM recommended to assess the oral health status, risk factors for oral diseases, and use and delivery of oral health services for older adults as well as to consider methods for performing oral cancer screenings in primary care settings.

Older adults frequently do not access oral health care. According to MEPS, only 42% of adults age 55 and older reported visiting a dentist in 1996, ranging from 46% of 55- to 65-year-olds to 32% of adults over age 75 years. Older adults are more likely to have serious medical issues and functional limitations, which can deter them from seeking dental care. Older adults who spend more on medication and medical visits are less likely to use dental services. Additionally, the more functional limitations an older person reports, the less likely he or she is to seek dental care. Admittance to long-term care (LTC) facilities creates a significant barrier to receipt of dental care. While federal law requires LTC facilities that receive Medicare or Medicaid funding to provide access to dental care, only 80% of facilities report doing so. Even when dental care is available, evidence indicates that many residents do not regularly receive dental care and many oral health problems go undetected. For example, according to a 1999 survey, only 13% of nursing home residents over age 65 received dental services in the billing year of their discharge. Multiple factors contribute to low access to oral health services for older adults. LTC facilities may underestimate the importance of oral health. For example, in a survey of Ohio nursing home executives, 49% rated their residents' oral health as fair or poor but 64% were still satisfied with the oral health care provided at their facilities. In addition, LTC facilities have difficulty finding dentists to care for their patients. One study showed that the perceived willingness of dentists to treat LTC residents either in the facility or in private offices was the greatest barrier to providing dental care in Michigan alternative LTC facilities. In the absence of dentists, nursing home staff must identify residents' oral health needs, but nurses and nursing assistants are not adequately trained to identify many oral health issues.

Another significant reason that older adults have difficulty accessing oral health care is the relative lack of training of the health care workforce in the special needs of older adults. In a 2008 report on the care of older adults, the IOM noted that in 1987 the National Institute on Aging predicted a need for 1,500 geriatric dental academicians and 7,500 dental practitioners with training in geriatric dentistry by the year 2000. By the mid-1990s, however, only about 100 dentists in total had completed advanced training in geriatrics and little has changed since then. Of the dental students graduating in 2001, almost 20% did not feel prepared to care for older adults and 25% felt the geriatric dental curriculum was inadequate. The American Dental Association (ADA) currently does not recognize geriatric dentistry as a separate specialty, board certification by the American Board of General Dentistry does not explicitly require questions on geriatric dental care, and none of the 509 residencies recognized by the American Dental Education Association are specifically devoted to the care of geriatric patients.

People with Special Health Care Needs

It appears that both children and adults with special health care needs (SHCN) have poorer oral health than the general population. Most, though not all, studies indicate that the overall prevalence of dental caries in people with SHCN is either the same as the general population or slightly lower. But available data indicate that people with SHCN suffer disproportionately from periodontal disease and edentulism, have more untreated dental caries, poorer oral hygiene, and receive less care than the general population. However, little high-quality data exists on the oral health of people with SHCN. People with SHCN are a difficult population to assess, in part because of their diversity, and also because they are geographically dispersed. Moreover, it is also difficult to analyze national data on this population because their numbers are not large enough to produce reliable statistics. The few available studies of people with SHCN are conducted with populations that are not representative of the SHCN community as a whole. Access to care for people with SHCN appears to vary with age. While children with SHCN receive preventive dental care at similar or higher rates than children without SHCN, adults with SHCN are less likely to have seen a dentist in the past year than people without SHCN. Despite the similar rates of dental care visits, dental care is the most commonly reported unmet health care need among children with SHCN, and children with SHCN are more likely to report experiencing a toothache in the last six months than children without SHCN, with more severely affected children more likely to report a toothache.

Disparities in oral health for people with SHCN are due to a variety of reasons. First, they often take medications that reduce saliva flow, which promotes dental caries and periodontal disease. Additionally, people with SHCN often have impaired dexterity and thus rely on others for oral hygiene. They also face systematic barriers to oral health care such as transportation barriers (especially for those with physical disabilities), cost, and health care professionals who are not trained to work with SHCN patients or dental offices that are not physically suited for them. In addition, the current oral health care system has limited capacity to care for children with SHCN. It is likely that children and adults with SHCN experience different barriers to care; however, not enough information exists to divide the populations.

Pregnant Women and Mothers

Oral health problems are common among pregnant women and follow similar disparities with respect to race, ethnicity, income, insurance, and age. However, pregnant women have several unique oral health needs. Pregnant women are susceptible to periodontitis, loose teeth, and pyogenic granulomas, also known as pregnancy oral tumors. Periodontal disease has been identified in observational studies as a potential factor contributing to adverse pregnancy outcomes, such as preterm birth and low birth weight.

The oral health of pregnant women is important not only for their own health, but because there is a strong relationship between the oral health status and oral health care habits of a mother and her children's oral health status and habits. The bacteria that cause dental caries are transmissible from caregivers, especially mothers, to children. Moreover, children of mothers with untreated dental caries and tooth loss are between two and more than three times as likely to have untreated dental caries compared to children whose mothers had no untreated dental caries or no tooth loss. Children enrolled in Medicaid are more likely to receive oral health care when their mothers have a regular source of oral health care. The provision of oral health services for pregnant women and mothers may include education about how their own oral health relates to their children's oral health as well as how to prevent dental caries in their young children.

Recently, states and health care organizations have promoted the importance and safety of oral health care for pregnant women. The American Academy of Pediatrics and the American College of Obstetricians and Gynecologists agree that it is very important for pregnant women to continue usual oral health care. Both the New York State

Department of Health and the California Dental Association have released evidence-based guidelines for treating pregnant women. Both sets of guidelines recommend that prenatal care providers educate women about the importance of oral health and refer them for oral health care, and that oral health care professionals provide routine and necessary oral health care to pregnant women. Recently, several randomized clinical trials of pregnant women with periodontal disease have been performed to examine the effect of receiving treatment during pregnancy or postpartum. Results of these trials suggest that periodontal treatment is safe for pregnant women and their fetuses and effective in reducing the level of periodontal disease. However, periodontal treatment during pregnancy does not necessarily reduce the incidence of poor birth outcomes. Although oral health care is considered both safe and effective for pregnant women and their fetuses, many women do not receive dental care during pregnancy. Even when women report having an oral health problem during the pregnancy, only about half of them visit a dentist. Among women with oral health problems, the likelihood of visiting a dentist during the pregnancy is associated with dental coverage status and timing of the first prenatal care visit. Although over 40% of all pregnant women have medical insurance through Medicaid, many of them are not covered for oral health care because only about half of state Medicaid programs pay for the oral health care of pregnant women. In addition, some women report being erroneously informed to not visit the dentist during pregnancy.

Racial and Ethnic Minorities

Racial and ethnic minorities experience significant disparities in oral health status and access to oral health care compared to the U.S. population as a whole. These disparities can be attributed to a number of complex societal factors, including lower incomes, a lower prevalence of dental coverage, and a dearth of dentists located in communities where racial and ethnic minorities live, among many other factors.

African Americans: African Americans have poorer oral health than the overall U.S. population throughout the life cycle. African American children and adolescents have slightly more dental caries and more untreated dental caries than White children and adolescents. African American adults (ages 20–64) have approximately the same prevalence of dental caries as White adults; however, dental caries in African Americans are much more likely to be untreated. In addition, African American adults are significantly more likely to have periodontal disease than White adults. African American older adults have, on average, fewer teeth than Whites. African Americans also perceive their oral health as worse than Whites; parents of non-Hispanic Black children are twice as likely as parents of White children to rate their child's oral health as fair or poor; and African American adults are less than half as likely as White adults to rate their oral health as excellent or very good. Encouragingly, the oral health of African Americans appears to be improving for many, though not all, of these measures. For example, 17% of African American adults had periodontal disease in the 1999–2004 NHANES survey, down from 26% in the 1988–1994 survey.

African Americans also experience disparities in access to oral health care. In 2003, 72% of African American children received preventive oral health care, compared to 84% of White children. In 2009, 53% of African American adults reported seeing a dentist or other dental professional in the past year, compared to 61% of the overall population.

American Indians and Alaskan Natives: American Indians and Alaskan Natives (AI/AN) also have poorer oral health than the overall U.S. population throughout the life cycle. In 1999, the Indian Health Service (IHS) surveyed its patients to determine the burden of dental caries on the AI/AN population and compare AI/AN oral health to the overall populations' oral health. The survey found that AI/AN children and adolescents, ages 2–19, are more likely to suffer from dental caries and are more likely to have untreated dental caries as compared to the overall population. The rate of dental caries for AI/AN children ages 2–5 years, for example, is five times the U.S. average, and more than two-thirds of AI/AN children suffer from dental caries.

AI/AN adults ages 35–44 also have more teeth with untreated dental caries, but fewer missing teeth, and about the same number of filled teeth as the overall population. AI/AN adults over age 55 have fewer teeth, higher rates of dental caries, and more periodontal disease, but fewer root caries than the overall population. AI/AN elders are more likely to be edentulous; two surveys found that at least 40% of AI/AN adults between the ages of 65 and 74 were edentulous, compared to 29% of the overall population.

AI/AN populations face complex barriers to attaining good oral health, including a lack of sources of fluoridated water, instability in IHS dental programs, and geographic barriers to care. Historically, IHS has supported water fluoridation on Indian reservations for the prevention of dental caries, but the number of reservation systems submitting fluoridation monitoring reports to IHS dropped from 700 in the early 1990s to fewer than 500 in 1995.

Asian Americans: Although Asian Americans make up a growing proportion of the U.S. population, they have received little attention in the oral health literature. Asian Americans comprise many ethnic subgroups with varying age, education, income, and nativity statuses, and varying abilities to access oral health care. Underutilization of oral health care among Asian Americans is associated with poverty, lack of dental coverage, and residing in the United States for less than five years.

Latinos: Latinos have poorer oral health and receive fewer dental services as compared to White populations. These disparities exist independently of income level, education, dental coverage status, and attitude toward preventive care. While Latinos are a diverse population, comprising numerous subgroups, more is known about the oral health of Mexican Americans than other subgroups because NHANES oversamples Mexican Americans. Thus, the focus here will be on the oral health status of Mexican Americans, but it should be noted that the experience of Mexican Americans may not be representative of all Latino subpopulations.

Both dental caries experience and untreated dental caries are significantly more prevalent in Mexican American children (ages 2–11) than in both non-Hispanic White and Black children. Mexican American adults have fewer dental caries experiences than White non-Hispanic adults; however, they have higher rates of untreated dental caries. Disparities in the oral health of Mexican Americans persist throughout the life cycle, in adolescents through older adults.

Latinos also experience disparities in access to oral health care. They are less likely to report any dental visit in the past year, either for preventive, restorative, or emergency care. Latino children are less likely than White children to have ever seen a dentist or to have seen a dentist in the last year. In 2003, only 67% of Latino children received preventive dental care, compared to 84% of White children. In 2009, 48% of Hispanic and Latino adults reported seeing a dentist or other dental professional in the past year, compared to 61% of the adults overall.

Acculturation is associated with disparities in Latino oral health, indicating that reducing oral health disparities for Latinos requires linguistically and culturally appropriate oral health care and promotion. (Surveys generally use language as a proxy for acculturation, treating individuals who regularly speak English as more acculturated than those who primarily speak Spanish.) Latinos who primarily speak Spanish at home are less likely to report a dental visit in the past 12 months than those who speak English and are also less likely to have a dental home. The association between acculturation and oral health disparities persists throughout diverse groups of Latino Americans. Less acculturated Mexican American, Cuban American, and Puerto Rican Americans are all significantly less likely to report receiving recent oral health care than those who are more acculturated. Acculturation is likely to be related to access to care rather than overall oral health, because acculturation is associated with missing teeth and untreated decayed surfaces but not with overall experience with dental caries.

Rural and Urban Populations

High-quality data on oral health status and access to care by geographic location are sparse. Some data indicate that rural residents have poorer oral health than urban residents, while others indicate that urban residents have more oral health needs. Similarly, some analyses indicate that rural residents access less oral health care or report more problems accessing oral health care than urban residents; however, that association disappears after controlling for supply of dentists. More complex, multivariate analyses are needed to assess whether oral health status and access to care are related to place of residence, or instead to income, education level, supply of dentists, or other predisposing factors.

Rural residents may not access oral health care for a number of reasons. Fewer dentists work in rural areas than urban areas. In addition, a smaller proportion of rural residents have dental coverage, which is a good predictor of receipt of dental care. Finally, the water in rural communities is less likely to be fluoridated than city water, which means rural residents are more susceptible to dental caries.

In 2005, the IOM examined the quality of general health care in rural communities. The committee specifically noted the role of IHS and the Health Resources and Services Administration (HRSA) in providing scholarships and loan repayment for practice in rural areas as well as the efforts of individual programs by dental schools and others in providing exposure to care in rural settings. The committee concluded that "fundamental change in health professions education programs will be needed to produce an adequate supply of properly educated health care professionals for rural and frontier communities." They recommended that schools (specifically including dental schools) make greater efforts to recruit students from rural areas, to locate a meaningful portion of the formal educational experience in rural settings, to recruit faculty with experience in caring for rural populations, and to develop education programs that are relevant to rural practice.

Section 63.3

Contributing Factors to Limited Oral Care Access

Factors That Contribute to Poor Oral Health and Lack of Access to Oral Health Care

Underserved and vulnerable populations experience significant barriers to accessing oral health care and improving oral health. Barriers that are unique or particularly significant to a specific population have been discussed, but others cut across demographic lines and affect the oral health of many different populations. Those are discussed here. This list is not intended to be exhaustive, but is intended to highlight areas the committee believes are of importance and where significant progress can be made.

Social Determinants of Oral Health

Social determinants also affect oral health and contribute to inequalities in oral health. The World Health Organization describes social determinants of health as a combination of structural determinants ("the unequal distribution of power, income, goods, and services") and daily living conditions ("the conditions in which people are born, grow, live, work, and age"). Social gradients in dental decay, periodontal disease, oral cancer, and tooth loss have all been reported. Income inequality has also been shown to be related to oral health. Recognizing the relationship between social determinants of health and oral health outcomes is important for developing interventions.

Social determinants of health create significant barriers to reducing and ultimately eliminating disparities in oral health. Progress will require changes in the social and physical environment, such as public education, working and living conditions, health system, and

557

the natural environment. Interventions will need to focus on the individual, families, and communities. Unfortunately, not enough is known about bridging the science, practice, and policy of social determinants of health so that scientific knowledge can be translated into practical policies that will reduce disparities in oral health.

Oral Health Literacy

This section provides a brief overview of oral health literacy. The Committee on an Oral Health Initiative was specifically charged to address oral health literacy, and thus a more complete discussion of oral health literacy can be found in its report *Advancing Oral Health in America*. The Committee on Oral Health Access to Services recognizes that oral health literacy is an essential component of access to care, and the brevity of the discussion here is not meant to deemphasize its importance. Nearly all aspects of oral health care require literacy (for example: realizing the importance of self-care, understanding that dental caries is an infectious disease, scheduling a dental appointment, completing insurance forms). However, little is known specifically about oral health literacy. The National Institute of Dental and Craniofacial Research Workgroup on Oral Health Literacy proposed a research agenda for oral health literacy in 2005, but little progress has been made since then. Available data indicate that the public's oral health literacy (and general health literacy) is poor. Poor oral health literacy is strongly associated with self-reported lower oral health status, lower dental knowledge, and fewer dental visits. The public has little knowledge about the best ways to prevent oral diseases. Fluoride and dental sealants have long been acknowledged as the most effective ways to prevent dental caries, yet the public consistently answers that toothbrushing and flossing are more effective. Although each year 30,000 Americans are diagnosed with oral cancers and nearly 8,000 people die from them, the public's knowledge about the risk factors and symptoms of oral cancers is low.

Chapter 64

Expenditures and Financing of Oral Health Care

Chapter Contents

Section 64.1

Overview of Expenditures

Health care costs and spending have been rapidly increasing in the United States in recent years. In 2009, overall health expenditures were $2.5 trillion, including the cost of hospital care, physician and dental services, home health care, nursing home services, prescription drugs, medical equipment and supplies, and public health direct services. This translates to more than $8,000 per person and accounted for 17.6% of the national gross domestic product. Growth in national health expenditures is expected to increase by 6.1% between 2009 and 2019. In contrast, expenditures for dental services in the United States in 2009 were $102.2 billion, approximately 5% of total spending on health care. While medical and dental spending both have been rising, the growth in medical expenditures has far outpaced the growth in dental expenditures.

The reported national expenditure levels undercount the total spent on improving oral health. Estimates represent only the costs associated with direct services delivered by dentists in traditional practice settings. Spending on public health initiatives (for example, water fluoridation and public education campaigns) and oral health services delivered in medical care settings are not included in estimates of overall expenditures. For example, there are approximately 3.6 million craniofacial cases (such as diabetes-related conditions, oral cancers, and injuries) treated in medical care settings each year, and the total costs for these treatments exceed several billion dollars.

Average Annual Dental Expenses

In 2007, the average annual expense for individuals who had any dental expenses was $643. Individual expenses varied by age, income, race and ethnicity, and insurance status. Annual dental expenses also varied by source of insurance. The average annual dental expense for individuals with private dental insurance was $662. Among individuals with public dental insurance (Medicaid or Children's Health Insurance Program [CHIP]), the average annual dental expense was $370. Individuals with higher incomes had higher annual dental expenses. The average annual dental expense for "high-income" individuals (greater than 400% of the federal poverty level [FPL]) was $710. Among "poor" individuals (less than 100% FPL), the average annual dental expense was $428. This difference in expenses may reflect the ability of individuals with higher incomes to pay for and use dental care. Finally, older adults (individuals 65 and over) had the highest average annual dental expenses at $776. By contrast, children and adolescents (individuals under age 18) had the lowest average annual dental expenses.

In 2007, the source of payments for dental care (private insurance, out-of-pocket, or public insurance) varied among individuals who had any dental expenses. For example, the percentage of annual dental expenses paid out of pocket varied by age, race and ethnicity, income, and insurance status. As would be expected, uninsured individuals pay the highest percentage—nearly three quarters—of their annual dental expenses out of pocket (74.7%) compared to individuals with private insurance and those with public insurance (44.3% and 28.5%, respectively). Older adults (individuals 65 and over) had the highest percent of total annual dental expenses paid out of pocket than any other age group (70.3%). By contrast, children, who are more likely to have public insurance that includes dental coverage, had the lowest percent of total annual dental expenses paid out of pocket than any other age group (23%). Working age adults (individuals between 18 and 64 years of age), who are more likely to have employer-based dental coverage, had lower costs than older adults. The lack of dental coverage in Medicare and the lack of employee-based dental coverage translate into higher out-of-pocket dental expenses for older adults.

Overview of Coverage

Dental Coverage

There is strong evidence that dental coverage is positively tied to access to and utilization of oral health care, although whether or not this relationship is causal is not clear. For example, it may be that those with greater demand for dental care are the ones most likely to purchase dental coverage. This suggests it is not clear if more coverage leads to greater use or greater demand leads to the purchase of dental coverage (and then greater use). The tie is clear, though: In 2007, 52% of adults with private dental coverage had at least one dental visit, compared to 31% of those without private dental coverage and 22% of uninsured individuals. Moreover, children who have dental coverage, through public programs (Medicaid or CHIP) or private insurance, use preventive care more routinely than their counterparts who lack coverage. Studies using quasi-experimental designs to assess the impact of dental coverage on access and utilization indicate that, once children acquire coverage through a public program, they are significantly less likely to have unmet needs for dental care. For example, after enrolling in CHIP, unmet needs for oral health care decline among adolescents. Another study found that, after enrolling in CHIP, children with special health care needs had significantly improved access to a broad range of health care services, including dental care. Overall, uninsured children are at least twice as likely as children with dental coverage to have unmet need for oral health care.

Millions of Americans lack dental coverage. Recent data from several sources underscore this deficiency among children, adults, and older adults:

- An estimated 130 million U.S. adults and children lack dental coverage (based on enrollment in private dental plans).

- Over 40% adults ages 21–64 lack private dental coverage.

- Approximately 70% of adults age 65 and older, lack any kind of dental coverage—public or private.

- Over 22% of children ages 1–17 lack dental coverage.

Section 64.2

Dental Coverage through Private and Public Sources

Excerpted from "Improving Access to Oral Health Care for Vulnerable and Underserved Populations," © 2011 National Academy of Sciences. All rights reserved. Reprinted with permission courtesy of the National Academies Press, Washington, D.C.

Private Sources of Financing

Dental care is financed primarily through private sources, including individual out-of-pocket payments and private coverage. For more than 50 years, these two sources have financed over 90% of all dental expenditures. Americans spend billions of dollars out of pocket for dental services each year. In 2008, dental services accounted for 22% of all out-of-pocket health care expenditures, ranking second only to prescription drug expenditures.

Variation in Coverage Rates by Employment and Income

Variations in dental coverage have been observed by employment status and income level. For example, data from the 2008 National Health Interview Survey showed that the percentage of individuals with private dental coverage increased as income levels increased. Similarly, higher-paid workers are also more likely to have access to and participate in stand-alone dental plans. The availability of dental coverage through one's employer is associated with the size of the establishment; that is, the larger the number of employees overall, the greater the likelihood that stand-alone dental plans will be available to employees. Employers can add a separate oral health product to their overall coverage package, but often they do not. In 2006, 56% of all employers offered health insurance but only 35% offered dental coverage. Employees are more likely to be offered options for medical insurance than dental coverage, and a higher percentage of employees will take advantage of available dental benefits as compared with the percentage of employees who take advantage of available medical

563

benefits (80% versus 75%). As noted earlier, with the exception of coverage of rare events, dental coverage differs from the typical insurance model; thus, employer-based dental coverage might be viewed as a fringe benefit that subsidizes oral health care utilization.

Publicly Subsidized Coverage

Access to dental care depends on a variety of factors; however, chief among these is having a provider available and having the ability to pay for services (either through insurance, direct out-of-pocket payments, or subsidies). In 2009, public subsidies or direct payments for dental services from public programs totaled $7.4 billion or less than 1% of national expenditures for dental services. The overwhelming majority (73%) of these public expenditures for direct services or coverage came from Medicaid.

Medicaid and CHIP

Medicaid

Medicaid is a federal-state entitlement program for medical assistance to low-income children and pregnant women, persons over age 65, and those with disabilities who meet income and resource requirements; at the state's discretion, certain persons who are considered medically needy based on their high medical costs may also be covered. The vast majority of state Medicaid programs now purchase at least some medical care services through contracts with managed care plans.

Medicaid's Early and Periodic Screening, Diagnostic, and Treatment (EPSDT) service provides a comprehensive child health benefit, which requires states to fund well-child health care, diagnostic services, and medically necessary treatment services to Medicaid-eligible children ages birth to age 21. Under federal EPSDT law, states must cover any Medicaid-covered (allowed under the federal Medicaid statute) service that is necessary to prevent, correct, or ameliorate a child's physical health, which includes oral health. Dental coverage is required for all Medicaid enrolled children under age 21. This is a comprehensive benefit, including preventive, diagnostic, and treatment services. At a minimum, these services must include relief of pain and infections, restoration of teeth, and maintenance of dental health. In contrast, states are not required to provide coverage for adults. For adults, states must only cover medical and surgical services furnished by a dentist to the extent those services can be performed under state law by either a doctor of medicine or a dentist. Beyond this, states' coverage of routine dental benefits for adults varies widely among the states, with a number of states limiting the benefit to emergency coverage.

Medicaid coverage can improve access to medical and dental care; however, health status, age, race and ethnicity, gender, routine source of dental care, amount of reimbursement, and availability of providers all factor into the impact of coverage. There are variations in the patterns of utilization for preventive, treatment, emergency, and specialty dental services associated with Medicaid populations compared to privately insured populations.

At the same time, low provider participation in the Medicaid program has a direct and generally negative impact on access to oral health care for Medicaid beneficiaries. For example, 74% of pediatricians cite the lack of dentists who accept Medicaid as a "moderate to severe barrier for 0–3-year-old Medicaid-insured patients to obtain dental care." In addition, a recent study in Illinois found that a child with public dental coverage (Medicaid/CHIP) was significantly less likely to obtain an appointment for an urgent oral injury than a child with the same injury with private dental coverage. This effect was found even among Medicaid/CHIP-enrolled practices. Increases in Medicaid reimbursement have been shown by some studies to increase dentist participation. Other approaches (training, administrative support, and quality improvement techniques) also have been shown to increase dentists' participation in Medicaid, particularly for children's services. Multidimensional, strategically planned initiatives that include provider outreach, increased financing, and consumer education show particular promise. State Medicaid programs are increasingly electing to reimburse primary medical care providers and dental hygienists for preventive oral health services, including the application of fluoride varnish, performing oral examinations, and providing anticipatory guidance.

Children's Health Insurance Program (CHIP)

CHIP is a federal-state grant program that provides resources to states to expand health coverage to uninsured, low-income children up to age 19, and pregnant women. Unlike Medicaid, it is not an entitlement, but it does help states provide publicly subsidized health coverage to uninsured children in households earning up to 200% FPL (and with federal approval, well above that level). Following its enactment in 1997, millions of children received coverage for medical care and a portion of those were covered for dental care under CHIP. CHIP plans either offer eligibility for children under Medicaid or create a separate children's health insurance approach managed by the state (and typically operated by private insurance companies). Non-Medicaid approaches must be equivalent to one of the so-called benchmark benefits packages (for example: Federal Employees Health Benefits Program [FEHBP], Blue Cross/Blue Shield, or the state employee benefit plan). If CHIP is part of Medicaid, then benefits must be comparable, including EPSDT dental benefits.

The Children's Health Insurance Program Reauthorization Act (CHIPRA) enacted in February 2009 requires all states to provide dental coverage under CHIP, including "coverage of dental services necessary to prevent disease and promote oral health, restore oral structures to health and function, and treat emergency conditions." States can meet this requirement in separate CHIP programs by providing dental coverage equivalent to one of three benchmark dental benefit packages: (1) the plan under FEHBP selected most frequently by employees seeking dependent coverage; (2) the state employee benefit plan selected most frequently by employees seeking dependent coverage; or (3) the commercial dental plan in the state that has the largest non-Medicaid enrollment of dependents. In addition, states were given the option to offer a stand-alone or dental-only supplemental coverage to families whose children meet income eligibility requirements for CHIP and have private, employer-sponsored medical insurance but lack dental coverage.

CHIPRA also included provisions related to the dissemination of dental education materials, data reporting on dental access and quality, and requirements to post lists of participating dental professionals. For example, Health and Human Services' (HHS) *Insure Kids Now* website was designed to provide families with more timely and accessible information about the participating providers in their communities and whether these providers are accepting new patients. However, a recent study by the Government Accountability Office (GAO) highlighted the significant deficiencies in the website's lists of dental professionals participating in Medicaid or CHIP including incomplete and inaccurate information (for example: disconnected phone numbers, providers not accepting new patients, and providers no longer in practice). In response to this report, HHS is taking steps to improve the *Insure Kids Now* website.

Factors That Influence Provider Participation in Medicaid and CHIP

According to the 2000 GAO report *Factors Contributing to Low Use of Dental Services by Low-Income Populations*, the primary reason individuals enrolled in Medicaid are unable to locate and use needed services is limited dentist participation in Medicaid. A recent report identified three main reasons given by dentists for not seeing more Medicaid patients: low reimbursement rates, administrative requirements, and patient-related issues (such as missed appointments).

Low reimbursement rates: Medicaid reimbursement rates are generally lower than dentists' usual and customary fees. This is often cited as a disincentive to providers' willingness to participate in these publicly funded programs. For example, a recent state-by-state comparison of average retail fees and Medicaid reimbursement rates for oral evaluation revealed that, overall, Medicaid reimbursement rates were about 55% of the average retail fees ($18.00 versus $33.00). While this comparison illustrates substantial variations by state, it should be noted that health care providers negotiate with insurers to determine discounts to retail fees. Since individuals without insurance have no one to negotiate such discounts on their behalf, they typically pay the full retail fee for services. Therefore, the only individuals who would be billed at the commercial rate would be the estimated 130 million U.S. adults and children who lack dental coverage. Furthermore, final negotiated rates depend on individual agreements; the larger the size of the insurer, the deeper discounts they may be able to negotiate. The impact of Medicaid reimbursement rates has also been observed in other health professions. For example, one study found a strong and significant correlation between low Medicaid reimbursement rates and low participation in Medicaid by pediatricians.

Before the recent economic downturn, a number of states had increased reimbursement rates for dentists in an effort to encourage broader participation of dentists in publicly funded programs and increase access to care. However, as states began to look for ways to address budgets shortfalls, many made cuts to dental reimbursement rates. In fiscal year (FY) 2010, 13 states made cuts to dental rates, and seven more states adopted cuts to dental rates in FY 2011.

Increases in reimbursement rates have shown promise in increasing dentists' participation in publicly funded programs. A recent study found that both dentist participation in Medicaid and the number of Medicaid patients treated increased in states that implemented reimbursement rate increases. Moreover, the study found that dentists who were already enrolled in Medicaid began treating more Medicaid patients following the rate increases. Finally, in one state, both the number of providers and the geographic distribution of providers expanded following the increase in reimbursement rates. As a result, the average distance that children had to travel for care in the participating counties served decreased from 24.5 miles to 12.1 miles. Efforts to improve access through financing strategies will necessarily be multifaceted and will be one component of broader efforts to improve access. For example, studies have demonstrated that increasing reimbursement rates alone is not sufficient in improving access to care. Without more comprehensive actions (including case management and streamlined enrollment and billing processes), barriers to oral health care persist.

Administrative requirements: The administrative processes and requirements associated with Medicaid are frequently cited as a barrier to provider participation. In particular, dentists point to excessive paperwork, complex billing and preauthorization requirements, difficult eligibility-verification processes, slow payments, denials of submitted claims, and complicated provider enrollment as procedural obstacles to providing care to Medicaid patients. This corresponds with research in other health professions. For example, a nationally representative survey of U.S. physicians in direct patient care found that after inadequate reimbursement (84% of respondents), billing requirements and paperwork (70.4% of respondents) and delayed reimbursement (64.8% of respondents) were the most frequently reasons provided for limiting the number of Medicaid patients they see. Many states have taken measures to reduce administrative burdens as a strategy to improve provider participation in public programs. These actions, in conjunction with rate increases and other supportive strategies (such as increased education and outreach to beneficiaries), can have a significant effect on increasing provider participation and patient utilization rates.

Medicare

Medicare coverage is available to most Americans 65 and over, regardless of income, and persons with disabilities.(Individuals who have not worked at all or have not worked enough to be eligible for Social Security are not eligible for Medicare.) Medicare has several parts. Part A covers hospital and other institutional care for all who receive Social Security benefits, without a premium. Part B covers physician and certain other clinical services for those who elect to enroll and pay a premium. Most Medicare beneficiaries have both Part A and Part B coverage. In addition, Medicare Part D provides coverage for prescription drugs through private plans for those who wish to enroll.

The Medicare statute explicitly excludes coverage for what is generally known as dental care, specifically, "for services in connection with the care, treatment, filling, removal, or replacement of teeth or structures directly supporting the teeth." Coverage is not determined by the value or the necessity of the dental care but by the type of service provided and the anatomical structure on which the procedure is performed. Medicare will not cover most dental care. For example, Medicare will not cover routine checkups, cleanings, fillings, or dentures.

The Centers for Medicare and Medicaid Services (CMS) has approved dental coverage in special situations that relate directly to medical needs. Currently, Medicare will pay for dental services that are an integral part either of a covered procedure (such as reconstruction of the jaw following accidental injury or removal of a facial tumor). Medicare also pays for extractions done in preparation for radiation treatment for diseases involving the jaw, which may be appropriate for patients with extensive periodontal disease and dental abscesses, but not for others who can be treated with less drastic interventions. Medicare will also reimburse for oral examinations, but not treatment, preceding kidney transplantation or heart valve replacement, under certain circumstances (for example, such examination would be covered under Part A if performed by a dentist on the hospital's staff or under Part B if performed by a physician).

As increasing numbers of baby boomers (individuals born between 1946 and 1964) become eligible for Medicare, considerable attention is being paid to how these aging adults will pay for and obtain oral health care. The relative size of this cohort—approximately 78 million in 2009—coupled with increases in longevity will create an unprecedented demand for oral health care for older adults.

Chapter 65

Head Start Promotes Oral Health Services

Note: Head Start refers to Early Head Start and Head Start throughout the document.

What is Head Start?

Head Start was established in 1965 to improve the school readiness of children ages three to five from families with low incomes. In 1994, Early Head Start was established to serve low-income pregnant women, with a focus on positive birth outcomes, and to promote healthy physical and cognitive development in infants and young children from birth to age three from families with low incomes. Both Early Head Start and Head Start provide education and health services in the context of family and community.[1]

Head Start is a federal program administered by the Office of Head Start, Administration for Children and Families, through grants to approximately 1,600 community-based organizations.[2]

Who participates in Head Start?

Head Start programs serve approximately 900,000 pregnant women, infants, and children each year in all 50 states, the District of Columbia, and most U.S. territories.[1]

Excerpted from "Medical Providers and Head Start: What You Should Know about Oral Health and How You Can Help," © 2011 National Maternal and Child Oral Health Resource Center, Georgetown University (www.mchoralhealth .org). Reprinted with permission.

At least 90% of children enrolled in each Head Start program must be from families with low incomes, and up to 10% can be from families with incomes that exceed the low-income guidelines who would benefit from Head Start services.[3] Up to 35% of each Head Start program's enrollment may also be children whose families' incomes are between 100% and 130% of the federal poverty level. Children are automatically eligible, regardless of family income, if they are homeless, or in foster care; or if their families receive Temporary Assistance for Needy Families or Supplemental Security Income.[4]

Of the 94% of children enrolled in Head Start who have health insurance, 82% are enrolled in Medicaid or in the Children's Health Insurance Program (CHIP).[2]

Why are Head Start children at higher risk for oral disease?

Head Start staff and parents report that the number one health issue affecting children enrolled in Head Start nationwide is lack of access to oral health services.[5]

Despite improvements in oral health status nationally, profound oral health disparities remain in certain population groups, including children enrolled in Head Start. These children, like other children from families with low incomes, experience more tooth decay (dental caries) and resultant pain and suffering than children from families with higher incomes.[6]

While oral health is emphasized in Head Start program performance standards, many infants and children enrolled in Head Start continue to encounter barriers to care. For example, there is a shortage of dentists serving the Medicaid/CHIP population. Furthermore, many dentists do not feel comfortable providing services to infants and young children, despite agreement within the oral health community (Academy of General Dentistry, American Academy of Pediatric Dentistry, and American Dental Association) as well as the medical community (American Academy of Pediatrics) that children should see a dentist by age one year.[7–10]

What oral health services does Head Start offer?

Head Start health services are based on the premise that a child must be healthy to be ready to learn. Good oral health is essential to a child's behavioral, speech, language, and overall growth and development.[5, 11]

Head Start program performance standards require that staff track the provision of oral health care and help parents obtain an oral examination and follow-up care for their child. Information about examination results, plans for followup care, treatment completed, and oral disease prevention activities (for example: fluoride varnish, fluoride supplementation) are kept in a child's health record.[12]

Head Start program activities also promote good oral hygiene in the classroom. Each day, staff wipe infants' gums and assist children in brushing their teeth with fluoridated toothpaste.[12]

Head Start staff help parents understand the benefits of prevention and proper oral health care, along with the importance of establishing a dental home early in life.[13]

References

1. Office of Head Start. 2010. *About the Office of Head Start.* http://www. acf.hhs.gov/programs/ohs/about/index.html.

2. Office of Head Start. 2010. *Head Start Program Fact Sheet: Fiscal Year 2010.* http://www.acf.hhs.gov/programs/ohs/about/ fy2010.html.

3. U.S. Department of Health and Human Services, Office of Human Development Services. 1998. Title 45—Public Welfare, Chapter XIII, Part 1305—Eligibility, Recruitment, Selection, Enrollment, and Attendance in Head Start. 1305.4: Age of children and family income eligibility. *Code of Federal Regulations.* http://www.access.gpo.gov/nara/cfr/waisidx_08/45cfr1305_08. html.

4. Office of Head Start. 2008. *Head Start Reauthorization P.L. 110-134 (ACF-IM-HS-08_01) Information Memorandum.* http://www.acf.hhs.gov/programs/ohs/policy/im2008/ acfimhs_08_01.html.

5. Brocato R. 2001. Head Start and Partners Forum on Oral Health. *Head Start Bulletin* 71:1–43. Washington, DC: Head Start Bureau. http://eclkc.ohs.acf.hhs.gov/hslc/resources/ ECLKC_Bookstore/PDFs/ 421CEF928C56391D1041DFCE-1F0119AC.pdf.

6. Edelstein BL. 2000. Access to dental care for Head Start enrollees. *Journal of Public Health Dentistry* 60(3):221–229.

7. Academy of General Dentistry. 2010. *Advocacy Policies 2009–2010.* Chicago, IL: Academy of General Dentistry. http://www .agd.org/files/ advocacy/9937advocacypolicies.doc.

8. American Academy of Pediatric Dentistry, Clinical Affairs Committee, Infant Oral Health Subcommittee. 2010. Guideline on infant oral health care. *Pediatric Dentistry 32*(6):114–118. http://www.aapd.org/ media/Policies_Guidelines/G_InfantOral HealthCare.pdf.

9. American Dental Association. 2010. *Current Policies: Adopted 1954–2009*. Chicago, IL: American Dental Association. http:// www.ada.org/ sections/about/pdfs/doc_policies.pdf.

10. Hale, KJ; American Academy of Pediatrics, Section on Pediatric Dentistry. 2003. Oral health risk assessment timing and establishment of the dental home. *Pediatrics 111* (5 Pt 1):113–116.

11. Office of Head Start. 2007. *Child Health Services*. http://eclkc. ohs.acf.hhs.gov/hslc/resources/ECLKC_Bookstore/Weaving%20 Connections%20%28Multimedia%20Kit%29.htm.

12. Office of Head Start. 2006. *Oral Health—Revision: ACF-PI-HS-06-03* [program instruction]. Washington, DC: Office of Head Start. http://eclkc.ohs.acf.hhs.gov/hslc/Program%20 Design%20and%20 Management/Head%20Start%20 Requirements/PIs/2006/resour_ pri_00109_122006.html.

13. American Academy of Pediatrics. Oral Health Initiative [website]. 2010. *States With and Without Medicaid Reimbursement for Primary Care Medical Providers to Perform Caries Prevention Services*. http://www.aap. org/oralhealth/fluoride.cfm.

Chapter 66

Fluoride and Sealants at School-Based Services

School-Based Fluoride Mouthrinse Program Policy Statement

Problem

Dental caries (tooth decay) is a chronic, progressive, multi-factorial, infectious disease that can begin in early infancy and that, by the time children reach adulthood, will affect over 92% of the U.S. adult population. A smaller proportion of the U.S. population will develop moderate or severe dental caries. Dental caries prevalence and severity varies by age, dentition, and type of tooth surface. In addition, dental caries and other oral diseases are highly related to socio-environmental determinants, with the greatest burden on disadvantaged and socially-marginalized populations. Historically, dental caries control has been addressed by daily brushing, modifying dietary practices, and improving the resistance of tooth enamel to acid attack. However, only fluorides and dental sealants demonstrate a high degree of scientific evidence for reducing dental caries in populations. Benefiting from

This chapter includes excerpts from "School-Based Fluoride Mouthrinse Programs Policy Statement," adopted March 1, 2011. © 2011 Association of State and Territorial Dental Directors (www.astdd.org). Reprinted with permission. Also, excerpts from "School Dental Sealant Programs Policy Statement," adopted December 15, 2010. © 2010 Association of State and Territorial Dental Directors (www.astdd.org). Reprinted with permission. The entire documents with references are available online at www.astdd.org.

fluoride in drinking water and fluoride toothpastes, the baby boomer generation will be the first in which the majority will maintain natural teeth over their entire lifetime, according to the Centers for Disease Control and Prevention (CDC).

Methods

Fluoride modalities are systemic and topical and include: drinking water (natural and adjusted levels), milk, salt, toothpaste, mouthrinse, and the professional application of concentrated fluoride in gels, foams, or varnishes. Caries protection, lifetime cost, and appropriateness for use in populations will vary by the fluoride method or combination of fluoride methods selected. Fluorides are most effective when used in combination with other modalities to prevent, control, and reverse early dental caries. Fluorides are more effective in preventing dental caries on the smooth surfaces of teeth than in the pits and fissures. However, for carious lesions that are limited to the pits and fissures of permanent molar teeth, dental sealants alone or combined with multiple fluoride applications are more effective than fluoride alone. Daily, multiple low exposures to fluoride facilitate the balance between remineralization and demineralization of tooth enamel, thus reducing caries incidence.

School-based fluoride mouthrinse programs have been used for many years as a community-based caries prevention strategy, recognized by the Association of State and Territorial Dental Directors (ASTDD) Best Practices Project as a Best Practice Approach for State and Community Oral Health Programs. Fluoride mouth rinses containing a concentration of 0.2% sodium fluoride are prescribed for weekly school fluoride rinsing programs. Other ingredients may include saccharin, potassium sorbate, purified water, flavor, citric acid, and coloring agents. Fluoride mouth rinses are approved as a caries preventive agent by the Food and Drug Administration (FDA), Centers for Disease Control and Prevention (CDC), and the American Dental Association (ADA).

Fluoride mouth rinses work in the same way as other topical fluorides by enhancing fluoride concentrations in saliva, plaque, and enamel. Current laboratory and epidemiologic evidence indicate that fluoride's predominant effect is post-eruptive and topical, and the effect depends on regular fluoride availability.

Use of fluoride mouth rinse by children ages six years and older does not place them at risk for enamel fluorosis. By age six, most children can rinse and spit with little to no ingestion, making a rinse a good method for topical fluoride. Fluoride rinses are not recommended for children under the age of six because some young children might swallow the rinse rather than spit it out. Substantial fluoride ingestion at this young age when the teeth are developing might result in enamel fluorosis, thus affecting the appearance of the teeth.

Not all people have regular access to optimally fluoridated community water supplies or other sources of fluoride. Schools provide an ideal setting for promoting oral health education and prevention activities with approximately 88% of U.S. children attending public schools. An integrated approach that combines school health policy, skills-based health education, a health-supportive school environment, and school health services can tackle major common risk factors and contribute to effective control of oral disease. School fluoride mouthrinse programs can be administered by school personnel trained in mouth rinsing procedures and safe storage of fluoride, according to individual state regulations.

Evidence from studies conducted before 1985 supported the effectiveness of 0.2% sodium fluoride mouth rinses in preventing coronal caries of permanent teeth in school populations. These studies collectively showed that regular use of sodium fluoride mouth rinses reduced caries increments in children by 20% to 35% over two to three years.

The National Preventive Dentistry Demonstration Program (NPDDP), conducted in ten U.S. cities to compare the cost and effectiveness of caries-prevention procedures in the late 1980s, found only a limited reduction in dental caries attributable to fluoride mouth rinse, especially when children were also exposed to fluoridated water. Benefits were more likely for children in high-risk schools.

U. S. studies on effectiveness of school fluoride mouth rinsing programs since the NPDDP have been limited. The 2003 Cochrane Review of fluoride mouth rinsing in schools found a 26% dental caries reduction in permanent teeth in their reviewed studies. In 2007, an observational study in Europe targeting at-risk schools demonstrated caries reductions of 20%. Two studies (1985–86) reported benefits of fluoride mouth rinsing programs approximately two and one-half and seven years after completion of school-based mouth rinsing programs, but a later study (1995) did not find benefits four years after completion of a mouth rinsing program. Fluoride mouth rinsing in school programs has been discontinued in some countries similar to the U.S. because of doubts regarding the cost-effectiveness for children with a low prevalence of dental caries. While dental caries have continued to decline, school mouth rinsing programs appear to be effective in populations at high risk for dental caries.

The proportion of states with fluoride mouth rinsing programs has decreased 15% since 2003. Of the 50 states and the District of

Columbia reporting to the 2010 ASTDD State Synopsis, 35 states have fluoride mouthrinse programs, primarily targeting high-risk schools in non-fluoridated communities. Increased effectiveness of fluoride mouth rinsing would be expected in schools with a high caries increment. Increased effectiveness is expected in communities with less use of other systemic and topical fluorides.

School fluoride mouth rinse programs are inexpensive compared to professionally applied fluorides, especially when volunteers are used. Cost estimates in 1988 ranged from $0.52 to $1.78 per child per school year for fluoride mouth rinsing, depending on whether paid staff or volunteers supervise the procedure. In a 2010 ASTDD survey, states reported fluoride mouth rinse program costs between $0.54 cents and $2.54 per child per year.

The single greatest risk factor predicting dental caries in populations is low socio-economic status. Programs based on populations selected for socio-economic status alone, without considering dental caries incidence, may result in increased costs compared to the benefits. Other population risk or protective factors to consider in school program planning include availability of dental care; proportion of the population who 1) are low SES, 2) are an ethnic minority, 3) speak English as a second language, 4) are homeless, 5) have limited education, 6) have special health care needs, 7) have high caries incidence and prevalence rates or advanced disease, and 8) lack access to fluoridated water. Additionally, school districts and schools need to be sufficiently involved to assure a majority of students achieve 30 applications a year for at least two years, ideally age six to 16, to achieve caries reductions in the erupting permanent teeth.

Policy Statement for Mouth Rinse Programs

ASTDD supports the use of fluoride mouth rinse programs in schools for children age six years and older, when exposure to optimal systemic and topical fluorides is low, populations of children are at high risk for tooth decay and there is demonstrated support by school personnel.

School Dental Sealant Programs Policy Statement

Problem

The CDC reports that dental caries (tooth decay) affects more than one-fourth of U.S. children aged one to five years and one-half of those aged 12 to 15, and is almost entirely preventable. Although dental disease may affect any child, children from low-income households experience more tooth decay than those from higher-income families. Data show that children aged six through 11 years from families living below the poverty threshold are almost twice as likely to have developed tooth decay in their permanent teeth as are children from families with incomes greater than two times the federal poverty threshold. Nearly 80% of decay is experienced by just 25% of U.S. school-aged children. Most decay occurs on the pits and fissures of posterior tooth surfaces for which dental sealants are the most effective preventive approach. Other factors that increase the incidence of tooth decay in children are poor dietary habits, lack of dental insurance and access to dental care, as well as inadequate exposure to the benefits of fluoridated water and dental sealants.

The Healthy People 2010 goal is for 50% of U.S. 8-year-olds (third graders) to have at least one sealant on a permanent molar, but more than 65% of these children do not. Children from low-income families were only half as likely to have sealants as children from higher income families. Data show that only 20% of children aged six through 11 years from low-income families have received sealants compared to the 40% of children from families with incomes greater than two times the poverty threshold that received sealants.

Methods

The U.S. Preventive Health Services Task Force has identified school-based dental sealant programs as an effective community approach to dental caries prevention. Systematic reviews have found strong evidence that sealants are effective in 1) preventing the development of caries on sound pit and fissure tooth surfaces in children and adolescents; 2) reducing the percentage of non-cavitated carious lesions that progressed to cavitation in children, adolescents, and young adults; and 3) reducing bacteria levels in cavitated carious lesions in children, adolescents, and young adults.

Dental sealants protect up to 90% of the pits and fissures where decay occurs in school-aged children's teeth. Resin-based sealants are preferred due to their high retention rates. Sealants are not only beneficial for permanent molars, but also on primary teeth when determined that the tooth, or the patient, is at risk for experiencing caries. Radiographs should not be obtained for the sole purpose of placing sealants; nor is the use of other diagnostic aids, including a sharp explorer recommended.

Dental sealants are most effective when placed on teeth of children at highest risk for tooth decay. "School sealant programs can be an important intervention to increase the receipt of sealants, especially among underserved children." Targeting higher risk schools to reach higher-risk children is a practical approach for increasing sealant prevalence through school-based sealant programs. Using the Free and Reduced Price Meal Program enrollment as risk thresholds provides the ability to reach higher-risk children. Sealant programs could reduce or eliminate racial and economic disparities in sealant use if programs were provided to all eligible, high-risk schools such as those in which 50% or more of the children are eligible for the Free and Reduced-Price Meal Program. Additionally, school-based sealant programs have the potential to link students with treatment services in their community and facilitate enrollment in Medicaid and the Children's Health Insurance Program (CHIP).

Access to dental sealants in school settings affords an opportunity for every child to grow, develop and learn free of pain from dental disease. The CDC estimates that if 50% of children at high risk for dental caries participated in school sealant programs, more than half of their tooth decay would be prevented, and money would be saved on their treatment costs. To ensure their effectiveness, school sealant programs should follow evidence-based recommendations, monitor sealant retention and reapply sealants if lost, if possible. A four-handed technique should be used when resources allow and teeth should be sealed, even if follow-up care cannot be assured.

Policy Statement for Dental Sealant Programs

The Association of State and Territorial Dental Directors (ASTDD) fully supports, endorses, and promotes expansion of school-based and school-linked dental sealant programs that follow evidence-based guidelines as part of a comprehensive community strategy to serve the greatest number of children and adolescents at highest risk for dental disease. The ASTDD recommends school-based and school-linked dental sealant programs as an important and effective public health approach that complements clinical care systems in promoting the oral health of children and adolescents.

Chapter 67

Finding Low-Cost Dental Care

The National Institute of Dental and Craniofacial Research (NID-CR), one of the federal government's National Institutes of Health, leads the nation in conducting and supporting research to improve oral health. As a research organization, NIDCR does not provide financial assistance for dental treatment. The following resources, however, may help you find the dental care you need.

Clinical Trials

NIDCR sometimes seeks volunteers with specific dental, oral, and craniofacial conditions to participate in research studies, also known as clinical trials. Researchers may provide study participants with limited free or low-cost dental treatment for the particular condition they are studying. To find out if there are any NIDCR clinical trials that you might fit into, go to "NIDCR Studies Seeking Patients." If you do not have access to the internet, you may need to visit your local library or ask a friend or family member for assistance. To see if you qualify for any clinical trials being conducted at the Bethesda, Maryland campus:

Clinical Center's Patient Recruitment and Public Liaison Office
Toll-Free: 800-411-1222
Website: http://clinicaltrials.gov

"Finding Low-Cost Dental Care," National Institute of Dental and Craniofacial Research (NIDCR), NIH Publication No. 12–6097, November 2011.

Dental Schools

Dental schools can be a good source of quality, reduced-cost dental treatment. Most of these teaching facilities have clinics that allow dental students to gain experience treating patients while providing care at a reduced cost. Experienced, licensed dentists closely supervise the students. Post-graduate and faculty clinics are also available at most schools. Dental hygiene schools may also offer supervised, low-cost preventive dental care as part of the training experience for dental hygienists.

Bureau of Primary Health Care

The Bureau of Primary Health Care, a service of the Health Resources and Services Administration, supports federally-funded community health centers across the country that provide free or reduced-cost health services, including dental care. For a list of centers in your area:

Bureau of Primary Health Care
Toll-Free: 888-Ask-HRSA (888-275-4772)
Website: http://findahealthcenter.hrsa.gov/Search_HCC.aspx

Centers for Medicare and Medicaid Services

The Centers for Medicare and Medicaid Services (CMS) administers three important federally-funded programs: Medicare, Medicaid, and the Children's Health Insurance Program (CHIP).

- Medicare is a health insurance program for people who are 65 years and older or for people with specific disabilities. Medicare does not cover most routine dental care or dentures. Visit http://www.cms.hhs.gov/MedicareDentalCoverage.

- Medicaid is a state-run program that provides medical benefits, and in some cases dental benefits, to eligible individuals and families. States set their own guidelines regarding who is eligible and what services are covered. Most states provide limited emergency dental services for people age 21 or over, while some offer comprehensive services. For most individuals under the age of 21, dental services are provided under Medicaid. Visit http://go.usa.gov/V2T.

- CHIP helps children up to age 19 who are without health insurance. CHIP provides medical coverage and, in most cases, dental services to children who qualify. Dental services covered under this program vary from state to state. Visit http://go.usa.gov/V2D.

CMS can provide detailed information about each of these programs and refer you to state programs where applicable.

Centers for Medicare and Medicaid Services
7500 Security Blvd.
Baltimore, MD 21244
Toll-Free: 800-633-4227
Website: http://www.cms.gov

State and Local Resources

Your state or local health department may know of programs in your area that offer free or reduced-cost dental care. Call your local or state health department to learn more about their financial assistance programs. Check your local telephone book for the number to call.

United Way

The United Way may be able to direct you to free or reduced-cost dental services in your community. Check your telephone book for the number of your local United Way chapter.

Part Eight

Additional Help and Information

Chapter 68

Glossary of Dental Care and Oral Health Terms

abnormal dental development: Altered tooth development, craniofacial growth, or skeletal development in children secondary to radiotherapy and/or high doses of chemotherapy before age nine.[1]

braces: See orthodontic appliance.

bruxism: A clenching of the teeth, associated with forceful lateral or protrusive jaw movements, resulting in rubbing, gritting, or grinding together of the teeth, usually during sleep; sometimes a pathologic condition. Condition when people grit or grind their teeth.

caries: See tooth decay.

complete tooth loss: Complete tooth loss (edentulism) is the loss of all natural teeth. It can substantially reduce quality of life, self-image, and daily functioning.[3]

crown: In dentistry, that part of a tooth that is covered with enamel, or an artificial substitute for that part of the tooth.

Terms in this chapter that are unmarked are from *Stedman's Medical Dictionary, 27th Edition*, Copyright © 2000 Lippincott Williams & Wilkins. All rights reserved. Terms marked with a [1] are from "Oral Complications of Cancer Treatment: What the Oncology Team Can Do," National Institute of Dental and Craniofacial Research (NIDCR), NIH Publication No. 09–4360, March 25, 2011. Terms marked with a [2] are from "What You Need to Know about Oral Cancer," National Cancer Institute (NCI), December 23, 2009. Terms marked with a [3] are from "Glossary," National Oral Health Surveillance System, Centers for Disease Control and Prevention (CDC), July 23, 2010.

curettage: A scraping, usually of the interior of a cavity or tract, for the removal of new growths or other abnormal tissues, or to obtain material for tissue diagnosis.

dental calculus: Calcified deposits formed around the teeth; may appear as subgingival or supragingival calculus.

dental implant: A metal device that is surgically placed in the jawbone. It acts as an anchor for an artificial tooth or teeth.[2]

dental plaque: The noncalcified accumulation mainly of oral microorganisms and their products that adheres tenaciously to the teeth and is not readily dislodged.

dental sealant: A dental material usually made from interaction between bisphenol A and glycidyl methacrylate; such sealants are used to seal non-fused, noncarious pits and fissures on surfaces of teeth.

dental visits: Regular use of the oral health care delivery system leads to better oral health by providing an opportunity for clinical preventive services and early detection of oral diseases. Infrequent users of dental services have more decayed teeth, more severe periodontal diseases, and are more likely to lose all of their teeth.[3]

denture: An artificial substitute for missing natural teeth and adjacent tissues.

edentulism: See complete tooth loss.

endodontics: A field of dentistry concerned with the biology and pathology of the dental pulp and periapical tissues, and with the prevention, diagnosis, and treatment of diseases and injuries in these tissues.

erythroplakia: An abnormal patch of red tissue that forms on mucous membranes in the mouth and may become cancer. Tobacco (smoking and chewing) and alcohol may increase the risk of erythroplakia.[2]

fixed partial denture: A restoration of one or more missing teeth which cannot be readily removed by the patient or dentist; it is permanently attached to natural teeth or roots which furnish the primary support to the appliance.

fluoridation status: Status of a community water system in regards to water fluoridation level. Most water contains some amount of natural fluoride. Fluoridation involves adjusting fluoride in the water to the level optimal for the prevention of dental caries. The recommended amount of fluoride in water systems is 0.7–1.2 ppm (parts per million), which is equivalent to 0.7–1.2 mg/L (milligrams per liter).[3]

Gingival-Periodontal Index (GPI): An index of gingivitis, gingival irritation, and advanced periodontal disease.

impacted tooth: A tooth whose normal eruption is prevented by adjacent teeth or bone; or a tooth that has been driven into the alveolar process or surrounding tissue as a result of trauma.

leukoplakia: An abnormal patch of white tissue that forms on mucous membranes in the mouth and other areas of the body. It may become cancer. Tobacco (smoking and chewing) and alcohol may increase the risk of leukoplakia in the mouth.[2]

oral hygiene: The cleaning of the mouth by means of brushing, flossing, irrigating, massaging, or the use of other devices.

oral mucositis/stomatitis: Inflammation and ulceration of the mucous membranes; can increase the risk for pain, oral and systemic infection, and nutritional compromise.[1]

oral prophylaxis: Thorough dental cleaning.[1]

oral surgery: The branch of dentistry concerned with the diagnosis and surgical and adjunctive treatment of diseases, injuries, and deformities of the oral and maxillofacial region.

oropharynx: The part of the throat at the back of the mouth behind the oral cavity. It includes the back third of the tongue, the soft palate, the side and back walls of the throat, and the tonsils.[2]

orthodontic appliance: A mechanism for the application of force to the teeth and their supporting tissues to produce changes in the relationship of the teeth and/or the related osseous structures.

orthodontics: That branch of dentistry concerned with the correction and prevention of irregularities and malocclusion of the teeth.

osteonecrosis: Blood vessel compromise and necrosis of bone exposed to high-dose radiation therapy, resulting in decreased ability to heal if traumatized and extreme susceptibility to infection.[1]

periodontal diseases: Periodontal diseases include gingivitis and periodontitis. Both are inflammatory conditions of the gingival tissues (gum tissues around the teeth). In more severe forms, periodontitis includes loss of supporting bone tissue which can lead to tooth loss.[3]

periodontics: The branch of dentistry concerned with the study of the normal tissues and the treatment of abnormal conditions of the tissues immediately about the teeth.

plaque: See dental plaque.

public water supply system (PWS): A public water system provides water for human consumption to the public through piped or other constructed conveyances. A PWS has at least 15 service connections or regularly serves an average of at least 25 individuals daily for at least 60 days out of the year. Ground water sources, surface water sources, or a combination of the two sources may provide water to a PWS. In some cases, one PWS may purchase all or part of its water from another PWS.[3]

radiation caries: Lifelong risk of rampant dental decay that may begin within three months of completing radiation treatment if changes in either the quality or quantity of saliva persist.[1]

root canal therapy: Dental therapy for damaged pulp by removal of the pulp and sterilization and filling of the root canal.

sealant: See dental sealant

subgingival curettage: Removal of subgingival calculus, ulcerated epithelial and granulation tissues found in periodontal pockets.

teeth cleaning: A dentist or dental hygienist removes soft debris, stain, and hard deposits (calculus or tartar) on the teeth that cannot be removed by brushing and flossing. Regular teeth cleaning by a dentist or dental hygienist helps prevent periodontal diseases.[3]

tooth decay: Tooth decay is the commonly known term for dental caries, an infectious, transmissible, disease caused by bacteria. The damage done to teeth by this disease is commonly known as cavities. Tooth decay can cause pain and lead to infections in surrounding tissues and tooth loss if not treated properly.[3]

trismus tissue fibrosis: Loss of elasticity of masticatory muscles that restricts normal ability to open the mouth.[1]

x-ray: A type of radiation used in the diagnosis and treatment of cancer and other diseases. In low doses, x-rays are used to diagnose diseases by making pictures of the inside of the body. In high doses, x-rays are used to treat cancer.[2]

xerostomia/salivary gland dysfunction: Dryness of the mouth because of thickened, reduced, or absent salivary flow; increases the risk for infection and compromises speaking, chewing, and swallowing. Medications other than chemotherapy agents, such as psychotropic and some antihypertensive drugs, can also cause salivary gland dysfunction. Persistent dry mouth increases the risk of dental cavities.[1]

Chapter 69

Directory of Local Dental Schools

Alabama

University of Alabama at Birmingham
School of Dentistry
1919 7th Ave. S.
Suite 406
Birmingham, AL 35294
Phone: 205-934-3000
Website: http://www.dental.uab.edu

Arizona

Arizona School of Dentistry and Oral Health (ASDOH)
ASDOH Dental Clinic
5850 E. Still Circle, #101
Mesa, AZ 85206
Phone: 480-248-8100
Website: http://www.atsu.edu/asdoh

ASDOH Dental Care West
20325 N. 51st Ave., Unit 156
Glendale, AZ 85308
Phone: 623-251-4700
Website: http://www.atsu.edu/asdoh

California

University of California at Los Angeles
School of Dentistry
10833 Le Conte Ave.
CHS-Box 951668
Los Angeles, CA 90095
Phone: 310-206-3904
Fax: 310-825-2951
Website: http://www.dentistry.ucla.edu/patient-care

Excerpted from "Local Dental Schools," National Institute of Dental and Craniofacial Research (NIDCR). Contact information was verified as correct in April 2012.

University of California at San Francisco

Student Dental Clinic
707 Parnassus Ave.
San Francisco, CA 94143
Phone: 415-476-1891
Website: http://dentistry.ucsf
.edu/patient-services

Loma Linda University

School of Dentistry
Loma Linda, CA 92350
Phone: 909-558-4675
Website: http://www.llu.edu/
dentistry/patinfo.page

University of the Pacific

Arthur A. Dugoni School
of Dentistry
2155 Webster St.
San Francisco, CA 94115
Phone: 415-929-6501
Website:
http://dental.pacific.edu/
Dental_Services.html

University of Southern California

Ostrow School of Dentistry
925 West 34th St.
Los Angeles, CA 90089
Phone: 213-740-2800
Website: http://dentistry.usc.edu/
patient-care/contact

Colorado

University of Colorado School of Dental Medicine

Mail Stop F831
13065 East 17th Ave.
Aurora, CO 80045
Phone: 303-724-6900
Website:
http://www.ucdenver.edu/
academics/colleges/
dentalmedicine/PatientCare/
Pages/BecomeaPatient.aspx

Connecticut

University of Connecticut

School of Dental Medicine
263 Farmington Ave.
Farmington, CT 06030
Phone: 860-679-3415
Website:
http://sdm.uchc.edu/patients/
students.html

District of Columbia

Howard University

College of Dentistry
600 West St. NW
Washington, DC 20059
Phone: 202-806-0456; or 202-
806-0008
Website: http://www.dentistry
.howard.edu/patientcare.htm

Florida

University of Florida
College of Dentistry
PO Box 100405
Gainesville, FL 32610
Toll-Free: 800-633-3953
Phone: 352-273-7950
Website: http://www.dental.ufl
.edu/Patients

Nova Southeastern University
College of Dental Medicine
3301 College Ave.
Fort Lauderdale-Davie, FL 33314
Toll-Free: 800-541-6682
Phone: 954-262-7500
Website: http://dental.nova.edu/
clinics/index.html

Georgia

Georgia Health Services University
1430 John Wesley Gilbert Dr.
Augusta, GA 30912
Phone: 706-721-7019 (office)
Phone: 706-721-2371 (clinic secretary)
Fax: 706-721-6276
Website:
http://www.georgiahealth.edu/
dentalmedicine/patientservices/
becomingapatient.html

Illinois

University of Illinois at Chicago
College of Dentistry
801 S. Paulina St.
Chicago, IL 60612
Phone: 312-996-7555
Website: http://dentistry.uic.edu/
depts/patientservices/index.cfm
E-mail: dentalclinics@uic.edu

Southern Illinois University
School of Dental Medicine
2800 College Ave.
Alton, IL 62002
Phone: 618-474-7000
Website: http://www.siue.edu/
dentalmedicine/patients.shtml

Indiana

Indiana University
School of Dentistry
1121 W. Michigan St.
Indianapolis, IN 46202
Phone: 317-274-7433 Option #2
Website: http://www.iusd.iupui
.edu/patient-services

Iowa

University of Iowa
College of Dentistry
100 Dental Sciences Bldg.
Iowa City, IA 52242
Phone: 319-335-7499
Website: http://www.dentistry.
uiowa.edu/missions/patientcare/
becoming_a_patient.shtml

Kentucky

University of Louisville
School of Dentistry
501 S. Preston St.
Louisville, KY 40292
Phone: 502-852-5096
Website: http://louisville.edu/
dental/patients
E-mail:
DENTALCA@louisville.edu

University of Kentucky
College of Dentistry
800 Rose St.
Lexington, KY 40536
Phone: 859-323-6525
Website: http://www.mc.uky.edu/
dentistry/service/dentalserv.html

Louisiana

Louisiana State University
School of Dentistry
1100 Florida Ave.
New Orleans, LA 70119
Phone: 504-619-8700
Website: http://www.lsusd
.lsuhsc.edu/patients.html

Maryland

University of Maryland
Baltimore College of
Dental Surgery
650 W. Baltimore St.
Baltimore, MD 21201
Toll-Free: 866-787-8637
Phone: 410-706-7101
Website:
http://www.dental.umaryland.edu

Massachusetts

Tufts University
School of Dental Medicine
One Kneeland St.
Boston, MA 02111
Phone: 617-636-6828
Website:
http://dental.tufts.edu/
1175090438731/
TUSDM-Page-dental2ws_
1176988224004.html

Boston University
Goldman School of
Dental Medicine
100 E. Newton St.
Boston, MA 02118
Phone: 617-638-4700
Website: http://www.bu.edu/
dental/patients

Harvard School of Dental Medicine
188 Longwood Ave.
Boston, MA 02115
Phone: 617-432-1434
Website:
http://www.harvarddentalcenter
.harvard.edu/asp-html

Michigan

University of Detroit
Mercy School of Dentistry
2700 Martin Luther King Jr.
Blvd.
Detroit, MI 48208
Phone: 313-494-6700
Website: http://dental.udmercy
.edu/patient

University of Michigan

School of Dentistry
1011 N. University Ave.
Ann Arbor, MI 48109
Toll-Free: 888-707-2500
Phone: 734-763-6933
Website: http://dent.umich.edu/
patientservices

Minnesota

University of Minnesota

School of Dentistry
515 Delaware St., SE, 7th Fl.
Minneapolis, MN 55455
Phone: 612-625-2495
Website: http://www.dentistry
.umn.edu/patients/index.htm

Mississippi

University of Mississippi

School of Dentistry
2500 N. State St.
Jackson, MS 39216
Phone: 601-984-6080
Website: http://dentistry.umc
.edu/patients/becoming_a
_patient.html

Missouri

University of Missouri–Kansas City

School of Dentistry
650 East 25th St.
Kansas City, MO 64108
Phone: 816-235-2100
Website: http://dentistry.umkc
.edu/Patient_Information/index
.shtml

Nebraska

Creighton University

School of Dentistry
2500 California Plaza
Omaha, NE 68178
Phone: 402-280-4080
Fax: 402-280-5013
Website:
http://www.creighton.edu/
dentalschool/informationfor
patients/index.php

University of Nebraska Medical Center

College of Dentistry
40th and Holdrege St.
Lincoln, NE 68583
Phone: 402-472-1301
Website: http://www.unmc.edu/
dentistry/patient_care.htm

Nevada

University of Nevada, Las Vegas

School of Dental Medicine
1001 Shadow Ln. Campus
MS 7410
Las Vegas, NV 89106
Phone: 702-774-2400
Website:
http://dentalschool.unlv.edu/
clinics.html

New Jersey

University of Medicine and Dentistry of New Jersey
New Jersey Dental School
110 Bergen St.
Newark, NJ 07103
Phone: 973-972-7370
Website: http://dentalschool
.umdnj.edu/patients/index.htm

New York

Columbia University
School of Dental and Oral Surgery
630 West 168th St.
New York, NY 10032
Phone: 212-305-6100
Website: http://dental.columbia
.edu/patients/index.html

New York University
College of Dentistry
345 East 24th St.
New York, NY 10010
Phone: 212-998-9800
Website: http://www.nyu.edu/
dental/patientinfo/index.html

University at Buffalo
State University of New York
School of Dental Medicine
158 Squire Hall
Buffalo, NY 14214
Phone: 716-829-2821
Website: http://dental.buffalo
.edu/Patients.aspx

North Carolina

University of North Carolina at Chapel Hill
School of Dentistry
CB #7450
Chapel Hill, NC 27599
Phone: 919-966-1161
Website: http://www.dentistry
.unc.edu/patient

Ohio

Case School of Dental Medicine
10900 Euclid Ave.
Cleveland, OH 44106
Phone: 216-368-8730
Website: http://dental.case.edu/
patients

Ohio State University College of Dentistry
305 West 12th Ave.
Columbus, OH 43210
Phone: 614-292-2751
Website: http://dent.osu.edu/
patients/index.php

Oklahoma

University of Oklahoma
College of Dentistry
1201 N. Stonewall
Oklahoma City, OK 73117
Phone: 405-271-6326
Website: http://dentistry.ouhsc
.edu/patients.php

Oregon

Oregon Health and Science University
School of Dentistry
611 SW Campus Dr.
Portland, OR 97239
Phone: 503-494-8801
Website: http://www.ohsu.edu/
xd/education/schools/school
-of-dentistry/patient-care/index
.cfm

Pennsylvania

University of Pittsburgh
School of Dental Medicine
3501 Terrace St.
Pittsburgh, PA 15261
Phone: 412-648-8616
Website: http://www.dental.pitt
.edu/patients/index.php

Temple University
School of Dentistry
3223 N. Broad St.
Philadelphia, PA 19140
Phone: 215-707-2880
Website: http://www.temple.edu/
dentistry/CA/patientinformation
.html

University of Pennsylvania
School of Dental Medicine
240 South 40th St.
Philadelphia, PA 19104
Phone: 215-898-8965
Website: http://www.dental
.upenn.edu/patient_care/
dental_school_clinics/patient
_information

Puerto Rico

University of Puerto Rico
School of Dentistry
Medical Sciences Campus
PO Box 365067
San Juan, PR 00936
Phone: 787-758-2525, x1174
Website:
http://www.rcm.upr.edu/
Servicios_Odontologia.htm

South Carolina

Medical University of South Carolina
College of Dental Medicine
173 Ashley Ave.
PO Box 250507
Charleston, SC 29425
Phone: 843-792-2101, option 2
Website:
http://academicdepartments.
musc.edu/dentistry/patient_care/
new_patient.htm

Tennessee

Meharry Medical College
School of Dentistry
1005 D.B. Todd Jr. Blvd.
Nashville, TN 37208
Phone: 615-327-6348
Website: http://www.mmc.edu/FAP

University of Tennessee
College of Dentistry
875 Union Ave.
Memphis, TN 38163
Phone: 901-448-6200
Website: http://www.uthsc.edu/
dentistry

Texas

University of Texas
School of Dentistry
6516 MD Anderson Blvd.
Houston, TX 77030
Phone: 713-500-4000
Website: http://db.uth.tmc.edu/
patient-care

University of Texas
Health Science Center
San Antonio Dental School
7703 Floyd Curl Dr.
San Antonio, TX 78229
Phone: 210-567-3217
Website: http://dental.uthscsa
.edu/becomeapatient.php

Baylor College of Dentistry
A Member of The Texas A & M
University System
Health Science Center
PO Box 660677
Dallas, TX 75266
Phone: 214-828-8100
Website: http://www.tambcd.edu/
resources/patientsvisitors.html

Virginia

Virginia Commonwealth University
School of Dentistry
PO Box 980566
Richmond, VA 23298
Phone: 804-828-9190
Website: http://www.dentistry
.vcu.edu/patients/Default.aspx
E-mail: dentalinfo@vcu.edu

Washington

University of Washington
School of Dentistry
Health Sciences Bldg.
1959 NE Pacific St.
Room B307
Seattle, WA 98195
Phone: 206-616-6996;
or 206-685-1022
Website: http://www.dental
.washington.edu/patient/
patient-care-guide.html-0

West Virginia

West Virginia University
School of Dentistry
WVU Health Science Ctr.
1 Stadium Dr.
Morgantown, WV 26506
Phone: 304-293-6208
Website: http://dentistry.hsc
.wvu.edu/Patient-Services

Wisconsin

Marquette University
School of Dentistry
PO Box 1881
Milwaukee, WI 53201
Phone: 414-288-6790 (English)
Phone: 414-288-1520 (Española)
Website:
http://www.marquette.edu/
dentistry/patients/Patients
Index.shtml

Chapter 70

Directory of Additional Dental Care and Oral Health Resources

Government Agencies

Administration for Children and Families
Office of Head Start (OHS)
8th Floor, Portals Building
Washington, DC 20024
Toll-Free: 866-763-6481
Website: http://eclkc.ohs.acf.hhs
.gov/hslc/hs

Agency for Healthcare Research and Quality (AHRQ)
540 Gaither Rd.
Rockville, MD 20850
Toll-Free: 800-358-9295
Phone: 301-427-1364
Website: http://www.ahrq.gov

Bureau of Primary Health Care
Toll-Free: 888-275-4772
Website:
http://findahealthcenter.hrsa
.gov/Search_HCC.aspx

Celiac Disease Awareness Campaign (CDAC)
National Digestive Diseases
Information Clearinghouse
2 Information Way
Bethesda, MD 20892
Toll-Free: 800-891-5389
Toll-Free TTY: 866-569-1162
Fax: 703-738-4929
Website:
http://www.celiac.nih.gov
E-mail:
celiac@info.niddk.nih.gov

Resources in this chapter were compiled from several sources deemed reliable; all contact information was verified and updated in April 2012. Inclusion does not imply endorsement. This list is not comprehensive, it is intended as a starting point for gathering of information.

Centers for Disease Control and Prevention (CDC)
1600 Clifton Rd.
Atlanta, GA 30333
Toll-Free: 800-CDC-INFO
(232-4636)
Toll-Free TTY: 888-232-6348
Website: http://www.cdc.gov
E-mail: cdcinfo@cdc.gov

Centers for Medicare and Medicaid Services
7500 Security Blvd.
Baltimore, MD 21244
Toll-Free: 800-633-4227
Toll-Free TTY: 877-486-2048
Website: http://www.cms.hhs.gov

Clinical Trials Center
Patient Recruitment and Public Liaison Office
Toll-Free: 900-411-1222
Website: http://clinicaltrials.gov

Head Start
Administration for Children and Families
370 L'Enfant Promenade, SW
Washington, DC 20447
Toll-Free: 866-763-6481
Website: http://eclkc.ohs.acf.hhs.gov/hslc/hs

Health Resources and Services Administration
5600 Fishers Lane
Rockville, MD 20857
Toll-Free: 888-275-4772
Toll-Free TTY: 877-489-4772
Website: http://www.hrsa.gov

Medicaid-CHIP State Dental Association
4411 Connecticut Ave., NW, #104
Washington, DC 20008
Phone: 508-322-0557
Fax: 202-248-2315
Website: http://www.medicaiddental.org

National Cancer Institute (NCI)
NCI Public Inquiries Office
6116 Executive Blvd.
Room 3036A
Bethesda, MD 20892
Toll-Free: 800-4-CANCER
(422-6237)
Website: http://www.cancer.gov

National Diabetes Education Program
1 Diabetes Way
Bethesda, MD 20814
Toll-Free: 888-693-NDEP (6337)
Toll-Free TTY: 866-569-1162
Fax: 703-738-4929
Website: http://www.ndep.nih.gov
E-mail: ndep@mail.nih.gov

National Diabetes Information Clearinghouse
1 Information Way
Bethesda, MD 20892
Toll-Free: 800-860-8747
Toll-Free TTY: 866-569-1162
Fax: 703-738-4929
Website: http://www.diabetes.niddk.nih.gov
E-mail: ndic@info.niddk.nih.gov

National Digestive Diseases Information Clearinghouse

2 Information Way
Bethesda, MD 20892
Toll-Free: 800-891-5389
Toll-Free TTY: 866-569-1162
Fax: 703-738-4929
Website:
http://digestive.niddk.nih.gov
E-mail: nddic@info.niddk.nih.gov

National Institute of Child Health and Human Development (NICHD)

Bldg. 31, Room 2A32, MSC 2425
31 Center Drive
Bethesda, MD 20892
Toll-Free: 800-370-2943
Toll-Free TTY: 888-320-6942
Fax: 866-760-5947
Website:
http://www.nichd.nih.gov

National Institute of Dental and Craniofacial Research (NIDCR)

National Oral Health
Information Clearinghouse
1 NOHIC Way
Bethesda, MD 20892
Toll-Free: 866-232-4528
Fax: 301-480-4098
Website:
http://www.nidcr.nih.gov
E-mail: nidcrinfo@mail.nih.gov

National Institute of Diabetes and Digestive and Kidney Diseases (NIDDK)

Bldg. 31, Rm. 9A06
31 Center Dr., MSC 2560
Bethesda, MD 20892
Phone: 301-496-3583
Website:
http://www2.niddk.nih.gov

National Institute of Neurological Disorders and Stroke (NINDS)

NIH Neurological Institute
P.O. Box 5801
Bethesda, MD 20824
Toll-Free: 800-352-9424
Phone: 301-496-5751
TTY: 301-468-598
Website:
http://www.ninds.nih.gov

National Institute on Aging (NIA)

Bldg. 31, Rm. 5C27
31 Center Dr., MSC 2292
Bethesda, MD 20892
Toll-Free: 800-222-2225
Toll-Free TTY: 800-222-4225
Phone: 301-496-1752
Fax: 301-496-1072
Website: http://www.nia.nih.gov
E-mail: niaic@nia.nih.gov

601

National Institute on Deafness and Other Communication Disorders (NIDCD)

Information Clearinghouse
1 Communication Ave.
Bethesda, MD 20892
Toll-Free: 800-241-1044
Toll-Free TTY: 800-241-1055
Fax: 301-770-8977
Website:
http://www.nidcd.nih.gov
E-mail: nidcdinfo@nidcd.nih.gov

National Institutes of Health (NIH)

9000 Rockville Pike
Bethesda, MD 20892
Phone: 301-496-4000
TTY: 301-402-9612
Website: http://www.nih.gov
E-mail: NIHinfo@od.nih.gov

NICHD Information Resource Center

National Institute of
Child Health and Human
Development
PO Box 3006
Rockville, MD 20847
Website: http://www.nichd.nih.gov
E-mail: NICHDInformation
ResourceCenter@mail.nih.gov

NIH Osteoporosis and Related Bone Diseases

National Resource Center
2 AMS Circle
Bethesda, MD 20892
Toll Free: 800-624-BONE (2663)
Phone: 202-223-0344
TTY: 202-466-4315
Fax: 202-293-2356
Website:
http://www.bones.nih.gov
E-mail:
NIHBoneInfo@mail.nih.gov

U.S. Department of Health and Human Services

200 Independence Ave., SW
Washington, DC 20201
Toll-Free: 877-696-6775
Website: http://www.hhs.gov

U.S. Environmental Protection Agency (EPA)

Ariel Rios Building
1200 Pennsylvania Ave. NW
Washington, DC 20460
Phone: 202-272-0167
TTY: 202-272-0165
Website: http://www.epa.gov

U.S. Food and Drug Administration (FDA)

10903 New Hampshire Ave.
Silver Spring, MD 20993
Toll-Free: 888-INFO-FDA
(463-6332)
Website: http://www.fda.gov

Private Organizations

Academy of General Dentistry

211 E. Chicago Ave., Suite 900
Chicago, IL 60611
Toll-Free: 888-243-3368, ext. 5300
Fax: 312-440-0559
Website: http://www.agd.org
E-mail: info@knowyourteeth.com

American Academy of Cosmetic Dentistry

402 W. Wilson St.
Madison, WI 53703
Toll-Free: 800-543-9220
Phone: 608-222-8583
Fax: 608-222-9540
Website: http://www.aacd.com

American Academy of Implant Dentistry

211 E. Chicago Ave., Suite 750
Chicago, IL 60611
Toll-Free: 877-335-AAID (2243)
Phone: 312-335-1550
Fax: 312-335-9090
Website:
http://www.aaid-implant.org
E-mail: info@aaid.com

American Academy of Oral Medicine

23607 Hwy 99, Suite 2C
Edmonds, WA 98020
Phone: 425-778-6162
Fax: 425-771-9588
Website:
http://www.aaom.com/patients
E-mail: info@aaom.com

American Academy of Pediatric Dentistry

211 E. Chicago Ave., #700
Chicago, IL 60611
Phone: 312-337-2169
Fax: 312-337-6329
Website: http://www.aapd.org

American Academy of Periodontology

737 N. Michigan Ave., Suite 800
Chicago, IL 60611
Phone: 312-787-5518
Fax: 312-787-3670
Website: http://www.perio.org

American Association of Endodontists

211 E. Chicago Ave., Suite 1100
Chicago, IL 60611
Toll-Free: 800-872-3636
Phone: 312-266-7255
Toll-Free Fax: 866-451-9020
Facebook: http://www.facebook
.com/endodontists
Website: http://www.aae.org
E-mail: info@aae.org

American Association of Oral and Maxillofacial Surgeons

9700 W. Bryn Mawr Ave.
Rosemont, IL 60018
Toll-Free: 800-822-6637
Phone: 847-678-6200
Fax: 847-678-6286
Website: http://www.aaoms.org

American Association of Orthodontists

401 N. Lindbergh Blvd.
St. Louis, MO 63141
Toll-Free: 800-424-2841
Phone: 314-993-1700
Fax: 314-997-1745
Website:
http://www.aaomembers.org
E-mail: info@aaortho.org

American Dental Assistants Association

35 E. Wacker Dr., Ste. 1730
Chicago, IL 60601
Toll-Free: 877-874-3785
Phone: 312-541-1550
Fax: 312-541-1496
Website:
http://www.dentalassistant.org

American Dental Association

211 E. Chicago Ave.
Chicago, IL 60611
Toll-Free: 800-621-8099
Website: http://www.ada.org

American Dental Hygienists Association

444 N. Michigan Ave.
Suite 3400
Chicago, IL 60611
Phone: 312-449-8900
Website: http://www.adha.org

American Diabetes Association

1701 N. Beauregard St.
Alexandria, VA 22311
Toll-Free: 800-DIABETES
(342-2383)
Website: http://www.diabetes.org

American Head and Neck Society (AHNS)

11300 W. Olympic Blvd., Ste. 600
Los Angeles, CA 90064
Phone: 310-437-0559
Fax: 310-437-0585
Website: http://www.ahns.info

Children's Dental Health Project

1020 19th St. NW, Suite 400
Washington, DC 20036
Phone: 202-833-8288
Fax: 202-331-1432
Website: http://www.cdhp.org
E-mail: cdhpinfo@cdhp.org

Cleft Palate Foundation;

1504 E. Franklin St., Ste. 102
Chapel Hill, NC 27514
Toll-Free: 800-242-5338
Phone: 919-933-9044
Fax: 919-933-9604
Website: http://www.cleftline.org

Cleveland Clinic

9500 Euclid Ave.
Cleveland, OH 44195
Toll-Free: 800-223-2273
TTY: 216-444-0261
Website:
http://www.clevelandclinic.org

FACES: The National Craniofacial Association
Toll-Free: 800-332-2373
Website:
http://www.faces-cranio.org

Health Physics Society
1313 Dolley Madison Blvd.
Suite 402
McLean, VA 22101
Phone: 703-790-1745
Fax: 703-790-2672
Website: http://www.hps.org
E-mail: HPS@BurkInc.com

Juvenile Diabetes Research Foundation International
120 Wall Street
New York, NY 10005
Toll-Free: 800-533-CURE (2873)
Website: http://www.jdrf.org

National Academy of Sciences
500 Fifth St., NW
Washington, DC 20001
Phone: 202-334-2000
Website: http://www
.nationalacademies.org

National Dental Association
3517 16th St. NW
Washington, DC 20010
Phone: 202-588-1697
Fax: 202-588-1244
Website:
http://www.ndaonline.org

National Eating Disorders Association
165 W. 46th St.
New York, NY 10036
Toll-Free: 800-931-2237
Phone: 212-757-6200
Fax: 212-575-1650
Website: http://www
.nationaleatingdisorders.org

Hispanic Dental Association (HDA)
3085 Stevenson Dr., Ste. 200
Springfield, IL 62703
Phone: 217-529-6517
Fax: 217-529-9120
Website: http://www.hdassoc.org/
E-mail:
HispanicDental@hdassoc.org

National Maternal and Child Oral Health Resource Center
Georgetown University
2115 Wisconsin Ave. NW
Suite 601
Washington, DC 20007
Telephone: 202-784-9771
Fax: 202-784-9777
Website:
http://www.mchoralhealth.org
E-mail:
OHRCinfo@georgetown.edu

Nemours Foundation
1600 Rockland Rd.
Wilmington, DE 19803
Phone: 302-651-4000
Website:
http://www.kidshealth.org
E-mail: info@kidshealth.org

Oral Health America
410 N. Michigan Ave., Ste. 352
Chicago, IL 60611
Phone: 312-836-9900
Fax: 312-836-9986
Website: http://www
.oralhealthamerica.org
E-mail:
info@oralhealthamerica.org

Simple Steps to Better Dental Health
Columbia University
College of Dental Medicine
Website: http://www
.simplestepsdental.com
E-mail: help@simplesteps.com

Sjögren's Syndrome Foundation
6707 Democracy Blvd., Ste. 325
Bethesda, MD 20817
Toll-Free: 800-475-6473
Phone: 301-530-4420
Fax: 301-530-4415
Website: http://www.sjogrens.org

Special Care Dentistry Association (SCDA)
401 N. Michigan Ave., Suite 2200
Chicago, IL 60611
Phone: 312-527-6764
Fax: 312-673-6663
Website: http://scdaonline.org
E-mail: SCDA@SCDAOnline.org

Support for People with Head and Neck Cancer (SPOHNC)
PO Box 53
Locust Valley, NY 11560
Toll-Free: 800-377-0928
Fax: 516-671-8794
Website: http://www.spohnc.org
E-mail: info@spohnc.org

TNA Facial Pain Association
408 W. University Ave., Ste. 602
Gainesville, FL 32601
Toll-Free: 800-923-3608
Phone: 352-384-3600
Fax: 352-384-3606
Website:
http://www.fpa-support.org

Index

Index

Page numbers followed by 'n' indicate a footnote. Page numbers in *italics* indicate a table or illustration.

609